THE
COMPLETE
—BOOK OF—

Vitamins
and
Minerals
for
Health

ALL–NEW
EDITION

THE COMPLETE
BOOK OF
Vitamins
and
Minerals
for
Health

ALL-NEW
EDITION

By the Editors of Prevention® Magazine

 Rodale Press, Emmaus, Pennsylvania

Printed in the United States of America on recycled paper
containing a high percentage of de-inked fiber.

Library of Congress Cataloging-in-Publication Data

The Complete book of vitamins and minerals for health/by the
    editors of Prevention magazine.—All-new ed.
        p. cm.
    Compiled by Lewis Vaughn; editor, Sharon Faelten.
    Includes index.
    ISBN 0-87857-749-1
    1. Nutrition. 2. Vitamins in human nutrition. 3. Minerals in
human nutrition. 4. Health. I. Vaughn, Lewis. II. Faelten,
Sharon.
RA784.C59 1988
613.2—dc19   87–32933
                                           CIP

ISBN 0-87857-749-1 hardcover

2 4 6 8 10 9 7 5 3 1 hardcover

Contributors

Compiled by Lewis Vaughn, Assistant Managing Editor,
Prevention® Magazine

Editor: Sharon Faelten, Senior Editor, *Prevention*®
Magazine Health Books

Executive Editor, *Prevention*® Magazine Health Books:
William Gottlieb

Contributors: Stefan Bechtel, Diane Drabinsky, R.D.,
Paul Facinelli, Denise Foley, Judith Benn Hurley,
Jane Kinderlehrer, Gale Malesky, Jeff Meade, Maria
Mihalik, Eileen Nechas, Kerry Pechter, Tom Shealey,
Charles B. Simone, M.D., Deborah Spitz, M.D.,
Marguerite Thomas, Debora Tkac, Lewis Vaughn,
Susan Zarrow

Designer: Sandy Freeman

Copy Editor: Dolores Plikaitis

Editorial/Production Coordinator: Jane Sherman

Research Chief: Carol Baldwin

Associate Research Chief, *Prevention*® Magazine Health
Books: Susan A. Nastasee

Assistant Research Chief, *Prevention*® Magazine Health
Books: Holly Clemson

Research Associates: Doreen Brill, Martha Capwell,
Ann Gossy, Alice Harris, Cemela Dee London, Paris
Mihely, Linda Miller, Sally Novack, Carole Piszczek,
Cindy Wagaman, Lisa Warner

Office Manager: Roberta Mulliner

Office Personnel: Kim Mohr, Kelly Trumbauer

Contents

Achieving the Nutrient-Rich Lifestyle   Part I

Facts and fictions about food and nutrition . . . The
missing vitamins and minerals in high-protein, low-
calorie vegetarian menus . . . Nutritional tips for people
who hate vegetables . . . A realistic look at calcium
needs . . . Nutrition on the run: how to ensure that your
family gets their fair share of essential vitamins and
minerals.

Causes and effects of marginal vitamin and mineral
deficiencies . . . Some symptoms to look for . . . The
three phases of a deficiency . . . The high prevalence of
nutritional problems . . . Why older people are at special risk . . . The role of zinc in a healthy pregnancy.

How men and women differ in nutritional needs . . .
Why many women aren't getting enough iron, folate,
vitamin B_6 and calcium and what they can do about
it . . . Why some men may be at high risk for vitamin C
deficiency.

Why men and women who live alone risk being undernourished . . . How singles cheat themselves out of key
vitamins and minerals . . . Tips on how to avoid nutritional traps of living—and eating—alone . . . Breaking
bad habits.

Why an occasional shortfall in your kids' nutrition is
nothing to worry about . . . Vitamins and minerals that
children lack most . . . Beat finicky eaters at their own
game . . . How to pack a kid's lunchbox with nutritious
goodies . . . Tips on how to prepare nutrient-rich meals
that kids will eat.

Take this quiz to find out how much you know about
vitamins and minerals—and how you can choose between foods that help or hurt you . . . Some answers
may surprise you.

Using Supplements Wisely   Part II

A close-up look at "typical" supplement users . . .
Which vitamins and minerals are most popular, and
why . . . Do people take too much? . . . Supplements
are only one part of a healthy lifestyle . . . How cost-
effective are supplements? . . . Dietitians speak up for
supplements.

How to determine if a multiple vitamin/mineral formula is complete, balanced and right for your body . . .
How to read and understand labels on vitamin/mineral
preparations . . . The value of "stress formulas" and
other special multiples . . . A caution about health
claims . . . Comparison shopping for multiple formulas
before going to the store.

**From A to Zinc: Part III
A Guide to Vitamins and Minerals**

cancer . . . How beta-carotene may be a "morning-
after" pill for people who are already exposed to
cancer-causing agents . . . Dramatic preliminary research on beta-carotene and lung cancer . . . Lists of
the best food sources of beta-carotene.

How to recognize the signs of possible B-vitamin deficiency . . . Niacin may help protect cells against cancer
and reduce cholesterol . . . How vitamin B_{12} and vitamin C team up to fight leukemia in mice . . . The role of
vitamin B_{12} in counteracting asthmatic reactions to sulfites in food . . . The link between folate deficiency and
cancer . . . Investigating the link between memory
problems in the elderly and thiamine deficiency . . .
How B_6 deficiency can lead to depression and "premature aging" . . . A list of the best food sources of B
vitamins.

A guide to recognizing the subtle but serious symptoms of thiamine deficiency . . . Why today's teens are
at risk for thiamine deficiency . . . How weight-
conscious young women often fail to get enough thiamine . . . How thiamine deficiency has been linked to
hypothermia, slow wound healing, loss of memory and
muscle control . . . Where to find thiamine in foods.

How B_6 has been used to treat schizophrenia . . . How
B_6 is being used against seizures in children . . . An
alternative to steroids for a rare form of herpes . . .
Reports on how B_6 may be able to improve athletic
endurance . . . The latest news on treating carpal tunnel syndrome with B_6.

An easy-to-take quiz to assess whether your body is
getting enough B_6 . . . A look at the lifestyle and dietary
factors that affect your B_6 levels . . . Solid guidelines for
ensuring that your B_6 status is A-Ok.

Calcium's pivotal role in stopping the bone loss caused
by osteoporosis...How calcium can lower high
blood pressure...A list of the best food sources of
calcium.

23. **Copper: Essential to Life and Health** 166

Why copper is crucial to nerves, blood vessels and
bones...How copper may play a role in our ability to
fight off infections...How to maintain the right zinc-
to-copper ratio in your diet...How to make sure
you're getting enough copper—but not too much...
A list of the best food sources of copper.

24. **What You Should Know about Iron** 176

Why your body can show symptoms of even mild iron
deficiency...How iron helps protect you from infections...Getting enough iron can help you better withstand cold, prevent psychological disorders and overcome anemia...Why so many people have iron
deficiencies...A review of all the diet and lifestyle
factors that can lead to lack of iron...Practical tips on
making sure your diet is iron rich...A list of the best
food sources of iron.

25. **Give Yourself the Iron Test**
    (and Rate Your Energy Reserves) 186

A quiz that will tell you if you're at risk for iron deficiency...A review of the factors that can help deplete—or restore—your iron reserves...Tips on how
to calibrate your diet for maximum iron potency...A
review of how exercise, diet, drugs, cooking methods
can affect your iron levels.

26. **The Health Power of Magnesium:**
    A Medical Roundup 195

A real-life story revealing how magnesium has helped
people with heart problems...How doctors are now
using magnesium to treat heartbeat irregularities, high
blood pressure, blood clots, migraines and epileptic
seizures...Why too many people aren't getting
enough magnesium...A list of the best food sources
of magnesium.

Special Nutritional Allies for Health   Part IV

Solving Health Problems with Nutrition   Part V

eye troubles ... A review of evidence that vision problems may respond to vitamins A, C, E and B₂ and the
minerals zinc, selenium and chromium.

A report on treating asthma with vitamin C ... Using
better nutrition against bedsores ... Combining vitamin C with a cancer drug ... A report on using vitamin
E to prevent chemotherapy-induced hair loss ... Low
selenium and celiac disease ... Zinc lozenges: treatment for colds ... A possible link between deafness
and vitamin D deficiency ... Lupus and vitamin A ...
Treating Wilson's disease with zinc.

A commonsense guide to maximum safe doses for
vitamins and minerals ... Sound advice on safe and
sane use of nutritional supplements ... A review of scientific evidence regarding using supplements to prevent or treat health problems.

Better Nutrition for the Stages of Your Life   Part VI

Commonsense steps that will help to ensure a healthy
baby ... How to maintain proper body weight ...
Healthful advice about alcohol and caffeine ... A sensible guide to vitamin and mineral intake.

How scientists are using vitamins and minerals against
neural tube defects (NTD) ... Scientific research on
using nutrients to prevent cleft lip ... Investigating the
link between zinc deficiencies and birth defects ...
Treating rare birth abnormalities with vitamins.

Tips on recognizing bad weight-loss diets and picking
out the good ones ... How easily people on low-

calorie diets can run a deficiency . . . Ways to diet and
still get enough iron, calcium and other nutrients . . .
How to keep your diet on track nutritionally.

Designing a safe, sane diet for people who exercise . . .
How active people can avoid nutrient deficiencies . . .
Ways to get enough energy-boosting iron . . . The facts
about minerals, sweat and athletic performance . . .
Avoiding a deficit of B's.

Practical tips on improving your brainpower . . . How
to improve your thinking by improving your posture . . .
What iron deficiencies can do to your intellect and
how to avoid them . . . How aerobic exercise can increase brainpower . . . What scientists say about lecithin and mental performance . . . Brainpower and B
vitamins . . . Getting rid of emotional mind clutter.

How using energy can give you more energy . . . Ten-
sion-releasing exercises that can pep you up . . . Losing
weight increases energy reserves . . . How to avoid the
"mineral blues" . . . Why a vitamin C deficiency can
sap your energy.

Why injured people need top-notch nutrition . . .
Amino acids that promise to speed wound healing . . .
Using vitamin C to boost immunity . . . Why burn vic-
tims may need vitamin A . . . Injuries call for more zinc.

Why malnutrition is so prevalent in hospitals . . . Why
nutrient deficiencies are all too common in nursing
homes . . . Why the elderly in institutions risk low levels
of vitamin D . . . A guide to ensuring good nutrition for
someone who enters a hospital or nursing home.

Cooking and Eating for Maximum Nutrition   Part VII

plan diets, dishes and meals high in potassium- and
calcium-rich foods.

Tips on how to make countless tasty and healthy variations on the sandwich theme . . . Recipes for our best
sandwich ideas.

A review of low-sodium dishes served at some great
American restaurants . . . How to get your share of low-
sodium meals even when you're traveling . . . A guide
to low-sodium prepared foods from soy sauce to
crackers . . . 20 tips for low-salt entertaining . . . Tasty
low-sodium recipes.

Ingenious ways to reduce your sodium intake—without letting your taste buds know it.

Cooking to conserve nutrients . . . The best—and the
worst—ways to cook . . . How to salvage vitamins and
minerals in your food.

A review of the 11 most useful and healthful kitchen
gizmos.

Inside tips on the nutritional bonus of microwave
cooking . . . Secrets to microwaving perfect vegetables,
tender fish, velvety sauces and super stews.

How various breads can differ in protein, fat content,
dietary fiber and magnesium . . . A comprehensive nutritional profile of selected variety breads . . . A winning
recipe for whole wheat bread.

Tables

Preface

Can the right dose of vitamins or minerals cure disease? Can nutrition head off health problems and extend your life? Can diet affect the mind as well as the body? Do megadoses of nutrients help or harm?

The Complete Book of Vitamins and Minerals for Health appears in part because questions like these matter a lot to people and because science is continually digging for the answers.

We answer many of those questions right here. This volume is a nutritional update you can use now to help you assess the value of vitamin and mineral supplements, to plan healthier meals for you and your family, to use nutrition to help confront disease and enhance health. It reflects a new awareness among many doctors and scientists: Food is not just fodder but a force for improved health and well-being.

Part I introduces you to the basics of nutrition and shows you how to use them to improve your health and nourish your family. It tells you who gets nutritional deficiencies and why, how to spot your nutritional weaknesses, how to create diets that meet the different needs of men and women, how to upgrade the junk-food diets of kids and how to customize meals for the singles life. There's even a quiz to test how much you really know about nutrition.

Part II helps put nutritional supplements in perspective. It reveals survey results that show who takes supplements and why, tells you how to select a multiple vitamin/mineral formula that's right for you, details the uses and abuses of vitamin tests and helps you decide when taking supplements makes sense and when it doesn't.

Scientists have been scrutinizing nutrients for decades, piling up mounds of data. Part III helps you sort through much of this evidence. It covers a promising anticancer vitamin, the facts and fallacies of B vitamins, the latest scientific news on vitamins C and E and exciting research into calcium, magnesium, iron, copper, selenium and zinc.

Part IV is a report on some upstart nutritional factors that have been making headlines lately—amino acids, fish oils, dietary fiber and others. It tells you how these substances are being used in preliminary research to fight high cholesterol levels, insomnia, depression and other health problems.

Part V is a comprehensive review of ailments—from alcoholism to zinc deficiency—and how scientists and doctors are using nutrition to try to counter them. It's a massive catalog of intriguing possibilities for the prevention and treatment of disease. It covers B vitamins and mental health, magnesium and heart trouble, beta-carotene and cancer, low-fat diets and heart disease, dietary regimens and high blood pressure, calcium and osteoporosis, nutritional formulas and gum disease, nutrients and vision problems and more. Plus, there's sound advice on taking supplements safely and charts listing the best food sources of specific vitamins and minerals.

Scientists know now that there's no such thing as the perfect, one-size-fits-all diet. They've known for years that what's good for one person may not be good for another. But now it's clear that what's good for someone in one situation may not even be good in the next. Part VI explains what science knows about this new "situational nutrition." It's a guide to calibrating diets to meet the special needs of dieters, exercisers, pregnant women, people in hospitals and nursing homes, people over age 50 and others.

Part VII is a manual on the art and science of healthful cooking and eating. It meshes what science knows about good nutrition with what culinary artists know about preparing great meals. It shows you how to select foods high in specific nutrients, how to store food for maximum nutrition, how to prepare nutritious gourmet dishes, how to concoct deliciously healthful meals using everything from arugula to zucchini. It teaches you how to master low-sodium cooking, healthful microwaving and nutritious, inventive sandwich making. It includes scores of recipes and consumer reports on the new healthier dairy products, America's new vogue foods and healthful cookware and kitchen aids.

Part VII—indeed the whole book—reflects a sound nutritional principle: The preferred source of vitamins and minerals is your food. That means that supplements, as the name implies, should not be used as substitutes for food or good dietary habits. So if you do take supplements, keep the following in mind as you read this volume:

• Vitamins and minerals have a wide margin of safety. Just the same, you should never assume that any nutrient is completely safe in amounts much larger than the Recommended Dietary Allowance (RDA). Be especially careful to avoid excessive amounts of the fat-soluble vitamins A and D.

• Researchers and clinicians may use higher doses of supplements to treat some medical conditions, but this does not mean these amounts are appropriate therapy for you. For the proper diagnosis and treatment of your medical problem, consult your doctor.

• For some people, multiple-vitamin supplements can be valuable dietary additions. Those that contain all major nutrients in amounts from 25 to 100 percent of the RDA are usually best. These amounts are considered more than adequate to meet the requirements of practically all healthy people. For information specific to your own medical needs, consult a knowledgeable physician or a registered dietitian.

Mark Bricklin

Editor
Prevention® Magazine

Part I

ACHIEVING THE NUTRIENT-RICH LIFESTYLE

Spotting Your Nutritional Danger Zones

Research shows that many Americans are increasingly concerned about what's in the 1,500 pounds of food they chow down each year. They're eating fewer frankfurters and less luncheon meat, sugar and candy, oils and fats. They're eating more chicken, cheese, dark green vegetables and citrus fruits.

Their concern is certainly a step in the right direction, but most still have a way to go, says Paul Lachance, Ph.D., professor of nutrition and food science at Rutgers University, New Brunswick, New Jersey. "The average American doesn't know where the nutrients are. He doesn't go shopping and pick up a vegetable and say, 'Here's my vitamin C.' He'll read the label on a prepared food, but won't know what it means. When it comes to details, most people just don't know much about nutrition."

Mealtime. Do you know where the vitamins and minerals are?

What You Don't Know Can Hurt You

Many people have false notions about food—misconceptions that can affect their nutritional status. Phyllis Havens, R.D., a Hampden, Maine, consulting nutritionist, says, "People think margarine is so much better than butter, but then they'll use twice as much of it, not realizing there's as much fat and calories in it as butter. And they think granola bars are a healthy snack, when they're actually loaded with fat and sugar."

Havens is "reeducating" the clients she sees in her private practice and at the Holistic Center in South Portland, using an updated version of an old teaching tool—the basic four food groups. "I am encouraging people to look at them again, as a guide, but with an emphasis on specific nutrients and whole foods— whole grains, low-fat dairy products, fresh fruits, dark green, leafy vegetables, and fish and poultry."

Poor diet, poor health.

Good advice. But why exactly is it that so many individuals score poorly on personal nutrition? Lack of knowledge is one reason. But certain patterns of eating, or even patterns of living, also predispose many of us to dietary problems. And these dietary problems can often turn into health problems. Let's check out several common eating patterns or diets and ask, "Where are the hidden danger zones? How can they be eliminated?"

The High-Protein Predicament

Jean and Jerry like the high-protein "quick-weight-loss" diet. It lets them fill up on their favorite foods—steak and shrimp—and still drop five pounds in a week. It also allows them to eat plenty of chicken, low-fat cheese, lean fish and hard-boiled eggs, and to drink as much diet soda and coffee as their kidneys can handle. It prohibits any other foods. No fruits or vegetables. No carbohydrates. It's a diet they go on again and again, every time they regain those five pounds.

What's wrong with this diet? Plenty.

What's wrong with this diet? For starters, it's high in fat. Fifty percent or more of its calories come from fat. "Anyone who's worried about heart disease or liver or kidney problems would want to avoid eating this way," Dr. Lachance says. "And it's also higher in sodium than is wise."

The amount of fiber in this diet would be minuscule. "You are begging for dependency on a laxative," Dr. Lachance says. Low-fiber intake could aggravate gallstones or diverticulosis, Havens adds. A high-protein diet may also shortchange you on calcium and other important vitamins and minerals. A high-protein diet would make your body excrete up to twice the calcium it normally would. "Unless you are eating a lot of low-fat dairy products [a good source of calcium], you could definitely increase the risk of osteoporosis [thin, weak bones], especially with older women, with this diet," Havens says.

Other important vitamins and minerals found mostly in fruits, vegetables and whole grains would be missing in this diet—vitamins A and C, magnesium, potassium, and, among the B complex, thiamine (B_1), B_6 and folate. "When you see the number of nutrients that aren't being delivered and the health risks involved, you have to ask yourself, 'Why should I use this diet?' " Dr. Lachance says.

Protein-only weight-loss diets starve your body of vitamins and minerals.

Adding insult to injury, much of that quick and highly encouraging weight loss on the high-protein diet is loss of water—water that gushes back into your body the minute you resume eating carbohydrates. Both nutritionists recommend a diet high in fiber and low in fats for people who want to lose weight. "I recommend a diet similar to the Pritikin diet [high in grains and vegetables, very low in fat] but one that allows about 20 percent fat," Havens says. Dr. Lachance likes the diet outlined in *The F-* [for fiber] *Plan Diet*.

Both diets allow you ample quantities of food (and vitamins and minerals) while minimizing the most concentrated source of calories—fat.

The Iron Impasse

Let's look at another dieter, Joan, who's proud of her superslim figure and admits she practically lives

Weight loss doesn't have to mean vitamin loss.

on a few low-cal staples—cottage cheese, yogurt, broiled chicken and fish, lettuce and tomato, zucchini and string beans. She's also a big tea and coffee drinker. She thinks caffeine helps dull her appetite and perks her up. The trouble is, Joan hasn't been feeling very perky lately.

Joan's big problem is iron. She's getting less than half of what she needs from her food, and her tea and coffee drinking further inhibit absorption of the little she does get, according to Havens.

A list of iron-rich, low-cal foods for the dieter.

"I would focus on lots of dark green, leafy vegetables like broccoli, spinach and even some of the more unusual greens like collard, mustard and kale," she says. "And I would try to convince her that some iron-rich legumes like beans and lentils aren't all that fattening. A half cup of cooked kidney beans has only 110 calories."

Dr. Lachance is very concerned about the difficulty of absorbing iron from grains and vegetables. "I'd suggest, instead, some of the very lean red meats, the muscle meats from the shoulder and rump." Women unwilling to eat much red meat will have to take an iron supplement, he believes.

How about someone who's eating no meat at all?

Meatless Menus

When they went vegetarian ten years ago, Tom and Tina had the best of intentions and enough information to get them started. They'd read Frances Moore Lappé's *Diet for a Small Planet* and shifted their preferences toward dairy products, eggs, grains and plenty of fresh fruits and vegetables. They even got to like tofu and miso. They were determined to avoid all the ills associated with the typical Western diet—obesity, high blood pressure, heart disease. But were they setting themselves up for unseen troubles?

Deficiencies of both zinc and iron can be a problem in a vegetarian diet, especially for women, researchers have found. And vegans, who eat no dairy products or eggs, often get less than the Recommended Dietary Allowance (RDA) for calcium. "No vegetable is a reliable source of zinc, and I'm very supportive of every vegetarian taking a zinc supplement," Havens says.

Vegetarians may miss out on zinc and other essential minerals.

"And I think it's worthwhile if they're not feeling the highest energy level possible to have a blood test to see if they are iron deficient." If they are, she will try adding iron-rich legumes, blackstrap molasses and dark green, leafy vegetables to their diet for three months, then have a second blood test done. If the dietary changes aren't working, she'll then suggest an iron supplement.

Vitamin B_{12} used to be considered an inevitable deficiency for strict vegetarians. Now, though, researchers have found significant amounts of vitamin B_{12} in cultured and fermented foods such as miso, soy sauce and tempeh.

Fermented foods can help prevent a vitamin B_{12} deficiency.

How about people who turn up their noses at vegetables? They may face an entirely different set of nutritional shortcomings.

Vegetable-Hater's Plight

As far as Frank is concerned, the only vegetable "real men" eat is potatoes—french-fried with a burger, boiled with a pot roast or hash-browned with eggs. Like the picky little kid he was, Frank finds most fruits and vegetables yucky. But his childish holdover could be making him deficient in vitamins A and E, folate and potassium.

Let's not knock potatoes. A medium baked spud with its skin has 944 milligrams of potassium (about a third of what most adults require), 30 milligrams of vitamin C (half the RDA) and 4 grams of fiber, about a third of what many people get in a day. The problem is in the way most of us cook potatoes, says Georgene Barte, associate professor of foods and nutrition at Oregon State University, Corvallis. We peel the nutrient- and fiber-rich skin off, and boil or fry away some

How to cook potatoes for maximum nutrition.

of the vitamin C. Frank and other meat-and-potato lovers should be eating a baked potato, skin and all.

And adding even a few fruits and vegetables—as snacks and salads—to his limited menu could raise the vitamin and mineral content of Frank's diet to a healthful level.

"I find that some adults who are really turned off by cooked vegetables do better with raw ones," says Havens. "If they don't like cooked spinach, I suggest they start eating it raw, mixed with iceberg lettuce, gradually increasing the amount. Or they might enjoy dips with carrots or green pepper strips."

Some vegetables may be served with maple syrup.

Like many children, some adults dislike strong-flavored vegetables like cabbage, broccoli and onions. Instead, they may enjoy sweet-flavored carrots, winter squash and sweet potatoes, served with a smidgen of butter and maple syrup. These vegetables would certainly solve Frank's vitamin A problem. A four-ounce serving of sweet potatoes or carrots would supply his RDA of 5,000 international units, as would a half cup of butternut squash.

Citrus fruits and juices would be Frank's best bet for vitamin C. Just one cup of orange juice would give him 124 milligrams of C and an additional bonus of 496 milligrams of potassium and 500 international units of vitamin A.

Calcium Countdown

Mary's daughter has been nagging her to get more calcium in her diet ever since Mary fell and broke her wrist a few years ago. Now she's 70 and unsteady on her feet. Her daughter fears she'll fall and break a hip one of these days.

Are you getting as much calcium as you think?

The problem is that Mary thinks she gets all the calcium she needs. She drinks about a cup of milk a day, with cereal and coffee, and usually eats a slice of cheese or half a cup of cottage cheese every day. Other calcium-containing foods boost her daily intake to the RDA of 800 milligrams.

But that's not enough calcium to prevent osteoporosis, researchers say.

"I think the RDA for calcium for women past 30 should be 1,000 milligrams, and for those past menopause, 1,200 to 1,500 milligrams," says Barte.

Getting that much calcium in your diet would mean getting the equivalent of four or five cups of milk a day. Each cup has 290 milligrams of calcium, or 36 milligrams per ounce. One big misconception is that people think one serving of cottage cheese, usually about a quarter cup, equals the calcium in a cup of milk. Actually, about *two cups* of cottage cheese equals one cup of milk, Barte says.

Cottage cheese is not as good a source of calcium as milk.

The only foods that surpass dairy products for calcium content are sardines and salmon, but only if you eat the soft small bones mixed in the flesh. Sardines have 124 milligrams of calcium per ounce; salmon, 63 milligrams.

No Time for Nutrition

What if you're concerned with getting an entire busy family to eat better?

Marcia and her family are lucky if they see one another long enough to nuzzle up and say, "Hello, stranger." Both she and her husband work, and he's on the road a day or two each week. When her two teenage sons aren't in school, they're at band practice or a swimming meet. Marcia gave up on sit-down meals when she realized the only family member willing to show up on a regular basis was the dog.

Now meals are whenever they're hungry and whatever they manage to scrounge out of the refrigerator. She tries to keep it stocked with foods the kids like and can easily fix themselves—ground beef, tuna, cheese, eggs, hot dogs and beans, bread, milk, cold cuts, frozen pizzas. And, of course, sodas, potato chips and ice cream. Her kids would mutiny if she didn't keep those things around the house. She's about the only one who eats the salad fixings she

Meals on-the-run can fall short of the B vitamins and two essential minerals.

brings home. She'd like her family to eat better, but where to start?

The dangers in this diet are too much fat and sugar and too little fiber, B and C vitamins, and minerals like magnesium and potassium, Havens says.

"If Marcia were willing to commit even a few hours a week to cooking, she could make a huge pot of nutritious soup with beans, brown rice and all kinds of vegetables, keep part in the refrigerator and freeze some for use later. I do that myself, and I'm a busy professional."

Planning ahead is the key to nutritious meals.

Planning ahead by making and freezing large batches of other good foods—chili, corn bread, beans (which could later be refried for tacos), pizzas cut up into individual slices—could actually save Marcia time in the long run. And having cut-up crunchies or low-sugar sweets like homemade oatmeal cookies within a hungry hand's reach might help wean her sugar-loving adolescents off their regular fix.

A more realistic solution, says Dr. Lachance, would be to simply supplement the family's fast foods with items to make a complete meal. "If you're eating a hamburger or a pizza, which is not such bad food, make sure you have a salad and a glass of skim milk, too, not a soda," he says.

And you can choose convenience foods with an eye toward more nourishment and less fat and salt.

Choose convenience foods carefully.

Look for stir-fry meat and vegetable combinations and dieter's dinners, and pick store-brand frozen vegetables without butter or sauces.

Anyone's eating habits may contain a nutritional danger zone or two. In the next chapters, we'll take a closer look at how these problems arise, their effect on health—and what you can do to fill in any nutritional gaps.

Confronting the "Secret Threat" of Marginal Deficiencies

Your doctor has had you tested for everything from strep throat to cancer, examined you from head to toe, and now he's scratching his head.

His notes on your chart tell all: "Patient reports irritability, diminished appetite and weight loss. Chronic insomnia. Apparent malaise. All tests negative. Cause of symptoms: unknown."

He suspects advancing age or excessive worry and wonders if he's overlooking something.

Maybe he is. Without even knowing it, your doctor could be staring at a textbook case of marginal nutritional deficiency—a middle ground where you're neither optimally nourished nor suffering from classic signs of severe vitamin and mineral depletion (like scurvy or beriberi). You feel lousy, but not lousy enough to go to a hospital. Or you feel normal, just a little under par. And whatever symptoms you have are too general (too nonspecific, as physicians say) to point directly to a particular disease.

Not sick, but not really well? Check for vitamin or mineral depletion.

The Mystery behind Hidden Deficiencies

"Generally speaking, doctors can't detect marginal, or subclinical, deficiencies through conventional techniques," says Myron Brin, Ph.D., a nutrition researcher at Hoffman La Roche in New Jersey. "Unless a doctor does appropriate biochemical testing

Subtle deficiencies are hard to detect.

[the kind designed to assess nutrient levels], he can't tell if the general symptoms indicate a marginal deficiency. Most often it is difficult to connect the symptoms to vitamin or mineral depletion—they're just not classic enough."

Yet for over ten years, scientists and clinicians have been documenting this middle realm and taking the terrain seriously. The accumulating evidence is changing ideas about what is and is not a deficiency—and demonstrating that ignoring marginal cases can be a big mistake.

There are many health problems associated with marginal nutrient deficiencies.

"Marginal vitamin deficiencies may have different effects on the body's metabolism, which depends on the stage of life and the demands facing its normal development," says D. I. Thurnham, a London expert on human nutrition. "Growth restrictions, degenerative changes in tissues, fetal abnormalities, interference with milk production or composition, increased susceptibility to infection, altered response to dietary constituents, diminished work ability are among the possible effects of chronic marginal restrictions in the diet" (*Proceedings of the Nutrition Society*).

But not everyone who feels out of sorts is bordering on nutritional deficiency, and most Americans seem to be getting all the food they want. So just how widespread can subclinical deficiencies be?

Vitamin and mineral deficiencies are more common than many people realize.

"The problem is much more pervasive than many people realize," Dr. Brin says. "Certainly you cannot assume that a person who isn't getting his Recommended Dietary Allowance [RDA] of a specific nutrient is in a state of marginal depletion, since it takes time for such a state to occur. But it is clear that the diets of large segments of the population are not meeting the RDA for certain vitamins and minerals. And such nutritional shortfalls can eventually lead to marginal status."

Indeed, several large-scale government surveys of nutritional well-being have already shown that nutrient deficits are surprisingly common. They revealed that approximately one-half the U.S. population gets less than the RDA of one or more vitamins and minerals and that the nutrients most likely to be marginal are magnesium, calcium and iron and vitamins A, B$_6$ and C.

Nongovernment studies tell a similar tale of nutritional poverty and confirm that some Americans are more likely than others to drop below the line. They show that menstruating women, expectant mothers, schoolchildren, teenagers and the elderly may be especially prone to low nutrient levels.

Certain people are at higher risk than others.

A Downward Slide in Vitamin and Mineral Levels

But researchers are doing more than merely demonstrating that marginal deficiencies may threaten a lot of people. They're also digging up data on exactly what such depletions can do to the human body—and they're burying an old nutritional notion along the way.

The traditional view has been that if you don't have scurvy or rickets or some other classic manifestation, you must be adequately nourished. So among doctors the idea of a marginal nutrient deficiency has been about as prevalent as belief in marginal broken legs. But now it's clear that a deficiency state—whether marginal or classic—is the result of a long chain of cellular reactions. And a reduced nutrient level can set off a whole series of dire reverberations long before classic symptoms appear.

You don't have to have scurvy to be low on vitamin C.

Much of the evidence for such biochemical cataclysms has come from so-called depletion experiments—studies in which people were monitored for changes in their body or mental state as certain nutrients were limited.

Several experiments revealed that when people were put on lowered intakes of vitamin C, thiamine

(B_1) or riboflavin (B_2), they actually developed behavior problems. Researchers reported cases of hypochondria, depression, hysteria and even psychopathic abnormalities, all of which disappeared when the subjects got adequate doses of the depleted vitamin.

Clues to Low Vitamin Levels

Meanwhile, Dr. Brin, one of the pioneers in such work, has been able to identify three consecutive phases of marginal vitamin deficiency in the body.

"In the preliminary stage," he says, "the tissue stores of the nutrient are gradually depleted." Because of either low intake, poor absorption or abnormal metabolism, the body's nutrient silos get secretly emptied, and there's no physical damage to signal the deficit.

"Then," says Dr. Brin, "there's the biochemical stage, in which tissue stores are sufficiently depleted to result in reduced rates of biochemical reactions, which require the presence of the particular nutrient."

In this phase comes silent destruction: Enzymes responsible for energizing bits of biochemistry break down because the crucial vitamin is missing. And there isn't the slightest clue in the body's appearance or growth to disclose the hidden ruin.

Such clues start showing up only in the next physiological stage. "Here," says Dr. Brin, "tissue and biochemical depletion become so severe that there are behavioral and psychological manifestations of nutritional inadequacy."

The symptoms range from sluggish thinking to psychoses—and can easily be mistaken for ordinary human frailties. Beyond this phase lies deep depletion, with all its classic insignia.

"The rate of depletion varies from nutrient to nutrient," Dr. Brin says. "For example, a person may reach the biochemical stage for thiamine in only two days of deprivation. For vitamin C it may take from two weeks to two months."

Studies show that too little B_1, B_2 or vitamin C may cause depression.

Silent destruction is the second step of vitamin deficiency.

Older, but Not Always Wiser

All this has looming implications for the diagnosis and treatment of disease, especially for mental ailments. It's hard to imagine a group for whom this deficiency/brain connection has more relevance than the elderly, who are known to be singularly prone to nutritional shortcomings.

James S. Goodwin, M.D., and his colleagues, of the University of New Mexico School of Medicine in Albuquerque, would second that. They recently inves-

---

Curbing Vitamin Deficiencies in the Elderly

Elderly people who live in retirement homes are at risk of developing nutritional deficiencies, according to a group of doctors who studied the residents of four homes. That is, if they don't take supplements. Of the 244 people the doctors examined, 62 percent of those who did not take vitamins had some deficiencies, but only 10 percent who used supplements had deficiencies. Thiamine deficiency showed up most frequently, followed by riboflavin and vitamins A and C.

What are the implications for these people? According to Douglas Heimburger, M.D., of the University of Alabama Medical Center, an expert on the nutritional needs of hospitalized patients, various nutritional deficiencies can have a dramatic effect on the well-being of the elderly.

"Vitamins A and C are important in wound healing," Dr. Heimburger continues, "especially for patients recovering from surgery. Lung and urinary tract infections are common in the elderly, and it is possible that vitamin C would have a role here. For instance, C plays a part in the function of white blood cells [scavenger cells] and also acidifies the urine to inhibit infection in the bladder.

"Thiamine deficiency is most implicated in the decreased mental capacity often seen in nursing home residents," adds Dr. Heimburger. "The confusion and meandering thoughts in the elderly are frequently attributed to Alzheimer's disease or the effects of just sitting around all day. But it can also be caused by a thiamine deficiency."

tigated the possibility that marginal deficiencies could impair the thinking of men and women age 60 or older, and their findings suggest ominous possibilities.

"We knew that institutionalized elderly people had been shown to improve mentally when supplemented with vitamins," Dr. Goodwin says. "But these subjects had severe nutrient deficiencies and serious mental impairments. We wanted to determine if *mild* deficiencies might also be connected with cognitive problems. The question is important because even mild dementia is associated with a striking increase in mortality in the aged."

So the researchers selected 260 healthy people (all of them living at home and showing no classic symptoms of deficiency), assessed their intake and blood levels of nutrients, and tested their memory and abstract thinking.

Fuzzy thinking in older people may be due to a mild vitamin deficiency.

Analysis of the data revealed that people with the lowest nutrient levels got lower scores on the cognitive exams. Subjects with low blood levels of vitamins B_{12} or C demonstrated both poor memory and abstract thinking skills. Subjects with low blood levels of riboflavin or folate showed poor abstraction skills only (*Journal of the American Medical Association*).

People with low levels of vitamin B_{12} or C had poor memory.

"The association between marginal deficiency and impaired cognitive functioning was impressive," says Dr. Goodwin, "though we cannot yet say for sure that the one causes the other. But considering previous evidence, I think it likely that in older people subclinical deficiencies can indeed lead to less-than-optimal mental performance."

Pregnant Women Are Most Vulnerable

And if marginal status can possibly harm the elderly, can it also threaten people even more nutritionally vulnerable—such as pregnant women?

Researchers at the University of California think so. Recently they conducted a study to find out what marginal zinc deficiency would do to pregnant rhesus monkeys. Previous studies had hinted that zinc deficiency may be harmful to pregnant women, but the cause-and-effect relationship had never been nailed down. The California investigators were hoping to clarify the causal connection by restricting the animals' zinc intake and gauging the results—an obviously unacceptable methodology for pregnant women.

Pregnant women need the best nutrition they can get.

The researchers fed the monkeys a marginal zinc diet throughout gestation, and by the third trimester the resulting damage was apparent.

Despite "otherwise optimal dietary and environmental conditions," say the investigators, the animals showed a "compromised physiological condition as reflected in inadequate weight gain; reduced circulating [in the blood] glucose, triglycerides and vitamin A; slight iron deficiency anemia and reduced immune response." As you would expect, a control group of pregnant monkeys that were fed an adequate zinc diet had fewer problems (*American Journal of Clinical Nutrition*).

Pregnant animals that were deprived of zinc developed a number of health problems.

These findings, say the researchers, have significant ramifications for humans, suggesting that even a not-so-classic zinc deficit can produce serious abnormalities during pregnancy. This is simply another piece of evidence that subterranean nutrition can be dangerous ground—and that life is safer in the higher dietary elevations.

Chapter 3

Nutrition for Women, Nutrition for Men

Studies show that men and women have different tastes in food—and different nutritional needs.

Food preference surveys, for instance, show that men are nearly twice as likely as women to eat whatever they want, and what they want is a tender but fatty cut of red meat. That's one reason that even in these health-conscious times, the typical man's diet is too high in fat and sometimes low in the vitamins and minerals that are found in fruits, vegetables and dairy products.

Men and women are not created equal.

Women like meat, too, but they also want fruits and vegetables. Their food shopping and cooking skills make them likely to be more nutritionally aware than men, but they also have special dietary demands, particularly during pregnancy. And they're twice as likely as men to be watching their weight, possibly eating too few calories to supply all the nourishment they need, especially during their childbearing years.

Men need more B vitamins than women—but half as much iron.

The National Academy of Sciences' Recommended Dietary Allowances (RDAs) reflect most, but not all, of the differences in nutritional requirements between the sexes. At every age men require 10 to 30 percent more protein, vitamins A, E and B_6, thiamine (B_1), riboflavin (B_2), niacin and magnesium than women. They require equal amounts of vitamins D, C and B_{12}, folate, calcium, phosphorus, zinc and iodine. They require only about half as much iron.

Women who are pregnant or breastfeeding have the highest nutritional requirements. They need vitamins and minerals in amounts equal to or greater than those required by men. In some cases—with folate and calcium, for instance—their needs jump dramatically. Not meeting those needs can result in low-birthweight babies or seriously impair the mother's health.

Are You Getting Enough Iron?

Iron is one nutrient women need more of than men, according to the National Academy of Sciences. Menstruating women require almost twice as much iron as men (18 milligrams compared to 10 milligrams). And pregnant women may need 30 to 60 milligrams of iron each day.

Nutritional surveys show that about 40 percent of women of childbearing age don't get enough iron, says Cecilia Davis, a registered dietitian and former president of the nationwide dietitian's referral service, the Consulting Nutritionist Practice Group.

"Women absorb only about six milligrams of iron per 1,000 calories of food in a typical diet," she says. "They would need to eat about 3,000 calories a day to meet their iron RDA. Few eat that much, so many women need supplemental iron."

Unless a woman eats 3,000 calories a day, she may need extra iron.

Teenage girls are even worse off, Davis contends. "I'd say 80 percent could be iron deficient. Some eat as few as 1,000 calories a day, and their food preferences are poor in iron."

Among teenagers, boys can also develop iron deficiencies, sometimes rather quickly when they start the rapid growth of adolescence. There is an enormous demand for blood-building materials at this stage. "And I'd say this is more likely to be overlooked in boys than in girls," Davis says.

Both men and women may sometimes become iron depleted during very strenuous athletic training, says Paul Zabetakis, M.D., a research physician at the

Athletes can risk low iron levels.

Institute of Sportsmedicine and Athletic Trauma in New York. In superathletes, strenuous exercise can actually break down red blood cells and lead to anemia (iron deficiency).

Dr. Zabetakis cautions that average runners as well as ultramarathon athletes may also develop "pseudo-anemia." Blood tests will show lower-than-normal iron levels, but the larger volume of blood they have developed as a result of their athletic activities means their oxygen-carrying capacity remains the same. They'll have no physical symptoms of anemia.

Overuse of aspirin or alcohol can cause blood loss—and iron loss.

When most adult men (and women past menopause) develop iron deficiencies, though, diet or exercise is rarely the cause, says Robert McGandy, M.D., a Tufts University professor of medicine and consulting doctor for the Boston-based Human Nutrition Research Center for Aging. Internal bleeding—ulcers, intestinal polyps, excessive aspirin or alcohol use, even hemorrhoids—are too often the cause. "In this case, it's important to be checked for blood loss and not to try to cure yourself with an iron supplement," Dr. McGandy says.

Too much iron is as bad as too little—but not nearly as common.

Anyone, but especially men, small children and postmenopausal women, can develop iron overload. They can take in so much iron that it builds up in their liver or spleen and begins to cause damage. (It can also make it difficult to travel by air. One man with this problem found it impossible to get by the metal detector at an airport. He'd been getting frequent blood transfusions for a medical problem.)

"Nobody is going to get an overload, though, unless he's getting at least five to ten times the RDA," Dr. McGandy says. "No man is going to get this just by taking his wife's multivitamin with iron."

Too Little Folate and B_6— Women Pay the Price

Sometimes what masquerades as an iron deficiency is actually a folate problem. One common nutritional problem in the United States is a low intake of this B vitamin. People just aren't eating enough folate-rich dark green, leafy vegetables, and women, especially, pay the consequences.

Dark green leafy vegetables are rich in folate.

Anemia can occur when there is not enough folate in the body to produce red blood cells. Among older women, especially, folate rather than iron may be the culprit in this problem. And folate deficiencies have been implicated in cervical dysplasia, a condition that can lead to cancer of the cervix. The vitamin has also been found to reverse the disease in some women.

Pregnant women need to double their folate intake from 400 to 800 micrograms, and those who are breastfeeding need 500 micrograms. "Folate is needed for the manufacture of all cells," Dr. McGandy says. That's why it's so important to fetal growth and growth of the newborn baby. In fact, both spina bifida, a birth defect in which the tissue around the spinal cord doesn't close properly, and cleft palates have been associated with low folate intake. In one study, women who had had one baby with spina bifida were much less likely to have a second baby with the same problem if they got adequate folate.

Pregnant and nursing women need folate.

Vitamin B_6 has been associated with "women's problems" for some time now. It's been used to treat fluid retention and other symptoms associated with premenstrual syndrome. It's also been prescribed for women taking birth control pills, who often have lower blood levels of this vitamin. Mood changes, like depression, that some women taking birth-control pills experience, have been attributed to lower levels of B_6, which some researchers speculate may lead to decreased production of the brain neurotransmitter serotonin. See your doctor if you think you need more than the RDA of B_6. High doses have been associated with neurological changes.

Taking birth control pills? B_6 may be low.

Building Better Bones

The RDA table (see pages 637–43) lists the same calcium requirements, 800 milligrams a day, for men and women. As we mentioned in chapter 1, this does not reflect the growing belief among nutritionists that women need more than this amount to prevent the brittle, porous bones of osteoporosis. Some feel that younger women need 1,000 milligrams and post-menopausal women up to 1,500 milligrams a day of calcium to help protect against this disabling disease of older women.

The problem is that many women don't even get 800 milligrams a day, Davis says. Calcium deficiencies among women are second only to iron. The average daily intake of calcium for women is 600 milligrams. Next to iron, calcium is the mineral women most often miss out on.

"Getting 1,000 milligrams a day of calcium means consuming three or four servings of high-calcium foods, mostly dairy products," Davis says. "Although you can get this amount of calcium through foods—and that's the best way—it does take quite a bit of attention to do so without taking in a lot of calories." Low-fat dairy products or calcium supplements provide bone-building material without the fat-building side effects.

Real Men Need Vitamin C

You might think scurvy disappeared along with pirates and wooden galleons, but that's not what some doctors have found.

It's true that in these days of year-round availability of fresh fruit and instant breakfast juices, scurvy is uncommon in the United States. Most people get at least the ten milligrams of vitamin C needed to ward off this disease.

Would your doctor recognize scurvy if he saw it?

Most, but not all, as doctors at the Veterans Administration Medical Center in Portland, Oregon, recently discovered. Each of the three men they saw had swelling, pain and purplish bruising of their legs, along with other symptoms like gum disease, fatigue, blood in the stools or, the classic scurvy tipoff, corkscrew hair. Two of them had undergone extensive medical testing to try to determine the cause of their symptoms.

But it was an analysis of their diet and a check of their blood levels of vitamin C that led to the correct diagnosis—scurvy. It turned out all three lived alone and cooked for themselves or ate out. Each admitted he rarely ate fresh fruits or vegetables. Supplemental vitamin C eliminated their symptoms in just a few days (*Journal of the American Medical Association*).

Men who live alone and cook for themselves may skimp on vitamin C-rich foods.

Because scurvy is rare, physicians may not recognize it when they see it, the Portland doctors say. Men who live alone and cook for themselves, especially the elderly or heavy drinkers, are among those at highest risk for developing scurvy, they point out.

The Nutritional Bonus in Fruits and Vegetables

Turning up their noses at fruits and vegetables can have other consequences for men. "We tend to see too little fiber in their diets," says Rebecca McCully, R.D., administrator of Greenhouse Diet Services and consulting nutritionist for the Cardiovascular Clinic in Oklahoma City. "Men who have very sedentary jobs and eat low-fiber diets are more likely to develop chronic constipation. Women are less prone to this problem because they tend to eat a lot more fresh fruits and vegetables."

Too little fiber—and too much fat—compound nutritional losses.

Admittedly, the men she sees may eat less well than some—after all, they've had heart problems. "The biggest problems I see in people's diets are excesses—too much fat, salt, calories," she says. Nutritional deficiencies are much less common, at least in the middle-class midwestern men she sees. In any case, her advice applies equally well to men and women.

"I tell my people that their doctors aren't responsible and their spouses aren't responsible for what they put in their mouths. They are, and they must accept that responsibility and learn to make healthy food choices and decisions."

Chapter 4

Vitamins and Minerals for Singles

I f you're one of the 23.2 percent of the American population living in what the census bureau calls a one-person household, it's a safe bet your diet makes World War II C-rations look like health food.

"What do I usually eat?" says a 31-year-old single personnel consultant in Washington, D.C. "TV dinners, M&M's, Haagen-Dazs ice cream every Sunday night. I wouldn't eat this way if I weren't single. I wouldn't be so careless. But I want you to know I've seen the error of my ways . . . all 20 pounds of the error of my ways."

Sad but true: Many singles are undernourished.

Like this reformed careless consumer, many singles atone for their dietary indiscretions only after they learn the direct relationship between their waist size and the number of disposable single-serving food packages in their trash. But the damage they do with their quickie over-the-sink meals and their fast-food feasts is far from merely cosmetic. Next to the poor, they may be the most undernourished people in America.

Living Alone? Nutrition Can Suffer

George Demetrakopoulos, M.D., M.P.H., is medical director of the Medical Nutrition Center of greater Washington, D.C. Among the patients who come to him for nutritional assessments are people who should know about nutrition: employees of several of the government's top health-regulation agencies. But, he says, it doesn't seem to give them an edge if they're single. In a study of 40 single men and women between 25 and 45, he found most were deficient in zinc, folate and B_6. The women were also deficient in calcium and were getting only 57 percent of their recommended daily allowance of iron.

"These are not typical people," says Dr. Demetrakopoulos. "These are nutrition-conscious people. They should have performed above average, but they didn't. Imagine," he says, "the ones who are not as informed."

Though the research is meager, it seems to show that living alone is a significant nutritional risk factor, even if you're nutritionally savvy. In fact, eating for one seems to be most perilous for young single women who are aware consumers and older single men who don't know their way around the kitchen without a guide.

Researchers at Auburn University took a look at the diets of 50 single professional women, most of whom usually made food lists and menu plans and avoided convenience foods. Despite those good intentions, their diets were low in calories, calcium, iron, vitamin A and thiamine (B_1). What's more, their good food habits seemed to be done in by their frequent lunches out.

Single professional women fall short on calcium, iron, vitamin A and thiamine, says one study.

In a study of 3,477 people between the ages of 65 and 74, researchers at the University of California and the University of Texas found that poor men living alone had the lowest intake of milk products, fruits, vegetables, meat, poultry and fish of any group. And they were more likely to be getting less than two-thirds of the Recommended Dietary Allowance (RDA) of protein, riboflavin, vitamins A and C, and other nutrients.

Why Singles
Don't Always Eat Right

Busy schedules, dieting, lack of motivation or cooking skills, even loneliness and depression can contribute to meager mealtimes for many singles, say the experts. And unfortunately, there's usually no immediate retribution for bad diet that might persuade a fast-food aficionado to change his ways.

"Most nutritional problems don't manifest themselves right away, so it's easy to cheat," says David Ostreicher, D.D.S., professor of nutrition at Bridgeport University in Connecticut, who is single. "If you're not getting enough vitamins A and C, you might not know until 20 years later when you develop cancer. If you're eating a diet high in saturated fats and salt—the staples of most convenience foods—you might not know until you have your first heart attack at age 50."

Don't let loneliness or a busy schedule rob you of good nutrition.

How to Upgrade a Singles' Diet

So what do you do? "Get married," jokes Dr. Demetrakopoulos. Or, failing that, simply steal some tricks from your wedded friends who are following a better diet.

Cook for four. "Never, never cook for one," says Dr. Ostreicher. "Cook for four, eat one serving and freeze the rest in individual servings. You'll be making your own convenience foods, you'll pay less for it and you will be eating better."

Make shopping lists. "All my married friends have lists; none of my single friends do," says Dr. Ostreicher. Why a list? First, it will make you plan your weekly meals. And it will keep you from straying into dangerous territory: the family pack of cookies that looks too good to pass up, 500-calorie-a-slice frozen pizza and the special on heavenly hash ice cream. Needless to say, don't go shopping when you're hungry and, advises Dr. Ostreicher, have regular shopping days, so you aren't tempted to dash into the deli for a hot pastrami on the way home because there's nothing in the fridge.

A shopping list reduces temptation and helps build nutrition into your menu.

Shop with a friend. Going on the premise that everything is better with a friend, try shopping on the buddy system. Your companion will be your conscience. "If you have a companion, you can discuss what you're going to buy and make with the other person," says Dr. Demetrakopoulos. "Alone, you'll wind up buying things you'd be better off without."

Two singles are better than one—shop with a friend.

Steer for the freezer section. Many singles have given up on fresh vegetables because they are forgotten and then grow moldy in the refrigerator before the week is up.

"Psychologically, that stops you from buying vegetables the next time," says Dr. Ostreicher. "But right next to the frozen convenience foods, you'll find plastic bags of vegetables with nothing added that are just as nutritious as fresh. You can reseal the plastic bags so you can use what you like and freeze the rest. You don't pay more, and they don't give you all that excess salt and fat."

Upgrade your diet with frozen foods.

Don't buy big. Those family packs and mammoth cans may be cheaper, but they're no bargain if you have to throw half of the food away. If you want to buy the bigger packages, consider sharing them with a friend. And if you see a cut of meat or produce you like in a larger package, ask a store employee to repackage it.

Develop good eating habits. If you have to, pretend you're eating with a friend. Would you eat a chicken leg over the sink or swig milk right out of the bottle if you had a dining companion? Then don't do it when you're alone. "Always set the table," says Dr. Ostreicher. "You decide how—with a tablecloth or place mats. Candlelight might be excessive, but get into the habit of having a place setting, even if you're just grabbing a piece of fruit.

Avoid "stand-up" meals and snacks.

"When you live alone, you often get into the habit, when you've got nothing to do, of standing in front of the open refrigerator snacking. Always eat at the table, always with a place setting."

Make Dining a Pleasant Experience

Make dining an adventure. And share meals with friends.

Lynn Shahan, author of *Living Alone and Liking It!*, says that during her first year eating alone, she became "a pretty skinny kid" because mealtime, previously spent with family and friends, lost its appeal. Her solution for happier soloing at the dinner table was to buy new and interesting foods and experiment with recipes, so eating became more of an adventure.

Share your meals. Invite friends or neighbors for dinner. Start a cooking club with your fellow singles. Call your local agency on aging to find out if your neighborhood provides free or low-cost meals for older people at community centers or churches.

Or join a group like Single Gourmet, a New York–based organization that tackles the problems of eating alone by arranging for up to 100 singles to eat out together seven to ten times a month.

Cofounder Art Fischer says that not only will it improve your social life and your outlook but it may also improve your digestion. "Doctors have told us that one of the problems with single people eating alone is they not only eat all the wrong food, they eat too fast, which can cause digestive problems," says Fischer, whose group numbers 3,000 members in the New York metropolitan area. "In a group like ours, you'll spend two to three hours eating a meal that, if you ate it alone, would be gone in a matter of minutes. People tell us that they've never been able to eat garlic before without getting indigestion, but when they eat it at a Single Gourmet dinner, it doesn't bother them at all. Really, it's the single lifestyle that doesn't agree with them."

The psychological boost of having pleasant companions and good food is inestimable. "One is a very lonely number," says Effie Seaman, a writer who joined Single Gourmet after the death of her physician husband. "This gives you a reason to get dressed and go out, wearing your finery, which is far better than sitting in front of the TV with a sandwich."

Dine Out Wisely

Ned Schnurman, executive producer of the acclaimed PBS television series *Inside Story*, regards eating out "as a form of theater."

"Eating is one of my principal interests. I eat out 300 nights a year," says Schnurman, who is in his midfifties and single. By all logic, Schnurman should be as wide as he is tall. Instead, even with his rigorous restaurant schedule, he managed to lose 25 pounds in the last few years. How? He eats out wisely. When he chooses a dinner spot to please his palate, he adjusts his other meals accordingly. A light breakfast and lunch are the perfect preludes to the "good saloon fare" he favors: simply grilled chicken, fresh vegetables and "a little wine . . . very little." He avoids heavy sauces and bypasses the dessert cart for fruit. "I don't think it matters where you eat," says Schnurman. "Even if you eat out as much as I do, you can make sure you're eating things of good nutritive value."

Choose light fast-food fare. "It's a real break for singles that most fast-food restaurants now have salad bars," says Dr. Ostreicher. "But if you want to have a burger, have a plain burger. Don't order the fancy burger with the special sauce. And especially don't order a cheeseburger." Keep in mind that almost 90 percent of the calories in cheeses and special sauces come from fat.

You may want to consider supplements, if necessary. "People will not make drastic changes in their diets, so I recommend supplementation," says Dr. Demetrakopoulos. Most women need calcium, he says. And most of the patients he has tested don't get even a third of the RDA of zinc (15 milligrams). But most single people are going to have to face up to it: A bad diet can't be rescued by pills entirely. "Going to the trouble of taking supplements when your diet is grossly inadequate," he says, "is like having a nicely painted house with no windows."

Dine out—but eat smart.

Don't rely on supplements alone to make up for poor eating habits.

Chapter 5

Better Nutrition for Kids

G etting kids to eat right is easier said than done. Ask any mother of a two-year-old who locks his jaw whenever she tries to spoon-feed him carrots. Meanwhile, his older brother trades his nutritious tuna-on-whole-wheat sandwich for a triple pack of cupcakes in the school cafeteria.

How can parents possibly know for sure whether children are properly nourished—getting at least the Recommended Dietary Allowances (RDAs) for vitamins and minerals?

It's unrealistic to expect kids to eat right every day. The overall diet is what counts.

"Everyone who has any kids knows that they don't eat right every day," says Lendon Smith, M.D., an Oregon pediatrician and author of *Dr. Smith's Diet Plan for Teenagers* and *Feed Your Kids Right.* "Even though we'd like them to, it's unrealistic to expect it. You should look at the overall diet. It's okay if your child doesn't get the RDA every day. But is he getting it every week?" (Consult Appendix A to find out how much of each nutrient children should be getting.)

Don't worry about occasional lapses.

Another thing to remember is that getting less than 100 percent of the RDA for a nutrient does not necessarily mean you will become instantly unhealthy. Scientifically, a nutrient isn't considered on the low side until your intake falls below 67 percent of the RDA, and even then, a deficiency disease isn't imminent. Knowing that alone should make you feel better if your child lives on nothing but bananas and graham crackers for a day or two.

Vitamins and Minerals Kids Miss Out On Most

Not surprisingly, certain vitamins and minerals are more likely than others to be in short supply in a child's diet. One study conducted at the University of Washington in Seattle tested a group of healthy children from the ages of 3½ to 9 to see how they fared on the RDA for vitamin C and the B vitamins thiamine (B_1), riboflavin (B_2), B_6, B_{12} and folate—all essential nutrients in normal childhood development. While intakes were adequate for most nutrients, some of the children showed intakes below 70 percent for folate and B_6 (*Journal of the American Dietetic Association*).

Dr. Smith feels that zinc, a trace element that aids normal growth, also is often low in the average child's diet. But it's iron, more than any other nutrient, he says, that is most commonly in short supply.

Alvin N. Eden, M.D., agrees. This practicing pediatrician in New York City and associate clinical professor of pediatrics at the State University of New York, Downstate Medical Center in Brooklyn, says iron is a very neglected area. "I think there's a large group of children out there who are iron deficient without being anemic. For this reason I think it's important for parents to consider giving their children an iron supplement. In fact, the most important thing I tell parents is to 'think iron.' "

A lot of kids lack iron but aren't actually anemic.

Meeting the Recommended Dietary Allowance

If children would eat liver, the biggest source of iron, there would never be a deficiency problem. Nor would a deficiency of zinc, selenium, chromium, vitamin A, riboflavin, B_{12} and folate ever occur. Unfortunately, when it comes to liver, most kids consider going to bed without any supper the better alternative.

(continued on page 32)

Getting Kids to Eat Better: A Doctor Shows How

Many a parent wonders how a kid can survive on peanut butter and more peanut butter. We asked pediatrician Lendon Smith, M.D., to assess a typical day's menu for two typical children—Josh, age 11, and his sister, Elizabeth, age 7. Menu A lists Elizabeth's intake for one day. Menu B lists Josh's. Neither meets the daily allotment for all nutrients. A computer analysis reveals that

MENU A

Menu of a Typical 7-Year-Old Girl	Dr. Lendon Smith's Improved Menu	Dr. Smith's Comments
■ Breakfast		
½ cup sugar-coated cereal with ½ cup low-fat milk ¼ cup orange juice (store brand)	½ cup Grape-Nuts with raisins and ½ cup low-fat milk 1 whole orange or ½ cup fresh orange juice	"The Grape-Nuts will provide more across-the-board nutrients (and less sugar!) and the raisins a little extra shot of this day's allotment of iron. A whole orange is more likely to have more vitamin C, bioflavonoids and fiber."
■ Lunch		
1 peanut butter and jelly sandwich on a potato roll 1 package cheese and crackers 1 cup cran-raspberry juice 3 Oreo cookies 1 peanut butter cup	1 peanut butter and banana sandwich on whole grain bread Thermos of homemade soup, such as chicken noodle or vegetable 1 cup apple juice 3 oatmeal cookies Celery stuffed with peanut butter	"It goes without saying that a banana is a far more nutritious choice than jelly. Whole wheat bread might be a better choice to help give her more B vitamins. The thermos of nutritious soup will help fill a child up and help eliminate her desire for cookies and candy. Apple juice will help bolster this day's low iron allotment, as will the oatmeal cookies."
■ Dinner		
About 1 ounce baked ham 1 bite steamed broccoli ½ cup scalloped potatoes, made with carrots and onions ¼ cup gelatin dessert with a bit of applesauce mixed in ½ cup low-fat milk	2 ounces baked ham 1 spear broccoli ½ cup scalloped potatoes, made with carrots and onions ½ cup applesauce 1 cup low-fat milk	"With the exception of the gelatin dessert, this is a decent meal, although the child may have eaten more had she not had such a large lunch or so much sugary food at breakfast and lunch."

both diets are on the low side for iron and zinc. Elizabeth's diet for this particular day is also low in some of the B vitamins, and Josh's falls short for vitamin A.

By making a few substitutions, adjustments and additions, Dr. Smith illustrates how easy it can be to naturally add extra nutrients to your child's diet. In fact, with Dr. Smith's revision, Elizabeth's total nutrient intake soared to over 100 percent. Josh's vitamin intake more than tripled, and his calcium, zinc and iron levels were boosted as well.

MENU B

Menu of a Typical 11-Year-Old Boy	Dr. Lendon Smith's Improved Menu	Dr. Smith's Comments
■ Breakfast		
½ cup orange juice 2 slices 7-grain bread with peanut butter	1 whole orange 2 slices 7-grain bread with "old-fashioned" peanut butter ½ cup low-fat milk	"The fresh orange is included for vitamin C, bioflavonoids and fiber. The milk will help increase calcium. Use homemade—"old-fashioned"—spread. It doesn't contain the salt and sugar that store-bought varieties contain."
■ Lunch		
1 peanut butter and jelly sandwich on 7-grain bread 1 peanut butter and chocolate granola bar 1 raspberry fruit bar	1 peanut butter and banana sandwich on whole wheat bread Trail mix (dried fruit, raisin and nut mixture) Carrot sticks	"As with his sister, this boy should be weaned from jelly to a more nutritious alternative—bananas. The trail mix, unlike granola, will go a long way in improving the RDA, particularly some of the B vitamins, vitamins A and E and magnesium. The carrots will help restore this day's vitamin A supply."
■ Dinner		
1 slice meat loaf, made with lean beef 2 new potatoes, made with herb butter ½ cup peas 1 potato roll 1 cup low-fat milk	1 or 2 slices meat loaf, made with extra-lean beef 2 new potatoes with herbs 1 spear broccoli 1 slice whole wheat bread 1 cup low-fat milk	"A little extra meat loaf will add extra zinc and iron, which are low on this day. The butter seems an unnecessary addition of fat to this diet and adds nothing in terms of nutrition. The broccoli helps increase the calcium intake."

Not to worry. There are plenty of other ways to get your liver-shy kids to eat right. If you include certain core foods in the diet each day, the doctors we spoke to say you'll be doing your best to help your children meet their RDA.

For breakfast, the most concentrated form of nutrition is a whole grain cereal and a fruit, either whole or as juice. "Hot oatmeal with applesauce and raisins tastes great and is very nutritious," says Dr. Smith. Or, for a change of taste, try serving leftovers from last night's dinner. "There's nothing wrong with a chicken leg for breakfast," he says. "It's protein."

Our experts also suggested it's best to pack a child's school lunch rather than depend on what's being served in the cafeteria. Whole wheat bread or another whole grain should always be used on sandwiches. It provides needed B vitamins. Peanut butter is just fine, but eliminate—or at least cut down on—the jelly. Instead, substitute a banana. Always include fruit in the lunchbox, too. For snacks, opt for carrot sticks or trail mix (an assortment of nuts, dried fruits and raisins).

For dinner, serve lean meat or fish, steamed vegetables and fruit for dessert. If you want to feed your kids pastry, think whole grains, and go for oatmeal cookies instead of brownies.

Allow your kids to drink only low-fat or skim milk. "Kids shouldn't drink too much milk," says Dr. Eden. "I think milk is a little overrated. Too much spoils an appetite, and it's too high in fat to be good for you. Two glasses a day is plenty."

Is there anything else you can do?

Dr. Smith suggests giving a multiple vitamin, "for insurance, not as a food substitute. It's good to remember that the RDA is only a minimum and an estimate at that," he says. "And keep in mind that every child is different. How each person absorbs nutrients and their degree of wellness can vary."

Breakfast tips for finicky eaters.

How to pack a lunch box with nutrient-rich goodies.

Supplements are not a substitute for food.

Chapter 6

Test Your Nutritional Know-How

D o you know how to make sure you're getting all the vitamins and minerals you need? Can you correctly choose between foods that help or hurt your body?

To test your nutritional know-how, we have compiled the following quiz. And here's a little help: There may be more than just one correct answer to each question.

Q. You are on medication for high blood pressure and your doctor told you to be sure to get lots of potassium. Which of the following drinks should you order at lunch? (a) new Coke, (b) mineral water, (c) iced tea, (d) orange juice, (e) a martini.

Which has more potassium, orange juice or mineral water?

A. (d). Orange juice is highest in potassium, with a six-ounce glass providing 354 milligrams. But other fruit juices are rich in potassium, too. Apple juice, apricot nectar, grapefruit juice and pineapple juice are all good sources of the mineral. Mineral water, despite its promising name, is a poor source.

Q. Your kids absolutely refuse to drink a glass of juice in the morning and rarely eat any fruit or vegetables, for that matter. Sometimes it seems like all they'll eat is meat and potatoes. You're concerned that they're not getting enough vitamin C. You should (a) consider brainwashing, (b) feed them more yogurt, (c) feed them more meat, (d) feed them cod-liver oil, (e) let them keep eating potatoes.

Should you worry about how much vitamin C your kids are getting?

A. (e). Luckily, potatoes are a very good source of vitamin C. One baked potato has 26 milligrams; a cup of mashed potatoes has up to 20 milligrams. Tomato sauce is another good source, and since most kids like spaghetti, that can help boost their vitamin C intake, too. But you should try to get them interested in at least *some* fruits and vegetables, because they're missing out on a lot of other vitamins and minerals— and fiber, too.

Q. You're either lactose intolerant, or milk just doesn't agree with you. Where else can you get vitamin D? (a) nowhere else, (b) from fresh air, (c) from a walk in the sun, (d) from leafy green vegetables, (e) from tuna fish.

How to get enough vitamin D—even if you can't drink milk.

A. (c) or (e). Fish and fish-liver oils do contain vitamin D. So do egg yolks and butter. But the amount varies. A walk in the sun, however, is a fairly reliable source. Just 15 to 20 minutes of summer-afternoon sun every other day can convert enough of the pro-vitamin D in your skin to vitamin D to fulfill your requirement.

Q. High blood pressure runs in your family. You've heard about the link between sodium and hypertension, and you want to keep the sodium in your diet to a minimum. As an inveterate snacker, which of the following is the best choice to mollify your craving for munchies? (a) celery sticks, (b) almonds, (c) regular twist pretzels, (d) cheddar cheese, (e) popcorn.

Snacks don't have to be salty.

A. (b) and (e). These snacks are the best choice, provided they are unsalted. A cup of unsalted popcorn has only 1 milligram of sodium. A cup of almonds has only 4 milligrams, and they're high in potassium, which may help fight off hypertension. They're fairly high in fat and calories, though, so you'll want to be careful not to overdo it. Celery has more sodium than you might expect—one stalk has 25 milligrams. That's okay as long as you don't have too much. Cheddar cheese is high in sodium: 176 milligrams in one ounce. Most other cheeses are high in sodium, too, although some low-sodium cheeses are now available. Forget the pretzels—they have 101 milligrams of sodium each.

Q. You want to get as much calcium as you can in order to prevent osteoporosis, but your lunch usually consists of a quick stop at a fast-food salad bar. Which items from the salad bar should you be sure to heap on your plate? (a) spinach, (b) broccoli, (c) chick-peas, (d) Swiss cheese, (e) croutons.

Calcium from the salad bar.

A. (b), (c) and (d). Surprisingly, spinach is not a very good source of calcium. It does contain calcium, but it's bound up chemically, so that it's unavailable to us. The lacy-leaf kale that's often used to decorate the salad bar, however, is actually a better source of calcium than the spinach in the salad bowl. One ounce of kale provides 38 milligrams of the mineral. Of course, spinach is a fine source of fiber, vitamin A and B vitamins, so you probably don't want to pass it up.

Q. To prevent osteoporosis, you faithfully take a calcium supplement every night before going to sleep. You've been (a) wasting your time, (b) taking it at the wrong time, (c) depleting your calcium reserves, (d) doing exactly the right thing, (e) sleeping on the job.

A. (d). According to Morris Notelovitz, M.D., medical director of the Climacteric Clinic in Gainesville, Florida, taking calcium supplements at bedtime prevents calcium from being leached from your skeleton in your body's attempt to maintain blood levels of the mineral, as would normally be the case. He also recommends taking the supplement with some milk or yogurt, because the lactose in them helps the body absorb more of the calcium.

Q. You've had a couple of bouts with iron-deficiency anemia and you want to prevent it from happening again, so you're trying very hard to get lots of iron. Which of the following should you look for on your trip down the cafeteria line? (a) orange juice, (b) green peppers, (c) cantaloupe, (d) tomatoes, (e) three-penny nails.

Where to look for iron.

A. All of them except the nails, but not because they're high in iron. Orange juice, green peppers, cantaloupe and tomatoes are all high in vitamin C, so they'll increase the amount of iron that you absorb from other foods you eat at the same meal. In a study done at the University of Goteberg, in Sweden, a glass of orange juice served with a meal of hamburger, string beans and mashed potatoes increased iron absorption by 85 percent. Some good sources of iron to look for at the cafeteria are beef liver, beef, poultry, fish, lima beans, broccoli and peas.

On the Pill? Watch out for B$_6$.

Q. You've been taking birth control pills for several years and you've just heard that they're a common cause of vitamin B$_6$ deficiency in women. Which of the following should you bring home from the supermarket if you want to stock up on B$_6$? (a) organ meats, (b) beets, (c) wheat bran, (d) brown rice, (e) brown sugar.

A. (a), (c) and (d). Besides these three, other good sources to stock up on are wheat germ, walnuts, salmon and blackstrap molasses.

Scoring: 7 to 8 correct answers: Congratulations, you're a Nutritional Merit Scholar. 4 to 6 correct answers: You've got the basics, now go for the fine points. 0 to 3 correct answers: Remedial nutrition study advised.

Part **II**

USING
SUPPLEMENTS
WISELY

Who Takes Vitamins and Minerals?

She's younger, smarter, more affluent, more self-reliant and more responsible than anyone expected. And to top it off, she doesn't even exist. She's an abstraction—a composite of the "typical" supplement user.

We can thank research surveys for bringing her to light and for giving us our first clear look at the profiles and purposes of people who use vitamins and minerals. Who are they? What nutrients do they take? Why do they take them? What does supplementation do for them? The answers to these questions and others like them are real eye-openers.

For instance: The people who take supplements (over half the adult population and most women) are usually college-educated careerists with a household income of $30,000 or more. The data come from a 1982 Gallup poll, as well as several other population studies. The conclusions are crystal clear: People with higher socioeconomic status are more likely to take supplements.

What kind of people take supplements?

"It makes perfect sense," states James P. Frackelton, M.D., a preventive medicine specialist in Cleveland. "People at the lower end of the socioeconomic scale are more apt to believe the traditional view that supplements are unnecessary. But those higher up the ladder—those more informed on nutritional matters—are more likely to reject that view and take the supplements they think they need."

What People Take and When

Are people who take supplements more nutritionally aware than those who don't? Theoretically, yes. But the theory gains some credence when you look at how people use supplements day to day.

According to a massive survey conducted by Simmons Market Research Bureau, the most popular supplements are multiple vitamin/mineral formulas, followed by individual supplements of vitamins C, E, B complex, B_{12} and A. And many people take their vitamins once a day.

As for how *much* of each vitamin or mineral people take, supplement users may show a strong streak of nutritional sophistication.

For one thing, most of them apparently know how to keep nutrient intakes at reasonable levels. Take two of the "star" vitamins, for instance. Research suggests that the most common daily intake of vitamin C is 500 milligrams or less; for vitamin E, it's 400 international units or less. A mountain of nutritional studies says that these levels are safe. What's more, the scarcity of nutrient-toxicity cases (instances of side effects caused by excessive supplement intakes) may be the best evidence that most people are keeping their intakes within rational limits.

Indeed, it seems that whatever supplementation levels are being used, most people are approaching supplements with far more savvy than once thought. When supplement users in the Gallup poll were asked how they determined proper vitamin intake, 48 percent of them said they scrutinized the label, and 29 percent said they relied on their doctor. When the poll's vitamin users were asked if they were aware of the Recommended Dietary Allowances (RDAs), about half of them said yes.

It's clear that most people *do not* think taking supplements can be a substitute for eating food. A 1978 survey of consumer attitudes and practices showed that 97 percent of those polled disagreed

Overdosing on vitamins is uncommon.

Supplements aren't meant to replace foods.

with the statement, "It is okay to skip meals as long as you take a vitamin supplement."

We'd need a large-scale, in-depth study to more accurately gauge how responsibly people use supplements. But it's already apparent that there are a whole lot of supplement users who know exactly what they're doing.

"Before I try a supplement, I discuss it with nutritional experts," says Barry Shapiro, a 34-year-old film

---

Dietitians Speak Up about Nutritional Supplements

Registered dietitians, as a group, have traditionally maintained that a well-balanced diet alone will support nutritional health for the vast majority of people.

Yet, in a survey of dietitians in the state of Washington, nearly 60 percent said that they take some form of nutritional supplements (*Journal of the American Dietetic Association*). In contrast, only 47 to 54 percent of Americans use nutritional supplements.

"The attitude of 20 years ago—'If you eat right, you don't need dietary supplements'—still prevails among most," says Bonnie Worthington-Roberts, Ph.D., of the University of Washington in Seattle, a coauthor of the survey. "But some dietitians today recognize that they themselves don't always get what they need, especially if they are dieting."

One Seattle dietitian says that her partner used to be strongly against the use of any supplements when she first joined their practice. Now, several years into it, she "encourages moderate use of supplements under certain conditions."

Adds Sue McFarlane, a registered dietitian in Spokane, "We cannot safely recommend dietary supplements to a group. But in many cases, after individual consultation, we may find a particular deficiency that an individual is unable to satisfy by diet alone."

"Even though meeting nutritional needs through diet alone is the ideal," says Dr. Worthington-Roberts, "use of multivitamin/mineral supplements may be supported for individuals (including dietitians) when personal dietary patterns fall short of this goal."

**Smart people read and
analyze labels.**

producer. "Then I check the label. I never take any supplement without that kind of deliberation."

"When I first start taking a vitamin or mineral, I use very low amounts," says Gerry Patrick, a 63-year-old homemaker. "I set intake limits for myself, based on what I've learned about the nutrient. Then, if need be, I slowly increase intake."

The Logic behind Supplements

But why are people taking vitamins and minerals in the first place? Is it because (a) they don't always eat right; (b) they believe supplements help them stay healthy; (c) they think there aren't enough nutrients in food; (d) they believe that nutrients help them feel better and more energetic; or (e) all of the above?

**Why do people take
supplements?**

The answer is (e), all of the above, according to a 1982 survey of 200 readers of *Good Housekeeping*. In fact, the poll disclosed about a dozen other reasons as well, and other surveys have come up with similar lists. People not only have rationales for supplementation in general but they also have specific reasons for taking particular nutrients. They may take vitamin A to maintain good eyesight, vitamin E to head off skin problems, calcium and vitamin D to strengthen bones.

So where do such judgments come from? It would take a lot more studies to figure that one out. But it's difficult to ignore the fact that almost all these rationales have been, in one way or another, bolstered by nutritional data from laboratories around the world.

**People who take their
health seriously take
their supplements
seriously.**

It's also true that supplement users have—as you might have guessed—a sincere interest in their own health. The Gallup poll revealed that people who take vitamins are more likely to watch their diet, exercise and refrain from smoking. And other studies suggest that among supplement users, nutrition is a priority concern.

But there's more to this pro-health attitude than meets the eye. Saying that supplement users only want health is an understatement. They apparently want far more than that.

Says Barry Shapiro, "To me health is more than not being sick. It's being able to perform at my peak potential day in and day out—optimum functioning all the time."

Wellness—that's what he's talking about, a positive state beyond the so-called norm of nondisease. It's what a growing number of physicians are advocating and what, according to a U.S. Food and Drug Administration survey of consumer health practices, supplement users are seeking.

What's the Payoff?

Are they finding what they're looking for? Or, more to the point, are supplements really doing them any good?

Evidence of the health-enhancing powers of nutrients has been trickling in for decades, and doctors' clinical experiences with supplements corroborates much of the research data. But for most people, the true test of supplementation is what it does for them personally. And most people who use supplementation seem to think it does a lot of good: 61 to 80 percent of supplement users say that their supplements are working or that they're satisfied with the results.

Supplements work, according to four out of five people who take them.

This is what formal surveys show, and judging from accounts by health-care professionals who use supplements to treat patients, these numbers are right on target.

James D. Heffley, Ph.D., a nutrition counselor in Austin, Texas, is one of many such professionals. "I conducted a survey of about 2,000 of my patients for whom I had recommended supplements. As it turned out, 85 percent of them reported that they were happy

Are supplements worth the money?

with the outcome of the therapy. And I discovered that 75 percent of those who weren't satisfied with the results didn't stick to the treatment program."

So for many people, it seems, supplements pay off in good health. But is the cost reasonable? According to Market Research Corporation of America, in 1981 people spent an average of $28 annually on vitamins—about eight cents a day. That's small change to most people—and a good bargain to supplement users.

How to Choose and Use a Multiple

Have you ever stared at a store shelf full of vitamin bottles, totally bewildered? With visions of brightly colored pills spinning through your head, you might well wish for an easier way. Could a multiple vitamin/mineral formula be just the thing you need?

A multiple combines many nutrients into one tablet or capsule. It's for people who don't want to take several different vitamin pills each day. Then, if it falls short here or there (you may have some special needs), it's easy enough to supplement with additional individual nutrients.

Choosing the multivitamin that's best for you requires a bit of comparison shopping. You need to know how vitamin and mineral supplements meet, or miss, your particular nutrient needs. Here's a step-by-step guide.

Start with the Essentials

One of the best things you can do is compare the list of nutrients on a vitamin bottle label with those in the U.S. Recommended Daily Allowances (USRDAs). Take the table on page 52 with you to the store. Compare the label with the table, item for item. Does the multiple include all of the vitamins and minerals listed in the table? It should. These are the basic ingredients of good nutrition.

Does your multiple contain all the essential nutrients in adequate amounts?

Some essential nutrients, especially trace elements, do not yet have USRDAs. They do have safe and accepted ranges, which are also listed in the table.

How many of these nutrients are in the multiple? You may not feel you need every one, but you should know which you want, and why. You may want chromium if you're concerned about diabetes, since chromium seems to play a role in glucose metabolism; selenium, a potent antioxidant, because of its possible role in cancer protection; copper if you're taking supplemental zinc. (Copper is important in the formation of red blood cells and capillary stability. Zinc may affect copper absorption. Look for a ratio of about 7.5 to 10 units of zinc to 1 portion of copper. For example, 15 milligrams of zinc should be taken with 2 milligrams of copper.)

Many ingredients may not be essential.

You may find many other ingredients—from bioflavonoids to tin—in multiple vitamins. While it's true that these substances are found naturally in food, research has not determined any of them to be essential to human nutrition, at least not yet.

Decide How Much You Need

You also should look at the amount of each nutrient in the supplement, measured in milligrams, micrograms (1/1000 of a milligram) or international units. Compare each with the USRDA amounts. In addition to amounts, most labels list a nutrient's percentages of the USRDA, and this may actually provide you with the best information regarding the product's potency and balance, as you'll see below.

The percentage of USRDA listed is a reliable benchmark.

How potent a multiple do you want? If your goal is "insurance," look for those providing 50 to 150 percent of the USRDA. The American Medical Association generally considers this a reasonable range, with one important exception: The vitamin D level should not exceed 100 percent.

Some, but certainly not all, "one-tablet-daily" types are in this category. If you want more than the USRDA, "high-potency" brands may provide it. But so will some other multiples without these labels, says Sheldon Hendler, M.D., Ph.D., formerly clinical instructor of medicine at the University of California at San Diego, author of *The Complete Guide to Anti-Aging Nutrients*.

One-tablet-a-day multivitamins may provide 50 to 150 percent of the USRDAs.

Check Nutritional Balance

Look at the percentage of the USRDA of each nutrient. If the formula is balanced by USRDA standards, each nutrient will have the same percentage of the USRDA. A balanced multiple may contain 100 percent of the USRDA for each nutrient, for instance. If it's not balanced, some percentages will be high, some low. That's not necessarily bad. But you should note how it varies and decide if that's something you want.

A "balanced" formula isn't necessarily the best.

Some "women's formulas," for instance, contain additional iron or calcium to accommodate increased needs for those nutrients among many women. Some "geri," or geriatric, formulas have additional antioxidants—vitamins A, E and C and selenium—nutrients believed to play a role in slowing some aspects of aging.

Most of the so-called stress formulas provide much more vitamin C and B complex, and sometimes zinc, than they do other nutrients (because of their purported role in beating stress). Other formulas, like B-100 types, provide nutrients in increments of 100 milligrams or 100 micrograms. As a result, the formulas may be far out of balance, since the USRDAs for some B vitamins are less than one-tenth that of other B vitamins.

"I personally think these products play on the fact that people don't know what 'balanced' is," says Annette Dickinson, technical counselor of the Council for Responsible Nutrition, a vitamin manufacturers' trade association. "It makes no sense to have some of the B vitamins present at 100 times the USRDA, others at only a fraction of the USRDA."

Beware of Advertising Claims

There are now supplement formulas for almost every medical condition you can imagine—arthritis, high blood pressure, heart disease, immunity, depression, fatigue, premenstrual discomfort and so forth.

"Be extremely wary of any formula that claims to counteract any particular disease," Dr. Hendler says. "Most of the special formulas I've surveyed are very poorly designed. I think you're better off sticking with a good basic regimen."

But, with your doctor's advice, you may want to take additional vitamins or minerals for a medical problem. If you're a woman, you may take additional iron for anemia or additional calcium to prevent osteoporosis.

Don't use multivitamins as over-the-counter medicine.

If you have a leg cramping condition called intermittent claudication, your doctor might suggest extra vitamin E. Or he may prescribe extra B_6 and magnesium to help prevent kidney stones or larger-than-normal amounts of vitamin C for bronchial asthma. In this sense, the vitamins are going beyond the role of nutrition. They are acting almost as drugs, in a therapeutic sense. Their advantage is that they often have fewer side effects than drugs used for these same conditions. But they still need to be used wisely and under a doctor's supervision. And typically, multiples are not the best way because the target nutrient is mixed with many others.

Does Your Multiple Have a Deficiency?

Some vitamin manufacturers add inadequate amounts of nutrients to their products just so they can list the nutrient on their label, Dr. Hendler says. And even the better products sometimes contain only small amounts of some nutrients. Here again, it's important to read the label.

The once-daily multiple vitamin/mineral supplements are often low in calcium and magnesium, because these two nutrients are bulky and make the pill big. There are many individual calcium supplements on the market to make up the difference, though. You can also find some good calcium/magnesium products, which provide what some researchers think is an important 2.5 to 1 ratio of these two minerals. (Magnesium is an important mineral for calcium metabolism.) If you are taking calcium to prevent or treat osteoporosis, you should know that some researchers think trace minerals, such as zinc and copper, are very important for bones, too.

Check the label: Some multiples may not contain enough of certain nutrients like calcium or magnesium.

Other Shopping Tips

Here are some other things to be aware of as you choose a supplement.

Check the expiration date. Many, but not all, vitamin manufacturers now include an expiration date on their products. It's a good idea to avoid a product beyond the expiration date, although most products retain their potency much longer. Oil-based supplements deteriorate more quickly than others. If you're selecting products from a store's discount bin, check to see that the vitamins aren't leftovers from the Stone Age.

Make sure your supplements are fresh.

Too much to swallow? Some manufacturers who try to cram everything into a once-daily tablet do so at the expense of your esophagus. Check the pill size before you buy. Sometimes the better choice is to get a just-as-complete, but smaller, multiple that must be taken not once but two or three times a day.

Some pills are too big.

More is not better. You may be tempted to think that if your multiple at its suggested dosage isn't good enough, you can just take it more often and not bother to switch to some better-balanced product.

**Taking more of an un-
balanced multiple
doesn't make it bal-
anced.**

You may want more calcium, for instance, but you would need to take three pills daily, rather than one, to get it from your present supplement. "Don't do that," Dr. Hendler emphasizes. "Taking an unbalanced supplement three times a day still may not provide the recommended doses of some nutrients,

What to Look For in a Multivitamin

Nutrient	USRDA (adults and children 4 or more years of age)
Vitamin A	5,000 I.U.
Thiamine (B_1)	1.5 mg.
Riboflavin (B_2)	1.7 mg.
Niacin	20 mg.
Vitamin B_6 (pyridoxine)	2 mg.
Vitamin B_{12}	6 mcg.
Folate	0.4 mg.
Biotin	300 mcg.
Pantothenate	10 mg.
Vitamin C (ascorbic acid)	60 mg.
Vitamin D	400 I.U.
Vitamin E	30 I.U.
Calcium	1,000 mg.
Copper	2 mg.
Iodine	150 mcg.
Iron	18 mg.
Magnesium	400 mg.
Phosphorus	1,000 mg.
Zinc	15 mg.

	Suggested Ranges*
Chromium	50-200 mcg.
Selenium	50-200 mcg.†

* These nutrients are considered essential, but they have no USRDA. Instead, they have ranges that are considered safe and adequate.

† Supplements of selenium should not exceed 100 mcg., since the average diet supplies about 100 mcg.

but you may end up taking too much of other nutrients, throwing things even further out of balance."

Do your homework. You can do some comparison shopping before you go to the store by looking through the *Handbook of Nonprescription Drugs,* published by the American Pharmaceutical Association, Washington, D.C. 20037, and found in the reference section of large libraries, especially those affiliated with medical schools. This book contains a table of many multiple vitamin products, their ingredients and amounts. The table is a good way to do some comparison shopping for supplements before you head for the store.

A convenient way to comparison shop for a multivitamin.

Chapter 9

Getting Vitamins and Minerals to Work Better

I f you eat three square meals a day or take vitamin supplements, you might think you're getting adequate nutrition. But you could be wrong.

Nutrition isn't that simple or direct. Your body doesn't always make the best use of all the vitamins you take in, either in food or in supplements. Some vitamins never get to where they could do the most good. Others sail through your system without being absorbed.

The same is true of minerals. In fact, when it comes to figuring out how to make the most of your vitamins, minerals are often part of the plan.

If you want to squeeze every available microgram from your vitamins and minerals, it helps to understand some of the ways in which nutrients help each other along.

A Booster Plan for Better Nutrition

Here are some tips to help you make the most of your nutrients.

Eat small, nutritious meals and snacks. All the nutrients your body takes in at a big meal can be hard to swallow, says John Pinto, Ph.D., assistant professor of nutrition and medicine at Cornell University Medical College and associate member at Memorial Sloan-Kettering Cancer Center.

Smaller, more frequent meals help your system absorb vitamins and minerals better.

"If you stop and think how some people eat a large amount of protein and carbohydrates at one meal, they really swamp their system with this influx of nutrients all at one time," Dr. Pinto says. "And many of those nutrients won't be absorbed. That's because it's easier for the gastrointestinal tract to absorb nutrients from small amounts of food over a small period of time."

If you want to squeeze more nutritional value from your diet, scale down your main meals and eat healthful snacks—like a piece of fruit, crisp, raw vegetables, a whole grain muffin or a glass of milk—in between. You'll give your body a chance to absorb nutrients most efficiently, says Dr. Pinto.

A nutritional nudge from snacks.

Take your vitamin C in small, divided doses. "The higher your dose at a single time, the smaller the percentage of vitamin C you absorb," explains Mark Levine, M.D., a researcher at the National Institutes of Health in Bethesda, Maryland. "If you take 100 milligrams at one time, you get something like 90 percent absorption. If you go up to a gram [1,000 milligrams], it's approximately 50 percent absorption, and so on."

Instead of taking one large tablet of vitamin C, then, divide the same amount into smaller doses to be taken throughout the day.

"Let's say you chose to take two grams [2,000 milligrams] of vitamin C," says Dr. Levine. "You would increase the percentage of absorption if you took 500 milligrams four times a day or 1,000 milligrams twice a day."

A little vitamin C now and then is better than one big dose at once.

If you want to make sure your iron is more fully absorbed, get more vitamin C. "Vitamin C will enhance absorption of other nutrients, particularly iron," says Dr. Levine.

Think of vitamin C as a booster rocket for iron.

When we talk about iron, most of us think of foods like beef, poultry, fish and eggs. But not all iron is the same. Only about 10 percent of the iron in vegetables and grain—called nonheme (nonblood) iron—is absorbed. In contrast, we absorb from 15 to

30 percent of the iron found in meats, which is called heme iron.

Vitamin C is what is known as an iron enhancer. It helps convert the nonabsorbed iron into a form the body can use. So to make the most of your iron, eat more foods that are rich in vitamin C, such as tomatoes and oranges, along with iron-rich foods like lean meat, fish, poultry, leafy green vegetables and whole grains.

Top off iron-rich meals with vitamin C-rich foods.

One way to improve the absorption of iron in your beef, fish or chicken dish might be to add a thick, spicy tomato sauce. A piece of fruit for dessert, instead of that slab of double-fudge cake you've been coveting, is a healthier alternative if you want to boost your absorption of iron from your meal. If you take an iron supplement, wash it down with a little orange juice.

Special Advice for Vitamins A, D and E

Vitamins A, D and E are absorbed in the intestine in the presence of fat. Consequently, if you take your fat-soluble vitamins on an empty stomach, you might flush out most of the vitamins before they can be absorbed.

Take fat-soluble vitamins with foods that contain fat. "It's reasonable to take fat-soluble vitamins with foods that contain a small amount of fat—for example, a glass of low-fat (1 or 2 percent) milk," says Cedric Garland, Dr.P.H., assistant professor of community and family medicine at the University of California, San Diego. "A moderate amount of fat would cause the secretion of digestive enzymes that work on fats, which would enhance absorption of the fat-soluble vitamins. Without a small amount of fat, a portion of the vitamins will wash right through the intestine without being absorbed."

Low-fat milk helps you absorb vitamins A, D and E.

What about those of us on low-fat diets? Not to worry, says Dr. Garland. "From a practical point of view, a diet containing 15 to 20 percent fat would still be sufficient to absorb fat-soluble vitamins."

Getting the Most Out of Calcium

How and when you get calcium is important.

To move calcium along, get plenty of vitamin D. You can take calcium supplements every day and still leave your bones and teeth crying out for more—if you don't get enough vitamin D along with the mineral. Without vitamin D, calcium is not absorbed.

Without vitamin D, calcium can't reach your bones and teeth.

If you want to make sure you're getting enough of both nutrients, says Dr. Garland, one convenient way to do so is to drink milk, which contains plenty of calcium *and* vitamin D.

But drinking milk is only one way to boost your vitamin D. Perhaps the easiest way for most of us to make sure we get enough vitamin D is to take a stroll in the sunlight. Your skin manufactures vitamin D on its own, but it needs ultraviolet rays from sunlight to start the wheels turning. How much sun do you need to make vitamin D? "Just 15 minutes a day, with sunlight on your hands and face, should be enough in most cases," says Dr. Garland.

The walk will do you good, too, since weight-bearing exercise enhances the movement of calcium to your bones.

Take your calcium with food. Not all of us consume enough dairy products to keep us in calcium balance. If you don't get enough dietary calcium, you might take a supplement, but merely taking a supplement doesn't guarantee you the best results. If you take calcium, it's important to get your gastric juices flowing because some calcium supplements are absorbed best in an acid environment. (This is also a problem for many people over the age of 60, whose

Don't take calcium on an empty stomach.

production of stomach acid may be lower.) The solution is to take your calcium with a meal, thus stimulating your stomach to produce enough acid.

Among healthy adults, pregnant and lactating women need the most calcium. The Recommended Dietary Allowance (RDA) for this group is 1,200 milligrams of calcium daily. To get this amount of calcium, you would have to drink four or five glasses of milk a day. People who are at risk for osteoporosis may need even more, though the precise amount hasn't been firmly established.

Three groups who need more calcium.

Food also helps improve the absorption of other nutrients. "It's best that nutrients be consumed with a meal," says Dr. Pinto. "The very sight of food begins to stimulate the appetite, triggering the release of various enzymes. Also, hormonal responses begin to register. With food in the mouth, insulin rises. Intestinal blood flow increases, preparing to help transport food through the body and move nutrients from the intestine into the bloodstream."

Take your calcium supplements before bed. The timing of the dose could improve your body's absorption of the mineral, too. Morris Notelovitz, M.D., medical director of the Climacteric Clinic in Gainesville, Florida, has suggested taking calcium supplements just before you turn in.

The calcium thieves work at night.

During the day, your body extracts the calcium it needs from food. At night, when no food is coming in, your body still needs to maintain normal blood levels of calcium, so it raids the only source available to it—your skeleton.

A calcium supplement just before bed should keep your blood levels near normal and protect your bones from this nightly pilferage. But if you're going to take calcium, remember the previous advice and swallow it with a glass of low-fat milk to stimulate the production of stomach acids.

What You Should Know about Vitamin Tests

C an medical tests tell you whether you have a vitamin or mineral deficiency—or excess? Is such information really useful to you and your doctor? And will the tests end up costing you more than they're worth?

The answers, as testing experts point out, are yes, maybe and sometimes.

Nowadays, doctors can indeed order laboratory tests for most vitamins and minerals (though medical labs are not equally equipped to assess nutrient levels). Usually your physician gets a blood or urine sample from you and sends it to the lab with instructions to measure the amount of certain nutrients in the sample. The test results may or may not reflect your intake of nutrients but will, in most cases, indicate whether you have high or low levels in your system.

Tests tell whether you have high or low levels of nutrients.

The usefulness of such testing depends, in part, on how widespread vitamin and mineral deficiencies really are. Classic deficiencies—those with unmistakable symptoms, like scurvy and beriberi—are few and far between. Other evidence, however, suggests that milder deficiencies may be more prevalent than people think. (See the table, A Guide to Deficiency Symptoms, on page 62.)

Mild deficiencies may be widespread.

A Useful Tool— or a Waste of Time?

One of the researchers who has helped uncover such nutritional deficits is Myron Brin, Ph.D., former adjunct professor at both Columbia Medical School and Cornell Medical School. "We have to be aware," he says, "that national nutritional studies like the Ten-State Survey, the Household Food Consumption Survey and the Health and Nutrition Examination Survey demonstrated that there are many population groups who consume appreciably below Recommended Dietary Allowance (RDA) levels for vitamins A, C and B_6, folate and other nutrients. Such biochemical inadequacy without classic deficiency symptoms is called marginal deficiency—a condition often marked by vague signs like irritability, insomnia and reduced appetite. It's this type of deficiency that nutrient tests can help detect."

But if a doctor suspects that a patient has a deficiency, why can't he forgo nutrient testing and simply prescribe the missing nutrient and see if the symptoms disappear?

He can and often does.

Prescribing a vitamin can sometimes substitute for nutritional testing.

"This technique is called a therapeutic trial," Dr. Brin says. "In some cases, it may be cheaper than nutrient testing. As long as physicians know precisely what symptoms are associated with the deficiency, they can easily assess the effects of the prescribed supplements. If symptoms disappear in about three months, that's evidence that the patient may have lacked the nutrients."

There's more to nutrient testing, however, than just spotting nutritional deficits. Doctors sometimes

Nutrient tests can sometimes reveal serious disease.

use it to help confirm the presence of serious medical conditions that may have little or nothing to do with deficiencies. Calcium tests, for example, can help doctors diagnose bone disorders and problems of the parathyroid gland. Magnesium tests can help them detect systemic poisoning, including drug abuse. And the vitamin E test helps them pinpoint the cause of anemia in infants.

None of which means that doctors find nutrient tests as useful as old standbys like routine urinalysis and the complete blood count (the most frequently performed lab test). The majority of physicians use most vitamin and mineral tests sparingly, not routinely. And the consensus in the medical world seems to be that performing nutrient tests on apparently healthy people is a waste of time.

Testing the Tests

And, of course, some nutrient tests can yield more useful data than others.

Calcium tests (done either on blood or urine) are among the more revealing, which may be why they're often included in standard multiple-test batteries. "They're helpful in diagnosing numerous conditions," says Edward R. Pinckney, M.D., a California specialist in preventive medicine and coauthor of *The Patient's Guide to Medical Tests*. "They're used primarily in evaluating suspected abnormalities of the parathyroid gland, memory problems, unusual sleepiness and nerve or muscle dysfunctions. But they can also yield information in the diagnosis of other gland problems (such as lack of adrenal hormones), unexplained bleeding, vitamin D poisoning, osteoporosis, even cancer."

The calcium test can help to diagnose over a dozen medical conditions.

Tests for iron and folate (done on blood only) are especially valuable because they help physicians diagnose anemias, usually those caused by lack of these two nutrients. Iron tests, generally included in multiple-test batteries, are also used to monitor patients on hemodialysis and for tracking down vitamin and other food deficiencies. And folate tests are sometimes used to distinguish between two deficiencies—folate and vitamin B_{12}.

Then there are those nutrient tests of dubious worth. The niacin urine test is one of them, says Dr. Pinckney. "The test is performed to confirm the diagnosis of pellagra, the classic niacin-deficiency disease," he says. "But the symptoms and signs of the disease, plus a successful therapeutic trial of niacin, allow a diagnosis long before the test is needed."

Some vitamin tests mean little.

A Guide to Deficiency Symptoms

Nutrient	Possible Deficiency Symptoms*	RDA for Adults (age 23–50)
Vitamin A	Night blindness; abnormal dryness of the eyeballs; dry, rough, itchy skin; susceptibility to respiratory infection	5,000 I.U. (men) 4,000 I.U. (women)
Thiamine (B_1)	Confusion; weakness of eye muscles; loss of appetite; uncoordinated walk; poor memory; inability to concentrate	1.4 mg. (men) 1.0 mg. (women)
Riboflavin (B_2)	Discolored tongue; anemia; cracks at corners of mouth; scaly skin; burning, itchy eyes	1.6 mg. (men) 1.2 mg. (women)
Niacin	Dermatitis; insomnia; headache; diarrhea; dementia	18 mg. (men) 13 mg. (women)
Vitamin B_6 (pyridoxine)	Depression; skin lesions; extreme nervousness; water retention; lethargy	2.2 mg. (men) 2.0 mg. (women)
Vitamin B_{12}	Anemia, accompanied by symptoms such as heart palpitations, sore tongue, general weakness; weight loss	3.0 mcg.
Folate	Anemia; dizziness; fatigue; intestinal disorders; diarrhea; shortness of breath	400 mcg.
Vitamin C (ascorbic acid)	Easy bruising; spongy, bleeding gums; dental problems; slow wound healing; fatigue; listlessness; rough skin	60 mg.
Vitamin D	Softening of bones (osteomalacia); bone pain; susceptibility to bone fracture (osteoporosis); excessive tooth decay	200 I.U.
Vitamin E	Muscle degeneration; anemia; nerve dysfunction	15 I.U. (men) 12 I.U. (women)
Calcium	Softening of bones (osteomalacia); susceptibility to bone fracture (osteoporosis); periodontal disease	800 mg.
Iron	Anemia, accompanied by symptoms such as weakness, fatigue, headache, heart palpitations, mouth soreness	10 mg.
Magnesium	Foot and leg cramps; muscle weakness; irregular pulse; nervousness	350 mg. (men) 300 mg. (women)
Zinc	Slow wound healing; skin and hair problems; poor resistance to infection	15 mg.

* These symptoms can, of course, suggest medical conditions other than nutrient deficiencies. For a proper diagnosis of symptoms, see your doctor.

The vitamin B_6 test (done on urine and blood) may have similar problems. "A vitamin B_6 deficiency is usually diagnosed long before a laboratory test confirms it," says Dr. Pinckney. Plus, even when there's no deficiency present, several drugs and diseases can change B_6 levels, rendering the test results suspect.

The Lowdown on Test Results

But regardless of what a test tells you, it's important to remember that test results do not a diagnosis make. They're only a piece of the diagnostic puzzle that your doctor tries to put together. The other pieces are your medical history, health habits, physical exam, age, sex, symptoms, use of medications and more.

What tests can and cannot tell you.

It also helps to keep in mind that no medical test is 100 percent reliable. In most medical tests it's always possible, usually in a small percentage of cases, to get "abnormal" test results and still be perfectly healthy or get "normal" results and be sick. "For this reason, you shouldn't worry if your test results do not at first appear to be normal," says endocrinologist Bernard Kliman, M.D., of Massachusetts General Hospital in Boston and coauthor of *What You Should Know about Medical Lab Tests.*

So if you suspect a vitamin or mineral deficiency, should you ask your physician to order nutrient tests? "First of all," Dr. Kliman advises, "don't try to diagnose yourself. That's your doctor's job. Your symptoms could be completely unrelated to a nutrient deficiency or be a deficiency syndrome caused by some secondary disorder. So maybe nutrient tests would be useless—or just what the doctor ordered."

Rule number one: Don't diagnose yourself.

Chapter 11

Answers to Your Questions about Nutritional Supplements

A lot of people want to know about vitamin and mineral supplements and have asked plenty of interesting questions about them. Here are the answers to some typical—and some not so typical—inquiries.

Using Vitamins A and D with Care

Q. I know that beta-carotene and retinoic acid are both forms of vitamin A. What I don't understand is the difference between them. Can you explain?

A. Beta-carotene is a dietary source of vitamin A, a raw material the body uses to make the vitamin. It's a natural pigment found in abundance in many green and yellow vegetables. Retinoic acid, on the other hand, is derived from vitamin A rather than being used to make it.

Both forms of the vitamin help the body's cells, particularly those in the protective linings (of arteries, for instance), grow and mature properly. But vitamin A has two other important functions—maintaining normal vision and reproductive cells—in which retinoic acid plays no known role.

The difference between beta-carotene and retinoic acid.

Q. I have noticed what appears to be a high dosage of vitamin A in several high-potency vitamin supplements. I was wondering if these supplements are safe.

A. You don't say how high is "high," but U.S. government guidelines are very clear on maximum dosage. They recommend that adults take not more than 25,000 international units a day of vitamin A. That figure is distinct from the official Recommended Dietary Allowance (RDA) of vitamin A—4,000 to 5,000 international units for adults—which is recommended to ensure that the majority of the population doesn't become deficient.

Toxic effects—drying of the skin, hair loss, bone pain and fragility, enlargement of the spleen and liver—have been seen in adults taking a daily dose of 50,000 international units or more a day over a long period of time. Remember, vitamin A is a fat-soluble nutrient that the body is able to store—quite efficiently—in the liver. Chances are the supplements you've seen don't approach the toxic doses. The U.S. Food and Drug Administration (FDA) Advisory Review Panel considers 10,000 international units safe for use in over-the-counter supplements.

Caution: Too much vitamin A does more harm than good.

Q. I'm excited by studies showing that beta-carotene may be responsible for lowering the incidence of certain forms of cancer. Could I replace my daily vitamin A supplement entirely with beta-carotene?

A. Yes, you could. Normally the body converts about one-third of the beta-carotene to vitamin A. Research is uncertain which form is responsible for lowering the incidence of cancer, so it would be a good idea to include both in your supplement program.

Consider that the foods we typically eat are estimated to provide about half the vitamin A preformed and half as beta-carotene. A supplement program based on that same 50:50 ratio seems to make the most sense.

How beta-carotene acts as a vitamin A supplement.

Q. I've been told that taking excess amounts of vitamin D may be dangerous. Is that correct?

A. Yes, it is. Vitamin D is the most potentially toxic of all vitamins. Large doses can result in the deposition of calcium in soft tissues such as the arteries, heart and kidneys and may lead to high blood pressure.

In the past, toxic doses for adults were noted at a level of from 25,000 to 50,000 international units daily, but new findings suggest that a safer level may be about 1,000 international units daily or less. There is probably little need to exceed the maximum RDA of 400 international units a day. At this level vitamin D is considered safe—and adequate to prevent a vitamin D deficiency.

A safe level for vitamin D.

All about B Vitamins

Q. What is the difference between folate, folic acid and folacin, or are they all the same?

A. Consider this a short course on biochemistry. Folacin is the generic term for folic acid and its related compounds. Folate is simply one form of folic acid.

Three names, one vitamin.

Q. A few months ago I read in the paper about cases of nerve damage in people taking too much vitamin B_6. Is it dangerous?

A. Not when taken in reasonable amounts. In the particular study that was reported, people were taking from two grams (2,000 milligrams) to six grams (6,000 milligrams) per day for 2 to 40 months. Those levels are far in excess (1,000 to 3,000 times) of the RDA. Unfortunately, there are always some who take abusive levels of vitamins as well as other substances.

The safety of vitamin B_6 has been thoroughly reviewed. No evidence of adverse effects was found in patients taking from 20 to 1,000 milligrams per day (10 to 500 times the RDA) for up to four years. Vitamin B_6, like most of the B vitamins, has a wide margin of safety. However, excessively high levels should not be taken. Commonsense supplemental levels range from about 5 milligrams to 50 milligrams a day.

Taking too much vitamin B_6 can be dangerous.

Q. My two teenage children and I have been taking a heaping tablespoon of brewer's yeast every day with our hot cereal. I believe it's made a difference in our health. But someone told me it would be simpler to take a B-complex tablet, and that the tablet would have even more nutritional potency. Is that true?

A. Depending on what dosage B-complex tablet you would take, you would probably get more of the B vitamins than in your heaping tablespoon of brewer's yeast.

When the University of Massachusetts Nutrition Data Bank compared the nutritional contents of yeast and a popular B-complex tablet, they found far more B vitamins in the tablet: 10 milligrams of thiamine (B_1) in the tablet compared to 1.25 milligrams in the yeast, for example. But don't give up your brewer's yeast yet. It packs quite a few more things in that small spoonful. It's about 50 percent protein and contains small amounts of a number of important minerals, including potassium, calcium and zinc.

Which has more nutritional value—brewer's yeast or a B-complex tablet?

Q. Is there B_{12} in brewer's yeast? If so, how much?

A. To find out, we went straight to the source—a brewer, Anheuser-Busch, in St. Louis. They told us that uncontaminated brewer's yeast, used in the manufacture of beer, does not contain B_{12} naturally. However, some brewer's yeast supplements are fortified with the vitamin and may contain as much as 50 micrograms per tablet. Your best bet is to read labels, which will tell you exactly how much B_{12} is in your supplement.

Some brewer's yeasts have more B_{12} than others.

Q. Do the B vitamins increase appetite? I'm on a diet and have been taking the vitamins to help me get the most out of my pared-down meals. But I've noticed that I'm hungrier than I usually am when dieting. The only thing I'm doing differently is taking a B-complex supplement.

A. To more intelligently—and accurately—answer your question, we should know what foods and the number of calories you're consuming. But there are a few things we can tell you.

B vitamins and appetite.

The B vitamins in and of themselves aren't increasing your appetite. Though this scenario is rare, this is what could be happening, our experts say: If you have been on a severely restricted diet over a period of time, you may have developed vitamin deficiencies. Taking a vitamin supplement such as a B-complex might stimulate the body to better absorb the available nutrients. That, in turn, can promote a feeling of well-being that leads to a perceived increase in appetite. Though taking B-complex supplements while dieting is probably an excellent idea, make sure your diet isn't too drastic—too low in calories or restricted to a few foods. Vitamins can't replace food.

Q. When I was anemic, my doctor gave me B_{12} injections. Couldn't I have taken a tablet? Are injections of vitamins more potent than pills?

B_{12} injections: better than tablets?

A. If you were suffering from pernicious anemia, the B_{12} shot was more potent because people with that serious condition lack something called intrinsic factor, which enables the body to absorb the vitamin from the diet. But with other nutrients, injections aren't necessarily more potent, just faster acting. Normally, vitamin injections are recommended only in those instances when nutrients cannot be taken orally or when a medical condition, like pernicious anemia or Crohn's disease, inhibits absorption.

Q. What is the difference between niacin and niacinamide?

The big difference between niacin and niacinamide.

A. Essentially, there is no difference from a nutritional standpoint. Niacin and niacinamide may be used interchangeably. Niacin can cause a flushing reaction in some individuals, however, characterized by redness in the face, neck and other areas, accompanied in many cases by itching. This usually disappears in about a half hour. If you experience this sensation, switch to a supplement containing niacinamide; it does not cause flushing.

Vitamin C at Work

Q. I take about 1,000 milligrams of vitamin C a day and I'm a diabetic. Will vitamin C affect the results of a urine diabetes test?

A. Yes. In fact, the results can go haywire if you're taking large doses of vitamin C. According to Tufts University experts, if you have diabetes and are taking large doses of vitamin C, you may get a false-negative result with the Testape urine test for sugar. In other words, the test results may show that there's no sugar there when there really is. On the other hand, large doses of vitamin C give you a false-positive reading with the Clinitest urine test, making it appear as though there is sugar in the urine when there isn't.

Large doses of vitamin C can actually skew the results of a diabetes urine test.

Q. Since vitamin C is an acid, can it cause or aggravate an ulcer? My husband used to take his supplement faithfully until he developed a gastric ulcer. Now he not only won't take any vitamin C but he even avoids orange juice because he's afraid it will cause him pain.

A. There is no evidence that *any* food substance can cause an ulcer. But you're right, vitamin C is an acid, a very weak one called ascorbic acid that, according to one specialist we talked to, is even less potent than your normal gastric juices.

So unless your husband has experienced some pain after taking his vitamin C supplement or drinking orange juice, he should be safe going back to his old habits. There are some people, however, who are sensitive to some foods—tomato juice may give them heartburn, for example—so your husband may want to start back slowly, testing his own reaction to both supplements and foods and beverages containing vitamin C. He also might want to try a vitamin C supple-

Vitamin C isn't acidic enough to cause stomach ulcers.

ment in buffered form (calcium or sodium ascorbate), which reduces the acidity to nearly neutral.

Q. Is it true that there is an increased risk of vitamin C deficiency if after taking high doses of vitamin C, you suddenly stop taking the vitamin?

A. What you describe is known as "systemic conditioning," and reports of this occurring are contradictory. Most researchers report that vitamin C is more rapidly broken down in both animals and man maintained on a high vitamin C intake, increasing the risk of vitamin C deficiency when vitamin C intake is stopped. It has been proposed that high doses of vitamin C result in the production of increased amounts of the enzyme needed to metabolize the vitamin. When vitamin C intake is suddenly stopped, the higher levels of enzymes are still around, theoretically using up the remaining vitamin C and thereby causing a deficiency.

One experiment dealing with this phenomenon does not support the theory, however. Animals fed high levels of vitamin C for seven months prior to being placed on a diet designed to promote scurvy (the vitamin C deficiency disease) did not show any increased development of the disease.

Q. I'm on a low-sodium diet for hypertension. Can I take vitamin C in the form of sodium ascorbate?

A. If you're cutting your sodium intake to the neighborhood of 500 to 1,000 milligrams a day, you might want to consider taking something other than sodium ascorbate as a vitamin C supplement. For every 1,000 milligrams of vitamin C as sodium ascorbate, you are also getting about 130 milligrams of sodium.

Taking calcium ascorbate is one alternative, or take ascorbic acid at mealtime with a little milk if you're concerned about the effects of the acidity on your stomach.

Q. I heard somewhere that vitamin C can enhance the effects of certain drugs. Is this true? What drugs are involved?

Can taking too much vitamin C lead to a vitamin C deficiency?

Avoiding sodium in vitamin C supplements.

A. What you are probably referring to is a study by researchers at Indiana University who found that vitamin C enhanced the effectiveness of haloperidol, a drug widely used in the United States to reduce the symptoms of schizophrenia and paranoid psychosis brought on by amphetamine abuse.

The scientists tested the drug on rats that were given amphetamines. What they discovered was that the drug dramatically reduced the number of motor responses triggered by the amphetamine—moving around, repetitive head movements and rearing, for instance. Even more dramatic was the action of the drug when administered with a large dose of vitamin C, which had no such effects when administered alone.

The researchers noted, however, that vitamin C at higher doses can block amphetamine responses directly, and therapy with large doses of vitamin C has been used to successfully treat some forms of schizophrenia. Nevertheless, the significance of this study is the possibility that by raising the blood concentrations of vitamin C (which is not synthesized in the human body), physicians may be able to increase the effectiveness of haloperidol and other similar drugs used to treat schizophrenics.

Vitamin C and drugs for schizophrenia.

Vitamin E for Better Health

Q. I have been taking 600 international units of vitamin E, with my doctor's approval, for three months. I'd hoped it would help my leg cramps, which keep me from walking anywhere. But it has not helped. Is 600 international units a day enough?

A. You may have to take a dose of patience as well. Studies have shown that vitamin E may ease cramps caused by a decrease in blood flow to the legs (intermittent claudication). But it's proof of the old adage, "Good things take time." The leading researcher in the area, Knut Haeger, M.D., of Sweden, says his patients show no signs of improvement until *at least* 3 to 4 months after they begin supplementa-

Vitamin E may relieve leg cramps, but it takes time to work.

tion. Significant changes in the arterial flow in the legs are even longer in coming—18 months.

Dr. Haeger originally gave his patients 600 international units of vitamin E a day but reduced it to 300 international units, given in three doses of 100 international units each, when he discovered that the concentration of the nutrient in the blood was the same at 300 international units as at the higher dose.

Also talk with your doctor about the importance of gradually increased walking: That was an essential part of Dr. Haeger's therapy.

Q. I've heard you can have an allergic reaction to vitamin E when you use it on the skin. Can you actually be allergic to a vitamin?

A. Some people do seem to get a reaction when they use the contents of a vitamin E capsule on their skin. But our experts tell us the culprit probably isn't the vitamin itself but other elements in the capsule—wheat germ oil, for instance. Most vitamin E capsules available on the market aren't pure vitamin E. If there is a reaction, say our experts, it might help to try a product that contains alpha tocopherol acetate and mix about half a teaspoon of it into three ounces of vegetable oil for a topical treatment.

Allergy to vitamin E capsules? Try this.

Calcium from Food and Supplements

Q. I'm 21 years old and concerned about my calcium intake. My grandmother, who is 75, seems to have osteoporosis pretty bad—she's about two inches shorter now than when she was younger. My hope is to avoid this with enough calcium and exercise. Right now, I eat yogurt every day and cheese maybe three times a week. They're my only dairy products. My multiple supplement supplies 300 milligrams of calcium. Is that enough?

A. Without knowing more about your diet, it's difficult to judge. If you're eating an eight-ounce serving of yogurt, you're getting about 300 milligrams of calcium daily. Two to three ounces of cheese supplies roughly 500 milligrams. With your 300-milligram supplement, you're getting 1,100 milligrams of calcium three days a week and about 600 milligrams for each of the other four days. That's about 5,700 milligrams of calcium a week.

According to the recent recommendations of a government panel, you should be getting 1,000 milligrams a day, or 7,000 milligrams a week. If you do some simple math, you'll see that unless the rest of your diet supplies an additional 185 milligrams or so a day, you're probably coming up short.

Are you getting enough calcium? Some simple arithmetic can tell.

Q. I've been taking extra calcium to prevent bone loss, but I'm concerned about calcium deposits. Are they caused by too much calcium, or too little?

A. In most cases, neither. Calcium in the diet, even when taken in supplements as great as 1,500 milligrams a day, doesn't create the calcium deposits sometimes found in the joints or the heart, or in kidney stones. Those deposits are caused by some underlying damage to the tissues or by a hormonal imbalance. Unless you have a history of kidney stones, there is no apparent hazard in boosting the amount of calcium in your diet. If you do have a history of kidney stones, consult the physician who has been treating you before you make any dietary changes.

Calcium intake does not cause calcium deposits.

Q. How much calcium am I actually getting in a 500-milligram calcium carbonate tablet? The label says 200 milligrams of calcium. Can you explain the difference?

A. You are actually getting 200 milligrams of the element calcium in each tablet. The 500 milligrams refers to the entire tablet—calcium weight plus the weight of the carbonate. The compound calcium carbonate is 40 percent calcium and 60 percent carbonate. When purchasing mineral supplements such as calcium, magnesium and zinc, look for the designated amount of the mineral itself. That is the best way to be

A 500-milligram calcium carbonate tablet may not contain 500 milligrams of calcium. Here's why.

sure of how much of a particular mineral you are receiving.

Q. I am a 41-year-old woman, convinced of the need to take supplemental calcium. I have seen advertisements for calcium supplements made from eggshells and oyster shells. Are these supplements good sources of calcium?

A. Although we don't ordinarily think of eggshells and oyster shells as food supplements, both are excellent sources of calcium. When the shells are cleaned and finely ground, the resulting product is almost pure calcium carbonate. Calcium carbonate is one of the richest sources of elemental calcium, containing 40 percent calcium, which is readily absorbed and utilized by the body.

Supplements made from eggshells and oyster shells are excellent sources of calcium.

Q. What's the best source of calcium—milk or calcium supplements?

A. Calcium in a glass is superior to calcium in a pill for postmenopausal women, according to researchers at Creighton University in Omaha.

Doctors there studied a group of healthy women aged 45 to 70 who drank 24 ounces (that's three glasses) of low-fat milk a day for two years. Their bone density was measured before and after the experiment and then compared with that of women who took calcium carbonate and others who didn't take any extra calcium at all. The result? Women who drank milk had healthier bones than the women in the other two groups.

Why milk is the best calcium "supplement" of all.

It may just be, say the doctors, that other nutrients in milk and milk products help bones metabolize calcium better—a factor important in controlling osteoporosis, the fragile-bone disease that strikes postmenopausal women (*American Journal of Clinical Nutrition*).

The Iron Distinction

Q. What's the difference between organic and inorganic iron? What kind do we get when we use iron cookware?

A. The iron we find in foods like meat, spinach and whole grains is considered organic. On the other hand, inorganic iron (primarily in the forms of ferrous sulfate, ferric orthophosphate and sodium iron phosphate) is usually added to foods for purposes of fortification. Both forms of iron are utilized by the body, and either form can be found in iron supplements.

What you should know about organic and inorganic iron.

When acid foods, such as tomatoes, are prepared in iron cookware, varying amounts of organic iron are formed. Spaghetti sauce, for example, cooked for about 20 minutes in an iron pot, contains six milligrams of iron per 3½ ounces. But iron levels in that same amount of sauce prepared in a glass pot amount to only three milligrams.

Clearing Up the Confusion over Amino Acids

Q. Since I rarely eat red meat, only chicken and fish, as well as some grains, should I be taking amino acid supplements?

A. Not to worry. All animal proteins are considered "complete." That means they contain all of the nine essential amino acids your body must get from what you eat.

Amino-acid supplements are not necessary on this diet.

Q. I've heard that lysine is effective in decreasing attacks of herpes simplex (cold sores), but no one has ever said what dosage is most effective.

A. Doctors at the Mayo Clinic have. In a study involving a group of 41 otherwise healthy patients, they found that an oral supplement of 1,248 milligrams a day of L-lysine monohydrochloride decreased the recurrence rate of herpes simplex attacks and, in fact, helped decrease the severity of symptoms such as burning, itching, redness, swelling and pain in two-thirds of the volunteers. The researchers had no such luck with a lower dose of 624 milligrams.

While that may at first appear to be good news for the 50 to 70 percent of the population who suffer from herpes simplex, the Mayo Clinic scientists—and

Lysine may squelch cold sores, but use this nutrient with caution.

we—urge you to approach those findings with caution. They are preliminary results from a relatively small sample population. In any event, women who are pregnant or lactating should not take lysine because of reports of growth suppression in baby chicks and rats fed the amino acid.

Thinking Zinc

Q. Sometimes I take as many as ten zinc lozenges a day when I have a cold. I use the flavored ones, and they really work. Is ten too many?

How many zinc lozenges are too many?

A. Probably not, if you limit your treatment to seven days or less. The researchers at the University of Texas who discovered this new use for zinc suggested that their patients be given one lozenge every two hours during the day, which meant the cold sufferers were getting a 100- to 200-milligram dose of zinc daily. This is considered excessive—after all, the recommended daily allowance for adults is only 15 milligrams a day—but it is far from toxic.

Though taking large doses of zinc can cause stomach upset and vomiting, it's regarded as noncumulative and nontoxic when taken for a brief time. In this case, the researchers defined "brief" as a week or less.

Bonus Questions

Q. I find it convenient to take my vitamins with my morning coffee. Is there anything wrong with this?

Don't take your vitamins with coffee.

A. In the case of at least two nutrients, it's a little like mud wrestling after a beauty treatment. Studies have shown that coffee can rob you of both the B vitamin thiamine and iron. You can lose up to 39 percent of the iron you take with your morning coffee, even more if your only iron source is in a multiple vitamin/mineral tablet that contains other nutrients that prevent your body from absorbing iron. Coffee also appears to destroy thiamine in the body. In this instance, it's not the caffeine that's stealing nutrients but chlorogenic acid, a coffee ingredient that isn't washed away in the decaffeinating process.

Q. I am confused. Can you explain the difference between RDAs and USRDAs?

A. Recommended Dietary Allowances (RDAs) are average daily amounts of vitamins and some minerals established by the National Research Council that will prevent the development of obvious nutrient deficiency in practically all healthy Americans. In compiling the RDAs, nutrient allowances are broken down for 17 population groups based on age and sex, including allowances for pregnancy and lactation.

The U.S. Recommended Daily Allowances (USRDAs) are based on the RDAs and are used specifically for the labeling of products that have added nutrients or make nutritional claims. For practical purposes, the many categories of dietary allowances for males and females of different ages were essentially condensed to one set of values for nutritional labeling. Usually the highest RDA value for a particular nutrient was used to establish the USRDAs.

Q. I am puzzled about glandular products. I cannot seem to find a clear-cut explanation of what they are and what they're supposed to do for me. Can you help?

A. It is difficult to convey a healthful image of products labeled raw prostate, raw ovary, raw pituitary, raw orchic (from animal testes) and raw tranquil (from the brains of cows). The word "raw" indicates that the products, which come from cow and pig glands, haven't been heated above body temperature. But the supplements are processed in various ways—they are often freeze-dried—before being packaged in capsules.

Glandular products simply don't work.

The theory is that eating a certain gland from an animal will somehow affect the corresponding gland in a human being. For example, ingesting dehydrated brains is supposed to calm a person down, and eating pituitary glands supposedly will help a person grow taller. But in most cases the theory makes no scientific sense. According to a researcher at Stanford University, "Most of the factors in the glands, especially if they are proteins, are either destroyed in the manufacturing process or digested by the stomach acids when orally ingested." So while you may ingest traces of proteins or hormones, there's nothing to steer them directly to the proper gland once they're in your body.

More Information about Supplements

Q. What is vitamin F? I saw a passing reference to it in an article I was reading, but I'd never heard of it before.

A. That's understandable, because it's an obsolete term for essential fatty acids, polyunsaturated fats the body needs for several important functions, but which it cannot synthesize. So, like vitamins, the body gets essential fatty acids from the diet. Three polyunsaturated fatty acids were once considered essential, but the most noteworthy—and the only one that seems to be truly essential—is linoleic acid, found in foods such as safflower, corn and soybean oils, margarine, walnuts, almonds, peanut butter and pumpkin seeds. As with vitamins, a lack of linoleic acid in the diet can produce symptoms of a deficiency state, usually drying and flaking of the skin. It is rare, seen in infants and hospitalized adults being fed exclusively fat-free formulas.

"Vitamin F" explained.

Q. Recently I saw an ad claiming that for a fee of $50 and additional payments of $100 per month, I could receive a monthly supply of supplements computer-designed for my personal metabolic needs. Does this offer sound legitimate?

A. No. Beware of any organization making exaggerated claims about the effects of supplements, asking outrageous prices for supplements or asserting that some expert can determine the only supplementation regimen right for your body. When in doubt, consult your personal physician, the Better Business Bureau, a consumer protection agency or your local district attorney.

Beware of ads for mail-order nutritional advice.

Part **III**

FROM A TO ZINC: A GUIDE TO VITAMINS AND MINERALS

Blocking Cancer with Vitamin A and Beta-Carotene

The scientific evidence is still far from conclusive, but that didn't stop the National Academy of Sciences from issuing an anticancer prescription in 1982 that sounded remarkably like something your mother once told you: Eat your vegetables.

The new anticancer formula includes vegetables.

Even some cancer researchers who won't be pinned down to anything more concrete than a "maybe" admit that they haven't waited for the final test results before changing their diets. "I've seen it in this business for the last seven years," says one researcher who studies vitamin A and skin cancer. "What I—and all my colleagues—eat has changed. I used to be a typical junk-food eater. Now I eat a vegetable-based, high-fiber diet. Does it prevent cancer? My scientific answer is that the data overwhelming suggest that diet makes a difference. My unscientific answer is that what I eat has certainly changed."

Scientists Say, "Eat Your Vegetables"

Even without the definitive proof in hand, the normally conservative scientific community has become the unabashed patron of the salad bar. What convinced them? A persuasive collection of studies from all over the world that suggest that people who heap their plates with green and yellow vegetables and fruit reduce their risk of cancer.

Why scientists are lining up at the salad bar.

• A Japanese study—one of the largest of its kind—found that people who ate green-yellow vegetables every day had a decreased risk of developing lung, stomach and other cancers. The 20-year-old ongoing study also indicates that the damage wrought by bad habits—spurning vegetables or smoking, for instance—is reversible. Ex-smokers who had their daily dose of green-yellow vegetables also experienced a reduction in their risk of lung cancer, and there was a more than 25 percent reduction in the number of deaths from stomach cancer among those who increased their vegetable consumption (*Dietary Aspects of Carcinogenesis*).

Elderly people who ate the most fruits and vegetables had the least cancer.

• A Harvard University study of more than 1,200 elderly Massachusetts residents found that those who reported the highest consumption of carrots, squash, tomatoes, salads or leafy greens, dried fruits, fresh strawberries or melon, broccoli or brussels sprouts had a decreased risk of cancer (*Community Health Studies*).

• A researcher comparing the diets of healthy people and those with gastrointestinal cancer in both the United States and Norway found that the healthy people ate more foods such as carrots, leafy green vegetables and fresh fruits.

More Than Just a Pretty Vegetable

What's in a carrot that seems to counteract cancer? Buoyed by this impressive data, the National Cancer Institute (NCI) is spending millions of dollars to find out.

Starting with the only thing they knew for sure—there's something about green-yellow vegetables that acts as a buffer against cancer—NCI scientists latched onto color as their first clue. What gives these vegetables their hue? A naturally occurring pigment called beta-carotene, now the subject of at least a half dozen studies funded by NCI.

Beta-carotene, a new contender against cancer.

Of course, beta-carotene is more than just a pigment. It is one of the dietary chemicals the body converts into usable vitamin A. Because so little is known about it, researchers are grappling with several questions. Does beta-carotene inhibit cancer by its own unique mechanism or simply because it is converted into vitamin A, which has been shown in laboratory studies to be a cancer preventive? If it has its own potency, and since it is the common dietary source of vitamin A, could some of the anticancer claims made for vitamin A be more rightly credited to beta-carotene?

What evidence there is suggests that beta-carotene provides its own form of protection against cancer. And one cancer researcher, Richard Peto of Oxford, England, believes it's a strong possibility that it could prevent about a third of the cancer deaths in the United States.

A Shock Absorber against Cellular Insults

One thing scientists do know is that beta-carotene acts as what one researcher describes as a "shock absorber," protecting the valuable genetic blueprints inside each cell from the damage caused by reactive molecules known as free radicals. Theoretically, the havoc wrought by those excited molecules, natural by-products of fat metabolism, can turn a healthy cell into a cancerous one.

And beta-carotene has two major advantages over other forms of vitamin A. First, it has no known toxicity. Vitamin A taken in doses over 50,000 international units daily can be dangerous. "With an overdose of beta-carotene, on the other hand, all you do is turn yellow," says Frank L. Meyskens, Jr., M.D., of the Larry Smith Cancer Center of the University of Arizona in Tucson.

Unlike vitamin A, an overdose of beta-carotene has no major side effects.

Second, the dietary sources of beta-carotene are unarguably healthful foods. (See the table, Best Food

Sources of Beta-Carotene, on page 91.) For most people, the main sources of the other major form of dietary vitamin A—the retinoids—are milk and cheese. "Unless you go with skim milk and low-fat dairy products, that can mean a very high-fat diet," says Judith Wylie-Rosett, Ed.D. Beef and chicken liver are also high in vitamin A: 3½ ounces of fried beef liver has 36,105 international units of vitamin A, and 3 ounces of cooked chicken liver has 10,461 international units.

Lower Risk of Cervical Cancer

Dr. Wylie-Rosett and her colleagues at the Albert Einstein College of Medicine in New York City are a few of the handful of researchers who are adding to the growing body of knowledge about this nutrient-come-lately.

When they examined the diets of a group of healthy women and women with abnormal PAP smears, they found that women with a low vitamin A or beta-carotene intake had a threefold greater risk of developing cervical cancer or severe cervical dysplasia, a precancerous condition (*Nutrition and Cancer*).

Is too little beta-carotene a factor in cervical cancer?

One of the reasons Dr. Wylie-Rosett and her associates looked at beta-carotene intake, aside from their interest in the nutrient, was extremely practical. "In our computer analysis, we have the ability to evaluate it," she says. "Not all nutrition surveys do, which is probably one reason why so little has been done on it. The interest in beta-carotene is relatively recent."

Vegetables have an edge over animal sources of this nutrient.

Interestingly, at almost the same time the American researchers were probing the connection between beta-carotene and cervical cancer, so were a group of doctors in Milan, Italy. Their findings were similar: Women who averaged 5,000 international units of beta-carotene daily, as measured by their consumption of carrots and green vegetables, had a reduced risk of cervical cancer. Significantly, the researchers found no such association with the retinoids—measured by the consumption of milk, liver and meats—when they compared the diets of 191 women with cervical cancer and 191 healthy women in the same age group (*International Journal of Cancer*).

A Step against Oral Cancer

Of course, asking someone to recall the amount of carrots or squash he or she ate over any given period doesn't give the kind of rock-solid results experimental scientists prefer. These so-called retrospective studies are often severely criticized. So researchers at the British Columbia Cancer Research Center in Vancouver made sure they knew exactly how much beta-carotene and vitamin A their test subjects were taking. They administered capsules of each twice weekly to 40 rural Filipinos living on Luzon, the largest island in the Philippines, who were chosen because of their habit of quid chewing.

A quid is a concoction made from the areca nut, the betel leaf, lime produced from heating and crushing snail shells, and dried tobacco leaf. It is believed responsible for several hundred thousand oral cancer deaths each year in Asia. The Filipino tribesmen selected for the trial, ranging in age from 30 to 60, admitted to chewing from 4 to 15 quids a day.

Working with medical missionaries in this poor community, where the daily fare was usually potatoes and rice, the researchers made sure their volunteers got 100,000 international units of vitamin A and 300,000 international units of beta-carotene each week—well above the Recommended Dietary Allowances (RDA). Because the study was so short (only three months), the scientists knew they wouldn't see cancers develop, so they looked for the earliest warning sign: cell damage inside the mouth.

Needless to say, among the quid chewers there were quite a few damaged cells in the tissue samples scraped from the insides of their cheeks at the beginning of the study. But at the end, 37 of the 40 had substantially fewer damaged cells than they did at the

Can beta-carotene head off oral cancer?

start. In fact, the number of damaged cells decreased dramatically—by about 40 percent a month. The remaining 3 had no increase in the amount of damage.

The researchers found their results so "striking" they suggested that it may be possible for people at high risk of oral cancer to lessen their risk by simply adding vitamin A and/or beta-carotene to their diets (*Lancet*).

"Morning-After Pill" for Cancer?

Like the 20-year Japanese study, the Canadian research appears to indicate that we have a grace period, a time when dietary intervention will save us from the consequences of our bad health habits. Several important animal studies are providing clues to just how long it lasts.

Eli Seifter, Ph.D., professor of biochemistry and surgery, and his colleagues at the Albert Einstein College of Medicine found out more about that critical grace period. They discovered the earlier beta-carotene is given, the better. When they gave a hefty dose (equal to dozens of times the RDA for men) to rats at intervals ranging from two to nine weeks after exposure to a cancer-causing chemical, the researchers discovered the grace period lasted for five to six weeks. Rats given beta-carotene more than a month after their exposure to the carcinogen did not develop tumors.

The sooner you begin to take advantage of beta-carotene, the more health damage you may prevent.

While the results can't yet be translated into a human timetable, they still provide some valuable information. "What our study really shows," says Dr. Seifter, "is that beta-carotene is protective against either late stages of tumor development or early stages of tumor growth.

Beta-carotene may fight tumors directly.

"That's very good, because it shows in a sense that it's a 'morning-after pill.' Even after exposure to cancer-producing doses of some toxic chemicals, beta-carotene still has its effect." For recent converts to health-consciousness and those who still haven't kicked their bad habits, it's not too late.

Dr. Seifter believes a daily intake of five to ten milligrams (25,150 to 50,300 international units) of beta-carotene—the equivalent of 8,375 to 16,750 international units of vitamin A—will provide good protection against some tumors. "People at high risk for developing cancer, smokers for instance, would require twice that amount," he says.

One doctor's Rx: For tumor protection, a diet supplying at least 25,150 international units of beta-carotene a day.

Can Vitamin A Fight "Cancer Stress"?

"Most chemotherapy makes some people sick," says Eli Seifter, Ph.D., professor of biochemistry and surgery at the Albert Einstein College of Medicine in New York City. "Cancer and cancer therapy are very stressful to the body, and those very stresses promote cancer growth."

The result is an increased breakdown of body tissue, weight loss, a suppressed immune system and increased production of hormones, such as adrenaline, which are associated with stress. But Dr. Seifter has found that in mice "stressed" through partial body restraint, vitamin A reduced the physical symptoms of stress. It shrank the size of the stress-enlarged adrenal gland and enlarged the thymus, otherwise shrunk by stress.

He believes stress reduction will give people a real edge in fighting cancer. "Vitamin A, in combination with conventional therapy that reduces tumor size, along with other nutritional, hormonal and psychological treatments that help relieve stress, may prove to be valuable in tumor treatment in the near future," he says.

A Force against Lung Cancer?

Richard B. Shekelle, Ph.D., a professor of epidemiology at the University of Texas Health Science Center in Houston, has explored another aspect of beta-carotene's reputed anticancer power.

Dr. Shekelle sent the cancer-research community into a spin with the results of his long-term study on beta-carotene and its effects on the deadliest of malignancies to man—lung cancer.

Dr. Shekelle's study actually began as a long-term investigation into coronary heart disease on 2,107 workers of a Chicago-based plant of Western Electric Company. One aspect of the study was to take dietary records of the participants. When it came to plotting vitamin A intake, Dr. Shekelle and his colleagues decided to divide the vitamin intake into that which came from animal sources (whole milk, liver, cream, butter and cheese) and that which came from beta-carotene-rich fruits and vegetables.

Over the next 19 years, 33 of the men developed lung cancer—all positively related to cigarette smoking. However, Dr. Shekelle and his colleagues noticed something else very significant in those who developed lung cancer. The rate was highest in those who ate the least amount of beta-carotene foods and lowest in those who ate the greatest amount. The result: an 8-to-1 difference in risk between the lowest and highest carotene-intake groups (*Lancet*).

Despite all this research, science can't yet tell us precisely how much vitamin A or beta-carotene we should get in our diets to avert cancer. But unless you're the strictly meat-and-potatoes type, shunting other vegetables to the corner of your plate, it's hard to avoid getting at least some beta-carotene in your diet. (See the table, Best Food Sources of Beta-Carotene, on page 91.) If you're taking your beta-carotene in its usual form (vegetables), you can even take more than 25,150 to 50,300 international units. But more than that—say, from eating pounds of carrots—is overdoing it.

Can beta-carotene stop the deadliest cancer of all?

Beta-carotene: How to make sure you're getting enough.

Best Food Sources
of Beta-Carotene

Food	Portion	Vitamin A Value* (I.U.)
Sweet potato, baked	1	24,877
Carrot, raw	1	20,253
Carrots, cooked, sliced	½ cup	19,150
Spinach, cooked	½ cup	7,370
Squash, winter, butternut, cooked, cubed	½ cup	7,141
Papaya	1	6,122
Kale, cooked, chopped	½ cup	4,810
Cantaloupe	¼	4,304
Turnip greens, cooked, chopped	½	3,959
Apricots	3	2,769
Broccoli, cooked	1 spear	2,537
Watermelon	⅟₁₆	1,762
Tomato, raw	1	1,530
Avocado	1	1,230
Broccoli, cooked, chopped	½ cup	1,099
Nectarine	1	1,001
Tangerine	1	773
Asparagus, cooked, sliced	½ cup	746
Lettuce, loose-leaf, shredded	½ cup	532
Peas, green, cooked	½ cup	478
Peach	1	465
Okra, cooked, sliced	½ cup	460
Lettuce, iceberg	¼ head	445
Beans, green, cooked, sliced	½ cup	413

SOURCES: Adapted from

Composition of Foods: Vegetables and Vegetable Products, Agriculture Handbook No. 8–11, by Nutrition Monitoring Division (Washington, D.C.: Human Nutrition Information Service, U.S. Department of Agriculture, 1984).

Composition of Foods: Fruits and Fruit Juices, Agriculture Handbook No. 8–9, by Consumer Nutrition Center (Washington, D.C.: Human Nutrition Information Service, U.S. Department of Agriculture, 1982).

Nutritive Value of American Foods in Common Units, Agriculture Handbook No. 456, by Catherine F. Adams (Washington, D.C.: Agricultural Research Service, U.S. Department of Agriculture, 1975).

Composition of Foods, Agriculture Handbook No. 8, by Bernice K. Watt and Annabel L. Merrill (Washington, D.C.: Agricultural Research Service, U.S. Department of Agriculture, 1975).

*Vitamin A value reflects the amount of vitamin A derived from the yellow, orange and green pigments, including beta-carotene, that are found in fruits and vegetables.

Chapter 13

Using the Healing Power of B Vitamins

Y ou can get to know the B vitamins intimately. Just skip a few meals or feast on candy bars and colas between work and your workout. The B team (by its absence) will introduce itself in no time flat— leaving you grouchy and tired.

If you're dragging as much as you're jogging, you may be a victim of what might be called "jock's syndrome." According to Jack Cooperman, Ph.D., director of nutrition at the New York Medical College, a subclinical, or marginal, vitamin deficiency is first signaled by a low blood level of B's—and it may be a hidden epidemic among the otherwise health conscious.

"Jock's syndrome"— the fitness buff's vitamin deficiency.

If you can't squeeze three squares a day in between your job and the gym, he says, you'll soon be running on empty. It takes only a few weeks for the B levels in your blood to drop. This increases the risk of a subclinical deficiency, which can occur after active forms of the B vitamins in the cells decrease.

The B's—there are 11 members of the B family, counting related compounds—help keep you going. Some of the best-known ones are thiamine (B_1), riboflavin (B_2), niacin, B_6, B_{12} and folate. They work together to help cells absorb and burn energy. Quite simply, without these pepper-uppers, you poop out.

The B's work in the body to help convert proteins, carbohydrates and fats into fuel, and in the brain to help synthesize the mood-controlling chemicals. That's why a B deficiency often manifests itself in

extreme muscle weakness and in psychiatric problems ranging from mild irritability to full-blown psychosis. Fortunately, severe cases are rare, but even a
marginal deficiency can leave you with the blues and
the blahs.

B vitamins are the spark plugs that ignite the body's fuel.

The after-work athlete, the erratic eater and the
dedicated dieter run the risk of marginal deficits because they're not replacing the B's they're using to
burn up energy. But deficiencies are also fairly common among the elderly and among people whose
diets are rich in refined foods and poor in nutrients.
Vegetarians, pregnant and nursing women and
women taking oral contraceptives also fall into the
serious risk category. (See the table, Best Food
Sources of B Vitamins, on pages 100–101, for a list of
foods that will help you beef up your intake of B's.)

But keeping you peppy and perky isn't the only
job of the B team. Certain discoveries offer some
promise that the B vitamins may also help you fight
cancer, cardiovascular disease and even the mental
deterioration of aging. Here are some of the latest—
and most intriguing—research results on the B's you
know best.

Can B vitamins fight cancer, cardiovascular disease and senility?

News about Niacin

Cancer researchers in Omaha, Nebraska, used
nicotinamide, a form of the B vitamin niacin, to counteract the toxic effects of a drug used to induce deadly
pancreatic cancer in hamsters. Niacin is an effective
antitoxin.

But what else it did surprised one of the researchers, Terrence Lawson, Ph.D., of the Eppley Institute
for Research in Cancer at the University of Nebraska
in Omaha.

"When we took the animals to term in 52 weeks,
we noticed there were no pancreatic tumors at all,"
says Dr. Lawson.

In another study, Dr. Lawson also discovered
that the animals treated with a dose of nicotinamide

Niacin as an antidote to cancer-causing toxins.

after a dose of the carcinogen had significantly less of the DNA damage usually caused by cancer. (DNA is a cellular molecule that carries genetic information.)

"It's reasonable to assume that somehow or other, the nicotinamide was cleaning up the damaged cells," he says.

Eventually, says Dr. Lawson, niacin may prove to be an effective "chemopreventive compound," a nutrient that doesn't cure cancer but prevents it.

Other research also suggests niacin may have some therapeutic uses in the treatment of blood clots that lead to cardiovascular diseases.

Using nicotinic acid (another form of niacin),

Niacin Reduces Post–Heart-Attack Risk

Sixteen years after 1,119 male heart attack survivors began taking niacin, the group had an 11 percent lower death rate than a similar group of men given a placebo (dummy pill), investigators found.

Overall, the men taking niacin lived about two years longer than those in the placebo group, reported Paul Canner, Ph.D., of the Maryland Medical Research Institute in Baltimore. Niacin, which protects against atherosclerosis by lowering blood lipids (cholesterol and triglycerides), was one of five lipid-lowering agents tested on over 8,000 male heart attack survivors in the Coronary Drug Project. Niacin was found to be the most effective of the five agents, which included

clofibrate, dextrothyroxine and two types of estrogen, or female sex hormones.

In the original trial, which lasted from 1966 to 1975, 8,341 male survivors aged 30 to 64 were placed on one of these five agents or a placebo. At the end of this period, the niacin group showed a modest benefit in terms of nonfatal heart attacks, but no clear advantage when it came to fatal attacks. But during a follow-up survey, conducted from 1981 to 1984, six to nine years after the conclusion of the study, niacin's protective power showed up clearly—perhaps, Dr. Canner suggests, because it slowed the progress of atherosclerosis (*Internal Medicine News*).

Ravi Subbiah, Ph.D., of the Lipid Research Center of the University of Cincinnati Medical Center, was able to suppress a process in atherosclerosis-prone pigeons that causes the clotting of blood platelets.

Niacin has an added bonus. It also reduces blood cholesterol and triglycerides—though at large doses—making it "potentially useful" as therapy for heart disease, says Dr. Subbiah.

Niacin, says one scientist, may even counter clot-forming blood fats.

B_{12} Teams Up with Vitamin C

Vitamin B_{12} is the vitamin that, with folate, helps produce red blood cells in bone marrow. Without it, red cell production diminishes and pernicious anemia results. Scientists believe that red cells are affected more than others by a B_{12} deficiency because B_{12} is part of the process that churns them out faster than other cells. Cancer cells are produced at the same quick pace, which is why doctors sometimes induce a B_{12} (and folate) deficiency in certain cancer patients to slow the growth of a malignancy.

Doctors sometimes manipulate B_{12} and folate in the body to slow cancer growth.

But there is also some recent evidence that B_{12} in conjunction with vitamin C is effective against cancer in a different way. The clues have turned up in animal studies conducted by Sister M. Eymard Poydock, Ph.D., a researcher at Mercyhurst College in Erie, Pennsylvania.

Dr. Poydock and her associates have had remarkable results with supplemental B_{12} and vitamin C in increasing the survival rate of mice with leukemia and several forms of malignant tumors, including one stubbornly resistant to other treatment. What is most remarkable is how fast the vitamins work.

"Even in the early stages, we see no increase of malignant cells," says Dr. Poydock. "After the seventh treatment, no tumor cells at all are present. The tumor cells just disintegrate. It's very exciting."

In laboratory animals, B_{12} and C disintegrate tumor cells.

Although the cancer-conquering process is still a mystery, Dr. Poydock suspects the vitamins work because they may alter the membranes of malignant cells so that the T-lymphocytes, the body's disease-fighting "killer" cells, recognize them as foreign and attack them. In fact, fluid extracted from their experimental mice was a veritable battlefield, littered with disintegrating tumor cells, lymphocytes and other disease-fighting cells (*Experimental Cell Biology*).

Though the day that B_{12} becomes a confirmed cancer therapy is probably still far off, the vitamin may be a lifesaver right now for the estimated half million asthmatics who are sensitive to the chemicals used to keep restaurant food looking fresh.

Can B_{12} save the lives of certain people with asthma?

The potentially dangerous substances are called sulfites. They can keep sliced potatoes from turning brown. They're also a common additive in wine and beer. Though there have been no documented deaths, at least one researcher believes that some restaurant fatalities written off as choking accidents may have been caused by allergic reactions to sulfites.

He is Ronald Simon, M.D., of the Scripps Clinic and Research Foundation in La Jolla, California. It was the research of Dr. Simon and his co-workers that originally piqued the interest of the producers of the CBS news program "60 Minutes," which first alerted the public to the dangers of sulfites.

The Scripps group research paid off in another way. They eventually discovered that an oral dose of vitamin B_{12} taken shortly before exposure to sulfites completely blocks asthmatic reaction. In fact, vitamin B_{12} worked better than three other drugs they tested on six sulfite-sensitive patients, and at a lower dosage, too.

B_{12} worked better than some drugs to stymie asthmatic attacks.

Apparently, says Dr. Simon, B_{12} enhances the chemical reaction that alters the sulfites in the body, quickly and efficiently converting them into an inactive substance.

Folate for Healthy Chromosomes

Folate works in partnership with B_{12} to form the red blood cells. It also helps dividing cells synthesize proteins, amino acids and nucleic acids. And research indicates that if your body isn't using folate properly, you risk serious damage to your chromosomes. That's important, because chromosome damage may be a catalyst for cancer.

"Many researchers believe that chromosome damage is an important part of the process that causes malignancy," says Richard Branda, M.D., a professor of medicine at the University of Vermont.

In fact, Dr. Branda has established a possible link between defects in the cells' use of folate, chromosome damage and cancer. The clue came from a study of a family with a history of chromosome damage and serious blood disease, including leukemia. Their cells weren't absorbing and using folate normally. In one family member with aplastic anemia, cell levels of folate were extremely low and remained low even after he took supplemental folate.

Folate may help keep chromosomes intact.

Dr. Branda believes the folate defect may have been the cause of the chromosome damage, which in turn precipitated the aplastic anemia. The case, though extremely rare, suggested to the researcher that it is folate that keeps the chromosomes from breaking.

There is other evidence linking folate deficiency to cancer. Researchers at the University of Alabama found that oral contraceptive users who had a precancerous condition along with folate deficiency were at less risk of developing cancer if they took folate supplements.

Women on the Pill, take note.

C. E. Butterworth, M.D., and his associates tested 47 young women taking birth control pills who had mild or moderate cervical dysplasia, a condition in which cervical cells can become malignant. Both folate deficiency and dysplasia are associated with the use of oral contraceptives.

A control group of contraceptive users who did not have the condition still had below-normal folate concentrations in their red cells. But the women with dysplasia showed an even more marked decline in

Folate kept precancerous growths in check.

folate levels. Folate supplements kept their precancerous condition from worsening.

The researchers believe that if their findings can be confirmed, it could provide important new information about the role nutrients play in controlling the growth of cancer (*American Journal of Clinical Nutrition*).

Riboflavin, the Exerciser's Friend

The 13-year-old patient posed a puzzling problem. At rest, her strength was normal. But when she moved her arms and legs, they grew weak. Her doctors at Academic Hospital Rotterdam in the Netherlands suspected and subsequently isolated a marginal enzyme deficiency that left her muscle cells unable to absorb the amount of energy they needed to work properly.

Although the teenager showed no signs of a vitamin deficiency, her doctors suspected her condition might respond to vitamin therapy anyway. So they gave her a supplement of riboflavin, the B vitamin crucial to the enzyme action that turns foods into fuel.

Riboflavin beat an enzyme deficiency and gave a teenager new strength.

Her doctors were right. Not only was her improvement "striking and sustained" but it wasn't long before she was riding her bike and active in sports again (*Lancet*).

Riboflavin, plentiful in dairy products, should be as much a part of your exercise gear as running shoes or tennis racquets. But it's easily lost from the body. In fact, you can literally sweat it away. And, like the fuel in your gas tank, you can lose it when you use it. Health-conscious women who exercise rigorously may be doing just that.

Very active women may need twice the Recommended Dietary Allowance of riboflavin.

Researchers at Cornell University discovered that very active women need about double the Recommended Dietary Allowance (RDA) of 1.2 milligrams of riboflavin a day. They learned this by testing the blood levels of the vitamin in a group of young female university students and staff eating a controlled diet and jogging 25 to 50 minutes a day for six weeks (*American Journal of Clinical Nutrition*).

Thiamine for Brain Power

A thiamine deficiency is characterized by severe fatigue and depression. In its most severe form, peripheral nerve damage and possibly paralysis appear. Rare in this country, it still has its victims, those whose calories are highly restricted and alcoholics who substitute drinking for eating.

In a study at the National Institutes of Mental Health, Bethesda, Maryland, researchers induced repeated thiamine deficiencies in a group of rhesus monkeys. Not only did the animals exhibit all the typical symptoms of human thiamine deficiency, they also suffered similar nerve damage, which the researchers found was reversible with supplemental thiamine. Their findings, the researchers said, point up the need for early detection and treatment of thiamine deficiency (*Annals of Neurology*).

Other scientists are interested in thiamine deficiency for a different reason. Resulting memory deficits closely resemble the mental deterioration of Alzheimer's disease, a degenerative brain disorder, and even normal aging.

Is thiamine the missing link in Alzheimer's disease?

Gary Gibson, Ph.D., of Cornell University's Burke Rehabilitation Center in New York, is involved in a long-term study of the biochemistry of thiamine deficiency in the hope that it can shed some light on the course of chronic brain deterioration. "We're looking for clues to see if there is some common element so we can get closer to what the biochemical deficit is and learn how to overcome it," he says.

B₆ Linked to Mood Swings

Vitamin B_6, also known as pyridoxine, is beginning to be recognized as nature's own antidepressant. In fact, there is evidence that a B_6 deficiency, even a marginal one, may be a cause of depression.

Without B₆, is depression inevitable?

Researchers at the Virginia Polytechnic Institute and State University tested the B_6 levels of a group of depressed patients and discovered that all had inadequate amounts of the vitamin. The scientists believe that without B_6 the brain is unable to produce an adequate supply of the mood-controlling neurotransmitter serotonin (*Nutritional Reports International*).

"Our research indicates that depression could be associated with inadequate B_6 levels," says one of the researchers, Carolyn Russ, currently a nutritionist and assistant director of the Clinical Nutrition Center at the University of California, Davis.

Best Food Sources of B Vitamins

Food	Portion	Thiamine (mg.)	Riboflavin (mg.)	Niacin (mg.)	B_6 (mg.)	B_{12} (mcg.)	Folate (mcg.)
Beef, round, full cut, separable lean only, cooked	3 oz.	0.086	0.195	0.430	2.53	3.540	9
Beef kidneys, simmered	3 oz.	0.162	3.450	0.440	43.60	5.110	83
Beef liver, braised	3 oz.	0.167	3.480	0.770	60.35	9.110	185
Brewer's yeast	1 tbsp.	1.250	0.340	0.200	0.00	3.000	313
Chicken, light meat, cooked	3 oz.	0.060	0.100	0.510	0.29	10.560	3
Chick-peas, boiled	½ cup	0.095	0.052	0.114	0.00	0.431	141
Egg, hard-cooked	1	0.040	0.140	0.060	0.66	0.030	24
Kidney beans, all types, boiled	½ cup	0.141	0.051	0.106	0.00	0.509	114
Chicken liver, cooked	3 oz.	0.130	1.490	0.500	16.49	3.780	654

SOURCES: Adapted from

Composition of Foods: Beef Products, Agriculture Handbook No. 8–13, by Nutrition Monitoring Division (Washington, D.C.: Human Nutrition Information Service, U.S. Department of Agriculture, 1986).

Composition of Foods: Breakfast Cereals, Agriculture Handbook No. 8–8, by Consumer Nutrition Center (Washington D.C.: Human Nutrition Information Service, U.S. Department of Agriculture, 1982).

Composition of Foods: Dairy and Egg Products, Agriculture Handbook No. 8–1, by Consumer and Food Economics Institute (Washington, D.C.: Agricultural Research Service, U.S. Department of Agriculture, 1976).

Composition of Foods: Legumes and Legume Products, Agriculture Handbook No. 8–16, by Nutrition Monitoring Division (Washington, D.C.: Human Nutrition Information Service, U.S. Department of Agriculture, 1986).

Composition of Foods: Nut and Seed Products, Agriculture Handbook No. 8–12, by Nutrition Monitoring Division (Wash-

What remains to be done, she says, is to test B_6 therapy on depressed patients whose B_6 levels are low. Whether or not more of the vitamin would help those who aren't deficient in it is uncertain. In any case, amounts over 50 milligrams a day should not be taken.

Can a B_6 deficiency make you older than you are? Two scientists at the University of Texas at Austin induced signs of premature aging in rats by feeding them diets deficient in B_6 or copper for two to three months. Without B_6, the delicate nerve branches, called dendrites, which receive nerve impulses, de-

In rats, B_6 deficiency produced premature aging.

Food	Portion	Thiamine (mg.)	Riboflavin (mg.)	Niacin (mg.)	B_6 (mg.)	B_{12} (mcg.)	Folate (mcg.)
Milk, whole	1 cup	0.090	0.400	0.100	0.87	0.210	12
Navy beans, boiled	½ cup	0.184	0.056	0.149	0.00	0.483	127
Peanuts, all types, dry-roasted	¼ cup	0.000	0.035	0.093	0.00	4.930	53
Brown rice, raw	¼ cup	0.170	0.030	0.280	0.00	2.350	8
Rye flour	¼ cup	0.200	0.070	0.100	0.00	0.880	17
Salmon steak, cooked	3 oz.	0.150	0.060	0.640	2.95	8.400	18
Soybeans, boiled	½ cup	0.133	0.245	0.201	0.00	0.343	46
Sunflower seeds, dry	¼ cup	0.820	0.090	0.450	0.00	1.620	85
Swiss cheese	2 oz.	0.010	0.210	0.050	0.95	0.050	4
Wheat germ, toasted	1 tbsp.	0.120	0.060	0.070	0.00	0.400	25
Whole wheat flour	¼ cup	0.170	0.040	0.100	0.00	1.300	16

ington, D.C.: Human Nutrition Information Service, U.S. Department of Agriculture, 1984).

Composition of Foods: Poultry Products, Agriculture Handbook No. 8–5, by Consumer and Food Economics Institute (Washington, D.C.: Science and Education Administration, U.S. Department of Agriculture, 1979).

"Folacin in Selected Foods," by Betty P. Perloff and R. R. Butrum, *Journal of the American Dietetic Association,* February 1977.

Nutritive Value of American Foods in Common Units, Agriculture Handbook No. 456, by Catherine F. Adams (Washington, D.C.: Agricultural Research Service, U.S. Department of Agriculture, 1975).

Pantothenic Acid, Vitamin B₆ and Vitamin B₁₂, Home Economics Research Report No. 36, by Martha Louise Orr (Washington, D.C.: Agricultural Research Service, U.S. Department of Agriculture, 1969).

generated and died, effectively short-circuiting the brain. The resulting damage closely resembled normal aging (*American Journal of Clinical Nutrition*).

But, says researcher Elizabeth Root, Ph.D., it's rare to find a B_6 deficiency without a drop in some or all of the other B vitamins and other vital nutrients. They are, after all, a team.

Taking advantage of the "B team."

"What we can safely say," Dr. Root says, "is that people, especially elderly people, should make sure that they get all of their minimum daily requirements of nutrients."

Thiamine: Preventing a Common Deficiency

Tony was a strapping teenager—tall, muscular and handsome. But likable he wasn't, at least for the past few months. His growing neurotic behavior and temper tantrums were making him lose friends fast. Then one day during a small spat with his mother, he knocked over a bookcase in a rage.

Mary lived the life of a typical professional woman: busy and on the go. Ever conscious of slipping her hips into her sizable size 7 wardrobe, she settled into a one-meal-a-day eating routine on the lunchtime restaurant circuit, subsisting mostly on salads or other diet-wise platters. Dinner, if there was one at all, was usually soup from a can or another salad—she was just too busy to do any real food shopping. Then one day she suddenly had no urge to eat at all, and she started to lose weight. Her friends urged her to see a doctor.

Three cases of thiamine-poor eating habits.

Billy was the star of his college soccer team. Back in shape after a summer of dieting and body building, he took his first loss on the chin—with a gaping wound to the jaw. But unlike the scrapes from his former fights, this one just didn't seem to be healing well. Worried, he went to see his doctor.

So, you wonder, what have we found to link a strung-out teen, an up-and-coming female executive and a college jock? It's thiamine (B_1). Yes, thiamine was needed to get this trio back in shape. Thiamine is the first of the B vitamins, and its importance to our health stems from the part it plays in the oxidation

Your body can't store thiamine, so dietary supplies are important.

process that takes place in each and every cell. Since our bodies don't store it, our need for thiamine is ongoing. A lack of it can cause nervous disorders, such as that experienced by teenage Tony.

Tony is a character closely aligned to a group of teens with neurotic behavior who were studied by Derrick Lonsdale, M.D., a former pediatrician who is now practicing preventive medicine in Westlake, Ohio.

Too Many Sweets

Dr. Lonsdale found many of the teens ate large amounts of junk food, particularly sweet soft drinks, candy and high-carbohydrate foods with little nutritive value. Since thiamine is essential to metabolize carbohydrates, a diet high in carbohydrates and sugars requires more of the vitamin. But these teens weren't getting enough.

Thiamine nourishes your nerves.

"These children displayed behavioral characteristics that we have come to accept as normal," Dr. Lonsdale says. "They complained of headaches, abdominal and chest pains and sleeping problems. They were irritable, and some were aggressive and hard to handle.

"What they were was nutritionally disoriented. Our blood test showed them to be deficient in a common form of thiamine. We changed their diets and gave them thiamine supplements. Of the ten we retested, all showed normal behavior." Some even lost their craving for sweets and soft drinks. Thiamine, Dr. Lonsdale notes, nourishes the nervous system, and a lack of it can cause abnormal behavior.

Consuming large amounts of sweets and soft drinks can rob teens of thiamine.

Dr. Lonsdale feels, however, the impact of this study goes beyond the importance of just thiamine in the diet. "There does appear to be a fairly large mass of kids in America who have behavior abnormalities because of a poor diet," he asserts. "The thing is that this is widely accepted as part of growing up. A high intake of carbohydrates, and caffeine and sugar in the form of soft drinks, increases the need for many vitamins and minerals," he says.

Other signs of thiamine deficiency are not quite as blatant as abnormal behavior. Such was the case with Mary. Her lack of appetite was also a sign of thiamine deficiency.

Crash Diets Lack Thiamine

Even the earliest studies of the vitamin pointed to its effects on the appetite. Since metabolism of carbohydrates depends on thiamine, a lack of it can slow the process down, leaving the victim with a loss of appetite.

Without thiamine, appetite plummets.

Mary could be a typical victim, in light of a study indicating that single professional women fail to get even two-thirds of their Recommended Dietary Allowance (RDA) of a number of essential vitamins and minerals. One of the nutrients found in low supply was thiamine. In fact, 36 percent of the women surveyed were falling short of this nutrient (*Nutrition Reports International*).

"Thiamine is a problem in young women because so many of them, particularly those going after the slender image, do not eat much. The amount of thiamine you get pretty much depends on the amount of food you eat," says Robert E. Keith, Ph.D., of the Department of Nutrition and Foods at Auburn University in Alabama, who studied the dietary habits of 50 well-educated career women in the area. Although their intake levels were marginal, the women were not showing obvious symptoms of deficiency.

Starvation diets sacrifice thiamine.

"They didn't eat a lot of meat, and calorie intake was generally low," reports Dr. Keith. "They ate a lot of salads, but salads are usually made up of iceberg lettuce, which isn't a good source of thiamine.

"Thiamine is well distributed in most foods. There aren't many things that contain a great amount of thiamine, although pork, organ meats and whole grains are good sources," he says. "Young women watching their diets don't eat a lot of those things."

Brewer's yeast and wheat germ are two good sources of thiamine that could fit into the diet of a weight watcher.

A lack of thiamine has also been found to cause hypothermia—a lowering of body temperature—in those suffering from the psychologically induced form of appetite loss, anorexia nervosa.

Lack of thiamine: A connection with lower body temperature?

This was illustrated in the case of a 32-year-old woman with a history of the disorder who was admitted to a hospital with a subnormal body temperature. Her thiamine level was found to be low, and she was put on 300 milligrams daily. After seven days, her temperature returned to normal, and she regained her appetite. Three months later, thiamine supplements were withdrawn. In two weeks her symptoms returned (*American Society for Clinical Nutrition*).

Aid for Wound Healing

And, as Billy's story revealed, thiamine is necessary not only for the metabolism of the foods that we eat. Research shows that it has an effect on the way our wounds heal, too. Animal studies showed that wound healing was significantly delayed in thiamine-deficient rats compared to those with normal thiamine levels (*Journal of Surgical Research*).

Thiamine helps long-term wound healing.

"We found increased levels of thiamine did not speed up the process, but it did do something significant. It made the wounded area stronger and more resilient after healing," says Oscar M. Alvarez, Ph.D.

Dr. Alvarez, former director of the Wound Healing Research Laboratory of the Cornell University Medical School, feels this finding could have an important impact for surgery patients. "The RDA for thiamine may be wrong in stressful situations such as wound healing, which is important in surgery," reports Dr. Alvarez.

Dr. Alvarez says he is not certain why thiamine is so important in the healing of wounds, but he feels that it has a lot to do with the overall reaction of the body to an injury.

Thiamine deficiency can block the metabolism of collagen, which is a protein of the body. "In order for a wound to heal, collagen must be produced, and energy is required for its production. Thiamine may be related to wound healing because of its direct relationship to energy production," Dr. Alvarez explains.

One more metabolic link in the chain of healing.

Other Nervous System Needs for Thiamine

Another new use for thiamine is showing up in the emergency room. At Bellevue Hospital Center in New York City, Lewis R. Goldfrank, M.D., and his emergency room staff are using thiamine in treating unconscious patients.

Thiamine at work in the emergency room.

The normal procedure in such a case is to give intravenous dextrose and water to the patient. "This is theoretically sound, but it can have disastrous practical consequences if a patient is thiamine deficient," says Dr. Goldfrank. "Since thiamine is needed to metabolize sugar," he says, "you simply cannot give glucose and expect to get a high energy yield unless thiamine is present."

This is particularly relevant with alcoholics, who are commonly thiamine deficient due to their generally poor nutrition and who often end up, unconscious, in a hospital emergency room. Symptoms of intoxication and thiamine deficiency are often similar—staggered walk, glazed eyes, loss of coordination and confusion.

"In light of this, giving supplemental thiamine to all alcoholics for whatever reason makes a lot of sense from the viewpoint of nutritional and preventive medicine, as does fortifying all alcoholic beverages," writes Dr. Goldfrank in *Emergency Medicine*.

Replacing lost thiamine can reverse some damage done by alcohol.

Severe thiamine deficiency can cause a loss of muscle control, loss of memory and even coma. "Many of these symptoms can be successfully reversed if thiamine is used promptly, before permanent damage takes place," says Dr. Goldfrank. "On the other hand, giving glucose without thiamine can result in a lifetime disability because you may precipitate Wernicke-Korsakoff's syndrome or considerably worsen a preexisting condition."

Wernicke syndrome is a nervous system disorder, characterized by loss of coordination, abnormal eye movement and delirium. It can progress to Korsakoff syndrome, which is permanent mental impairment.

The importance of thiamine was discovered about a century ago when a disease called beriberi, which debilitated the Japanese navy, was found to be the result of a diet containing a lot of polished (refined) rice. When grains are refined, much of the thiamine is removed. Researchers soon discovered that a person who eats large amounts of white flour, cornmeal, polished rice and refined cereals and sugars is more likely to wind up sick than one who eats unrefined foods.

Beriberi—the thiamine-deficiency disease—may not be as rare as many people think.

Although beriberi is rare, Japanese researchers have reported a reappearance of the disease over the past decade, this time in the nation's population of young people.

The importance of thiamine should not be overlooked. Without it we can lose our appetite, get depressed and develop other psychological problems. With it, our energy level is up, our minds are sharp and our emotions are high. So, when it comes to the basics of nutrition, thiamine should be at the top of the list. (To increase your intake of thiamine, see the table, Best Food Sources of B Vitamins, on pages 100–101.)

Vitamin B₆: More Reasons to Make Sure You're Getting Enough

I t began as just another offbeat case of side effects from medical treatment, but that's not how it turned out.

A 65-year-old woman was being treated for heart trouble with a drug (amiodarone) that causes an odd physical reaction. Doctors call the side effect photosensitivity, a malady where even short exposure to sunlight gives way to itching, rashes or, in the woman's case, sunburn.

This time, however, an unusual antidote was prescribed: vitamin B_6. When the woman was given daily doses of the nutrient along with her heart medication, her photosensitivity lessened.

B_6 lessened drug-induced photo-sensitivity.

The same thing happened with two other coronary patients who mixed B_6 and the same heart drug. And according to the medical investigator of these three cases, the B_6 "in no way impaired the desired pharmacological effects of amiodarone" (*Lancet*).

The Many Tasks Done by B₆

Is anyone surprised by such findings? Certainly not researchers who know B_6 well. To them this report is one outcropping of B_6 data in the landscape of nutritional research, an expanse already dotted with evidence of the nutrient's influence. They've seen studies hinting that B_6 may relieve asthma and hyperactivity in children, ease premenstrual tension and swelling, help prevent recurrence of bladder cancer,

B_6 has been suggested as a treatment for everything from asthma to cancer.

decrease depression in women taking birth control pills, reverse the nerve disorder called carpal tunnel syndrome and help impede the development of atherosclerosis.

Perhaps more than any other vitamin, some scientists say, B_6 is multifunctional and multifaceted.

"It's not at all astonishing that vitamin B_6 can affect so many different physical conditions that seemingly have nothing to do with one another," says Alan Gaby, M.D., a Maryland physician and author of *A Doctor's Guide to Vitamin B_6*. "The nutrient is a cofactor [biological activator] for at least 50 enzymes responsible for hundreds of biochemical tasks. Without B_6 the enzymes couldn't do their jobs, and body chemistry would break down in countless ways. With B_6 the biological functions can be activated and maintained."

Adults and infants, pregnant and menstruating women, body and mind—B_6's range of operations stretches far and wide. And researchers have been busy documenting it inch by inch.

B_6 for the Mind

And sometimes case by case. One example is a case report from doctors at Arlington Hospital in Arlington, Virginia—a scientific account that lends support to some B_6 studies done more than ten years ago.

Behind the scenes, B_6 research is going full tilt.

The subject: schizophrenia. "An 18-year-old male entered the hospital emergency room and was diagnosed as having acute catatonic schizophrenia," says Lawrence D'Angelo, M.D., one of the investigating doctors. "He showed signs of restlessness, insomnia, mental confusion, anorexia, hallucinations, psychomotor retardation and other symptoms. However, we could find no evidence of organic brain damage, drug toxicity or any other specific cause for his condition—even after about three weeks of intensive medical investigation."

The doctors tried antipsychotic drugs on the patient, discontinued them because of severe side effects, tested the patient some more, then considered B$_6$. "We knew about other psychiatric case reports involving B$_6$," says Dr. D'Angelo. "So we started the patient on a daily B$_6$ regimen."

After other attempts failed, the doctors tried vitamin B$_6$.

The dosage was 150 milligrams three times a day, then 500 milligrams per day—a therapeutic intake far above normal levels. The Recommended Dietary Allowance (RDA) is 1.8 to 2.2 milligrams. (Because evidence suggests very large doses can be dangerous, you should never exceed 50 milligrams daily unless you are advised to do so by a knowledgeable physician.) Within 48 hours after the dose was increased, the patient started to improve—and he kept improving as long as he stayed on the nutrient therapy.

"Over a period of seven months, most of the patient's symptoms went away," Dr. D'Angelo says. "He thought more logically and clearly and didn't demonstrate any of the abnormal behavior he had when he first came to the hospital."

B$_6$ caused dramatic improvement in a schizophrenic.

But when he reduced his B$_6$ intake, it resulted in relapse. He was virtually back where he started. And only the high therapeutic dose of the nutrient could bring him back toward normal.

Do the investigators understand why B$_6$ had such a profound effect? Not yet, but they do know that B$_6$'s power could not be due to a single biological action. Vitamin B$_6$, they say, causes a whole spectrum of biochemical actions in the brain, and such multiplicity is required to affect the bundles of symptoms known as schizophrenia (*Biological Psychiatry*).

An Attempt to Control Seizures

No doubt it was news of B$_6$'s brain work that prompted scientists to test the nutrient against seizures, those neural disturbances that dim consciousness and foment convulsions.

At Kobe University in Japan, researchers admin-

B₆ has been tested as a treatment for seizures—with dramatic results.

istered high doses of B₆ to 19 children suffering from uncontrollable seizures, and 17 of them improved. Three had complete relief from seizures, 6 showed short-term absence of seizures and 8 experienced fewer seizures and improved brainwaves. Overall, it took only 2 to 14 days for the B₆ to have a positive impact (*Brain and Development*).

Unfortunately, because of the high doses involved, some of the children had temporary side effects. But a report from David S. Bachman, M.D., then at Columbus Children's Hospital in Columbus, Ohio, suggests that such high intakes may not always be necessary.

Dr. Bachman documents a case of an eight-month-old boy with a history of seizures who did not respond to standard antiseizure medication. The boy did, however, respond to something not so standard.

Antiseizure medication couldn't help one seizure-prone boy, but B₆ did.

"He was given 50 milligrams of intravenous pyridoxine [B₆]," says Dr. Bachman, "and the seizures stopped within minutes. He remained seizure free for the next six days, when seizure activity recurred and again promptly stopped with intravenous administration of pyridoxine."

For the next 22 months, the boy got 25 milligrams of oral pyridoxine daily and had no seizures at all. Then his nutrient therapy was discontinued, and the seizures began all over again. When he was put back on pyridoxine, the seizures vanished (*Annals of Neurology*).

"At age six," Dr. Bachman concludes, "he remains seizure free on a daily dose of 25 milligrams of pyridoxine."

Soothing Mother and Child

Can vitamin B₆ reduce herpes during pregnancy?

In B₆ research there's a growing number of such upbeat conclusions. Here's one that reveals a side of B₆ that most people have never seen. "This case represents another anecdotal report of the amazing result of pyridoxine therapy in the treatment of herpes gestationis.''

So says Craig G. Burkhart, M.D., a dermatologist practicing in Toledo, Ohio. The problem he's referring to is a rare skin disorder that afflicts pregnant women, bringing blisters, severe itching and—no one knows why—an increase in fetal mortality. And the case in question is that of a 26-year-old expectant mother who had the blisters on her abdomen and thighs.

The usual treatment for the disease is steroid drugs, like prednisone, but such therapy can be risky for mother and fetus. So this time Dr. Burkhart prescribed large daily doses of vitamin B$_6$, and within two weeks new blisters stopped forming and old ones receded.

In this case, B$_6$ seemed to work as an alternative to steroid drugs.

The woman continued her B$_6$ intake right up to the birth of her healthy baby girl, then stopped—and the blisters started. She then got back on the B$_6$, and the herpes went into another remission (*Archives of Dermatology*).

In the past, a few other doctors have tested B$_6$ against this malady and also found it effective. It's necessary to watch out for side effects from large doses of B$_6$, says Dr. Burkhart, but the nutrient is still much safer than steroids.

B$_6$ for VO$_2$ Max

That's something athletes might want to remember—especially since some researchers have suggested that B$_6$ may improve stamina.

B$_6$ may boost stamina.

One link in the B$_6$/stamina connection comes from the University of Geneva in Switzerland. There, researchers were trying to find out if giving people B$_6$ along with a derivative of amino acid metabolism could increase their bodies' ability to burn oxygen. Scientists call this capacity VO$_2$ max, and it's one of the most critical measures of your body's cardiovascular and respiratory performance. A high VO₂ max means you can transport and use a lot of fuel (oxygen) and put out a lot of peak effort in the process.

So the researchers selected 20 young men in excellent condition and assessed their VO₂ max. Then they divided the subjects into two groups, gave one group the B₆ plus derivative every day for 30 days, gave the other group a placebo (dummy pill) for the same length of time, then tested all the subjects again.

B₆ improved oxygen metabolism in men.

The result: The placebo group experienced almost no change in VO₂ max, but the supplemented group had a 6 percent increase. "Such an increase," say the researchers, "is moderate, but it is highly statistically significant" (*European Journal of Applied Physiology*).

To boost VO₂ max 10 to 20 percent, the average person would have to train for up to ten weeks. A 6 percent boost in VO₂ max in 30 days for men already in perfect shape looks very good indeed. Whether B₆ by itself could increase oxygen utilization remains to be seen.

B₆: Better than Medicine?

Clinically, the condition is referred to as carpal tunnel syndrome, but to those who suffer with the swollen fingers, the stiffness, numbness and tingling in their hands, relief is more important than labels. The usual treatment is anti-inflammatory medication or cortisone injections to reduce swelling. If the drugs fail, surgery is recommended, which sometimes doesn't relieve the pressure on the median nerve that's causing the problem. Vitamin B₆ may offer some hope.

Use of B₆ for carpal tunnel syndrome is still controversial.

The connection between B₆ and carpal tunnel syndrome has been a topic of heated debate within the research community for years. Britain's medical journal *Lancet* fanned the embers by reporting the successful use of B₆ to treat carpal tunnel syndrome.

A West Coast neurologist has added even more tinder to the B$_6$ fire. Allan L. Bernstein, M.D., chief of neurology at Kaiser Hospital, Hayward, California, has found that 150 milligrams a day brings improvement in 3 to 4 months, with the daily dosage dropping to about 25 milligrams after 6 to 12 months. "It took longer for the older patients to respond because their systems had to be resaturated with B$_6$, and their degree of compression was greater, whereas the younger ones had a less severe injury and responded in a shorter amount of time," he says.

While there have been no side effects from the dosages, Dr. Bernstein cautions that excessive B$_6$ can be toxic and cause neurological problems. (Don't take more than 50 milligrams a day without medical guidance.) He advises that people who suspect they are suffering from the syndrome discuss B$_6$ therapy with their physician, especially if more drastic measures—especially surgery—are suggested.

B$_6$ therapy should always be pursued with caution.

For a list of foods that are high in vitamin B$_6$, see the table, Best Food Sources of B vitamins, on pages 100–101.

Chapter 16

Test Your Vitamin B$_6$ Status

A re you getting enough B$_6$? The Recommended Dietary Allowance (RDA) is just 2.2 milligrams, but some people have trouble getting even that much. And some people have increased needs for B$_6$.

Take this quiz to find out if it's likely that you're meeting your B$_6$ needs. It's just a rough guide, so if you have serious symptoms or suspect that you have a B$_6$ deficiency, check with a qualified medical professional.

Review each of the following factors that can affect your vitamin B$_6$ status, add or subtract points for each factor as indicated, then tally your score and read what it means at the end of the quiz.

1. You take birth control pills (−3). Oral contraceptives are a common cause of B$_6$ deficiency in women. In one study, half the women taking birth control pills were low in B$_6$.

2. You eat at least four servings a week of any of these B$_6$ rich foods (+4). At least three servings a week (+3). At least two servings a week (+2): wheat bran, walnuts, wheat germ, peanuts, organ meats, avocados, brown rice, salmon, blackstrap molasses.

3. You're depressed for no apparent reason. You may also have tingling in your hands (−4). In one study, one-fifth of the people treated for depression at an outpatient clinic had low B$_6$ levels. Doctors have successfully treated some cases of depression with B$_6$.

The Pill can steal your body's reserves of B$_6$.

B$_6$ may be the answer for some people with depression.

4. You get plenty of magnesium-rich beans and nuts, plus soy products like tofu and tempeh (+3). B₆ and magnesium work hand in hand.

5. You suffer premenstrual syndrome (−3).

6. You're under a lot of stress (−3).

7. You have carpal tunnel syndrome, a nerve disorder that produces numbness, tingling, pain and weakness in the hand and fingers (−4). Additional B₆ may be an alternative to surgery for some people with this condition, studies show.

8. You smoke cigarettes or drink: Heavily (−5). Moderately (−3). You're a heavy smoker and drinker (−10). About half of the heavy drinkers tested showed signs of B₆ deficiency. Moderate drinking doesn't cause severe problems, but it may strain B₆ metabolism. In a study of pregnant women, twice as many smokers as nonsmokers were deficient.

If you drink heavily, you may be deficient in B₆.

9. You're careful to limit fried foods that contain substances that interfere with B₆ metabolism (+2).

10. You're pregnant or nursing a baby (−2). There's good evidence to show that higher amounts of B₆, up to 20 milligrams a day, may be needed to ward off deficiency in pregnant women, and lactating women also need increased amounts. A B₆ deficiency may affect birth weight and nervous system development in infants.

If you're pregnant or lactating, you may need more B₆.

11. You experience Chinese restaurant syndrome: You get a headache or flush shortly after eating MSG-containing foods (−2).

What's Your B₆ Status?

If your pluses and minuses total:

+3 to +9. Both your diet and lifestyle are keeping your B₆ levels high. Congratulations. No need for changes.

−5 to +3. Your B₆ intake may be borderline. Watch for symptoms and lifestyle habits that deplete B₆. Get more through foods.

−5 to −15. You're at risk for a B$_6$ deficiency. Stop drinking or smoking or taking birth control pills. Add B$_6$-rich foods to your diet. (See the table, Best Food Sources of B Vitamins, on pages 100–101.)

−15 or more. You're at high risk for a B$_6$ deficiency, and you may have additional nutritional problems. See a nutrition-knowledgeable doctor for the special help you need.

Chapter 17

Folate Gives Birth to Better Health

When Miriam L., a coal-miner's wife in the village of Gwent, Wales, gave birth to a healthy girl, she experienced all of the joy and relief that a woman feels at the end of a successful pregnancy, and then some. Her previous child had been born with spina bifida, a crippling neural tube defect (NTD), and the 5 percent risk of having another handicapped child had hovered over her second pregnancy like a malignant cloud.

The two deliveries couldn't have been less alike, and yet the difference between them may have been nothing more than a few hundred micrograms a day of a B vitamin called folate. Miriam had taken part in a study conducted by Welsh researchers, who asked her and more than 100 women like herself to eat a good diet including high-folate foods before and during their next pregnancies. Like her, every woman who followed the researchers' advice later gave birth to a healthy baby.

Seldom has so little gone so far, and these results seemed to support something that's long been suspected: Folate (also called folic acid) is the single most important nutrient for pregnant women and their developing children. In fact, eating fresh fruit and vegetables (which are rich in folate) from conception until the due date might be the best policy a woman can adopt to ensure that her pregnancy will be a happy and healthy one.

Did daily doses of folate head off a mother's nightmare?

Folate, the "Molecular Midwife"

Why folate? Because, on the cellular level, folate is a kind of "molecular midwife." It is one of the catalysts that helps bring new cells into this world. It is a key element in an enzyme that makes possible the

Folate fosters the birth of healthy new cells.

Things a Mother Should Know about Folate

When it comes to protecting the health of the mother as well as her child, folate also plays a role. Deficiency, in or out of pregnancy, increases the risk of cervical cancer, gum inflammation and anemia.

As for anemia, researchers say, "In pregnancy, unless folate supplementation is provided, the extra requirement for folate frequently produces folate deficiency." In some cases, this progresses to anemia, which is sometimes accompanied by sleeplessness, irritability or depression (*American Journal of Clinical Nutrition*).

Some women who use oral contraceptives have a localized folate deficiency in the cervix. One sign of this deficiency is cervical dysplasia—abnormalities among the cells in that region. Dysplasia often leads to cancer, but folate supplements may help arrest or reverse that tendency (*American Journal of Clinical Nutrition*).

Then there's gum disease: Many pregnant women have gingivitis, or inflamed gums. But a Swedish study has shown that gargling twice a day for one minute each time with a high-folate mouthwash can reduce that inflammation considerably (*Journal of Clinical Periodontology*).

duplication of DNA, which in turn enables one cell to split into two, then two into four, and so on. Without folate, growth simply slows down. Or it may be distorted and produce birth defects.

Besides NTDs, cleft palate and low birth weight or even miscarriage can come of a low-folate pregnancy. Aside from that, a woman may develop anemia or an inflammation of the gums called gingivitis as a result of the unborn infant's demands on her folate supply. When it comes to folate, a pregnant woman is truly eating for two, and the National Academy of Sciences has decreed that pregnant women need twice as much folate a day as other adults.

If you're pregnant, you need twice as much folate as other adults.

Preventing Neural Tube Defects

It was to find out whether or not folate could prevent a second NTD delivery that the investigators, headed by Dr. K. M. Laurence, of the Welsh National School of Medicine, chose to study several hundred women in Wales. These women had, for the most part, delivered children with spina bifida or anencephaly, two potentially crippling or fatal NTDs in which the spine or skull fails to form around the spinal cord or brain. On the average, 15 of every 10,000 women in the United States deliver NTD babies. But in this group, because of their history, the risk was 1 in 20.

Dr. Laurence and his assistants made a two-part study of these women. First, they took a survey and discovered that fully half of them had had a poor diet during the pregnancy that ended with an NTD birth. Then they counseled 103 women to improve their diets in time for their next pregnancies. An additional 71 women were given no special dietary counseling.

Of the women who did improve their diets, none delivered a second handicapped child. All eight of the NTD children (out of 186 newborns) were born to women who ate a poor diet during their first six months of pregnancy (*Nutrition and Health*).

In birth defects, diet made the difference.

When high-risk pregnant women take folate, they boost their chances of delivering healthy babies.

"It seems likely that the main cause, in the British Isles at least, is a lack of folate available to the developing embryo," says Dr. Laurence, adding that the results of earlier work by himself and others "suggest that folic acid given to high-risk women greatly reduces the [NTD] recurrence rate," when taken before conception and continued until the end of the first trimester. Although Dr. Laurence concludes that some of the women in this latest study obtained enough folate from their diet alone to prevent a second NTD birth, he previously used a supplement of four milligrams a day—much more than would be available or advisable in the usual daily diet—for women at high risk for an NTD baby.

A Broader Role for Folate

Cleft palate, another birth abnormality, may also yield to a high-folate diet. Cleft palate occurs when an unborn child's facial bones fail to form properly, creating a distorting split in the roof of the mouth. Though not as traumatic as NTD, cleft palate can be socially crippling.

Folate may deter the birth defect known as cleft palate.

On hearing about the results of the English NTD studies, doctors in Czechoslovakia asked over 80 women who had already had a child with cleft palate to take ten milligrams of folate a day, along with a multivitamin, for at least three months before conception and then until at least the end of their first trimester. In 85 pregnancies, only one child was born with a cleft palate. In 212 pregnancies among a similar group where there was no supplementation, 15 cleft palates occurred (*Lancet*).

There are even references in the medical literature linking low folate in a mother's diet to unwanted abortion and to low birth weight. As long ago as 1977, British researchers found that mothers with low folate levels at the time of delivery were more likely to deliver low-birth-weight children (*Archives of Disease in Childhood*).

As for spontaneous abortion, Carl C. Pfeiffer, M.D., Ph.D., director of the Brain Bio Center in Princeton, New Jersey, writes that "Many women with histories of abortion and miscarriage have been able to complete successful childbirth subsequent to folate supplementation (*International Journal of Environmental Studies*).

Folate fights spontaneous abortions.

Fragile-X Syndrome: Handle with Folate

Sometimes folate can help repair the effects of birth defects after they occur—perhaps even long after they occur. Folate supplements have been used to improve the mental function and quality of life among mentally retarded children who suffer from what is called fragile-X syndrome. This syndrome, which appears under the microscope as a breakage in certain chromosomes, affects about 1 in every 1,000 newborns. In some cases, folate—if given early enough and in the right amounts—can raise the IQs of these children. In borderline cases, it might enable them to return to the mainstream of life.

Much work in this area has been done at the Children's Hospital Child Development Unit in Denver. Tad Jackson, a clinical researcher there, and Randi Hagerman, M.D., gave ten milligrams of folate a day to a group of boys with fragile-X syndrome. In the most remarkable case, one boy's IQ rose from 63 to a near-normal 86, then fell to 83 after folate was withdrawn. When the supplement was reintroduced, his IQ stabilized at 93.

After taking folate, the IQ of a retarded boy went from 63 to 93.

"It's not a cure," says Jackson, "but in most cases folate seems to improve the interaction between these children and the world around them. They talk more; they make better eye contact.

"The most encouraging sign has been that the parents of seven out of the eight boys under age 12 could tell by their behavior when their sons were taking folate, or not. In the boys over 12, however, not much improvement was seen."

Requirements Rise with Pregnancy

How much folate does a pregnant woman need? The National Academy of Sciences sets the Recommended Dietary Allowance (RDA) of folate for expectant mothers at 800 micrograms (0.8 milligram) a day and at 400 micrograms for other adults. These figures are low compared to the 4 milligrams some studies have suggested for NTD mothers.

Guidelines for folate intake.

Folate taken in even normal amounts can mask the symptoms of megaloblastic anemia, which is an early sign of vitamin B_{12} deficiency. Testing their patients for vitamin B_{12} deficiency before prescribing greater-than-RDA doses of folate is one way that doctors avoid this problem.

A checklist of folate robbers.

Certain drugs can deprive us of folate and increase our need. Drugs for epilepsy, such as Dilantin, as well as barbiturates and methotrexate, an antipsoriasis drug, have this effect. Oral contraceptives, estrogen and alcohol are also known to reduce body folate levels.

Keep in mind, too, that the folate in foods can easily decrease during cooking or processing. Heating or merely storing foods at room temperature can cut their folate content in half. And beware of the folate vicious circle. A folate deficiency can actually make it more difficult for the walls of the intestines to absorb the folate it badly needs. Supplementation can interrupt this cycle.

The top food sources of folate.

You may already be getting the folate you need from your diet, however. If fresh vegetables, especially spinach, romaine lettuce and asparagus are a part of your diet, you are halfway there. Lentils and dried beans, two foods that are high in fiber, also contain large amounts of folate. So does brewer's yeast, whole wheat bread and orange juice. (See the table, Best Food Sources of B Vitamins, on pages 100–101, for more information on folate-rich foods.)

Looking Ahead

"At this point, we're not ready to recommend folate supplements to all women," says M. J. Adams, M.D., of the U.S. Centers for Disease Control in Atlanta. "We can't say for sure whether they are helpful or harmful. Some women may need more or less than others. But it's an exciting hypothesis, and I think women who are at risk for an NTD should become familiar with the uses of multivitamins that include folate before their next pregnancy."

A promising future for stopping birth defects.

Chapter 18

Vitamin C Research: New Hope for Health

S cientists have been delving into the biological secrets of vitamin C for years. Here's a summary of what they've discovered. Some of the data are surprising; some of it expected. All of it is preliminary (and requires more research)—but suggests tantalizing possibilities for health.

A Treatment for Gum Disease

Vitamin C: a new force against dental disease?

This problem affects gum tissue and jawbone, leading ultimately to the loss of teeth. Hopefully it won't go that far, though, not when vitamin C could help turn it around. That's what a team of researchers from the University of Alabama School of Dentistry found when they compared the gum health of a group taking 300 milligrams of vitamin C with a group taking a placebo (dummy pill) for 21 days. Each volunteer also received a thorough cleaning and polishing of the teeth (prophylaxis) on one side of the mouth at the beginning of the experiment.

As one might expect, the research showed there was no significant change in the gums not receiving prophylaxis or vitamin C. Improvement was greatest with prophylaxis plus C, which led to a 58 percent reduction in gum inflammation. Vitamin C alone and prophylaxis alone also improved gum health, but the researchers concluded that combining the two treatments worked best of all.

In another study, from Yugoslavia, researchers found that supplementation with 70 milligrams of vitamin C may be enough to initiate gum tissue regeneration in people whose C intake is low—between 20 and 40 milligrams per day (*International Journal for Vitamin and Nutrition Research*).

Can vitamin C help re-grow deteriorated gum tissue?

Boosting Immunity

Lymphocytes (white blood cells) have a high concentration of vitamin C and use up vitamin C rapidly when fighting infection. Vitamin C may possibly increase the metabolism of some kinds of lymphocytes, making them react faster, says Benjamin Siegel, Ph.D., of the University of Oregon's Department of Pathology. Vitamin C may also increase the number of what are known as receptor sites on a lymphocyte's membrane, making it easier for the lymphocyte to latch onto bacteria or a virus. "We're not exactly sure *how* vitamin C works, but these are some theories," Dr. Siegel says.

Vitamin C may help your body fight germs.

Doctors in Brussels found that even in the elderly, who often have a weak immune response, 500 milligrams daily of vitamin C stimulated their production of lymphocytes (*Gerontology*).

Dr. Siegel's own studies have shown that 250 milligrams of vitamin C daily in the drinking water of mice significantly increased the level of interferon in their blood and reduced their susceptibility to leukemia. Interferon is produced by a cell that has been invaded by a virus. It induces surrounding cells to produce proteins that protect them from the virus.

Wounds That Heal Faster

Vitamin C is an important ingredient in a wound-healing nutrient solution developed by Anthony N. Silvett, M.D., formerly of the Wound Healing Intensive Care Unit at West Lake Community Hospital in Mel-

Vitamin C: part of a solution to bedsores.

rose Park, Illinois. At the time, the unit specialized in treating severe bedsores.

"Bedsores are caused by the pressure of lying immobile for long periods of time," Dr. Silvetti explains. "The skin and tissues on which the body rests are deprived of nourishment because the tiny blood vessels that provide it are squeezed shut by the body's weight, and they eventually clot. The tissue in that area dies, and an ugly crater forms in the skin."

Dr. Silvetti provides the nutrients—a mixture of essential amino acids, vitamin C and complex sugars—directly in a solution or in powder form. "Vitamin C helps to stimulate skin cells called fibroblasts to produce new tissue in wounds," Dr. Silvetti says. "It also helps fight infection by providing a slightly acid environment that discourages bacterial growth."

A mixture containing vitamin C puts healing in high gear.

The doctor reports his results have been "excellent." Within 24 to 72 hours after treatment begins, infection diminishes. Within a few days, fresh tissue full of tiny blood vessels begins to grow over the wound. Small or medium-size bedsores (up to six inches wide) heal in about two months; large wounds take slightly longer and may require grafting.

Fighting Heat and Cold

In research by S. D. Livingstone of the Defence and Civil Institute of Environmental Medicine, Downsview, Ontario, vitamin C relieved the constriction of blood vessels in the skin that comes with exposure to cold.

Livingstone gave four people 2,000 milligrams of vitamin C each day for a month, then monitored the skin temperature of one finger that was immersed in ice water or exposed to cold air (−9°F) for 30 minutes. After six weeks with no supplementation, he repeated the tests.

Can vitamin C protect your skin from the cold?

He found that the skin temperatures tended to remain higher during supplementation. Skin temperatures were as much as 15 degrees higher during the air exposure test. Vitamin C could have caused an increased blood flow that warmed the surface of the skin (*Lancet*).

At the other end of the thermic scale, studies have shown that vitamin C helps people adjust faster to hot weather. In a study by researchers in South Africa, mining workers not previously exposed to heat were given either 250 or 500 milligrams of vitamin C or a placebo. Then they exercised in an "acclimatizing room" at a temperature of 90°F. Both groups of men receiving vitamin C adjusted to the heat a full day faster than those not supplemented.

Vitamin C may counter-act the stress of high temperatures.

The researchers say vitamin C may counter some of the stressful effects of working in high-temperature conditions by delaying fatigue in the adrenal glands (*Journal of Applied Physiology*).

All of which goes to show that while our indoor environment may respond to the flick of a switch, our internal thermostat needs proper nutrition.

Asthmatics May Benefit

Wheezing or bronchial constriction brought on by exercise is something most asthmatics have come to expect. Typically, sufferers will experience chest tightness and trouble breathing within 3 to 5 minutes after exercising, and it will get progressively worse over the next 30 minutes.

With vitamin C, however, there is now hope for improving that condition, according to two doctors from New Haven, Connecticut. In their experiment, Alan Schlesinger, M.D., and Neil Schacter, M.D., gave 12 asthmatics either a placebo or 500 milligrams of vitamin C six hours or less before exercise testing. Using measurements of airflow, the researchers found that the group treated with vitamin C had significantly less chest tightness than the placebo group.

Wheezing lessened with vitamin C.

Fertility Restored

When infertility is due to sticky sperm, vitamin C may be the answer. Normally, sperm should swim

Best Food Sources of Vitamin C

Food	Portion	Vitamin C (mg.)
Orange juice, freshly squeezed	1 cup	124
Grapefruit juice, freshly squeezed	1 cup	94
Papaya	½ medium	94
Guava	½	83
Kiwi fruit	1 medium	75
Orange	1	70
Brussels sprouts, raw	4	65
Green peppers, raw, chopped	½ cup	64
Cantaloupe	¼	56
Watermelon	⅟₁₆	47
Tomato juice	1 cup	45
Strawberries	½ cup	42
Broccoli, raw, chopped	½ cup	41
Grapefruit	½	39
Cauliflower, raw, chopped	½ cup	36
Potato, baked	1 medium	26
Tangerine	1	26
Tomato, raw	1	22
Lemon	1 wedge	21
Turnip greens, cooked, chopped	½ cup	20
Cabbage, raw, chopped	½ cup	17
Blackberries	½ cup	15
Raspberries	½ cup	15
Banana	1	11
Blueberries	½ cup	9
Spinach, raw, chopped	½ cup	8
Snap beans, green, boiled	½ cup	6
Cherries, sweet	½ cup	5
Mung bean sprouts	¼ cup	3

SOURCES: Adapted from

Composition of Foods: Fruits and Fruit Juices, Agriculture Handbook No. 8–9, by Consumer Nutrition Center (Washington, D.C.: Human Nutrition Information Service, U.S. Department of Agriculture, 1982).

Composition of Foods: Vegetables and Vegetable Products, Agriculture Handbook No. 8–11, by Nutrition Monitoring Division (Washington, D.C.: Human Nutrition Information Service, U.S. Department of Agriculture, 1984).

singly. When more than 20 percent stay clumped together (called sperm agglutination), it's virtually impossible for conception to occur.

To test the effectiveness of vitamin C, Earl B. Dawson, Ph.D., and his colleagues from the Department of Obstetrics and Gynecology at the University of Texas Medical Branch in Galveston selected 35 men who could not impregnate their wives because more than 20 percent of their sperm stuck together. Each was told to take one 500-milligram capsule of vitamin C every 12 hours for one month. By the end of the first week, fertility was restored, since clumped sperm had dropped to 14 percent. By the end of three weeks, clumping was down to only 11 percent.

After taking vitamin C for one month, the men's fertility was restored.

In another study, Dr. Dawson says that pregnancy occurred in the wives of each of 12 men whom his group placed on a 60-day vitamin C regimen, while the wives of 8 subjects not given vitamin C did not become pregnant (*Journal of the American Medical Association*).

Stopping Colds Short

There is no firm evidence yet that extra doses of vitamin C can cure or prevent the common cold. But C may be able to reduce the misery that a cold brings.

Vitamin C can't cure a cold but may ease its symptoms.

Researchers of the University of Sydney in Australia separated 95 pairs of identical twins into two groups. One twin from each pair took a placebo every day, and the other took 1,000 milligrams of vitamin C every day for a total of 100 days. The researchers found that the vitamin C group had a significantly shorter average duration of colds (*Medical Journal of Australia*).

To help plan a diet rich in vitamin C, see the table, Best Food Sources of Vitamin C, on page 130.

Chapter 19

Vitamin C: Other Helpful Discoveries

Although you may have considered vitamin C, or ascorbic acid, essential to everyday good health, a growing body of medical evidence suggests this versatile nutrient may play a more important role in the prevention of disease. Consider these reports from the medical news grapevine.

• Eighty women seeking Pap smears at the Bronx Municipal Hospital Center may have helped medical science narrow down one of the causes of cervical cancer.

• At a medical research institution in Philadelphia, a laboratory experiment turned up unexpected results that may someday lead to much-needed relief for rheumatoid arthritis sufferers.

• A leading cancer journal has reported evidence supporting the role of a key food element in relief of certain kinds of cancer.

• From 1964 to 1978, consumption of vegetables and fruits high in a particular nutrient increased. At the same time, cardiovascular deaths declined. And at least one medical researcher thinks that it was no coincidence.

A new ally in preventing disease.

The surprising common denominator, in all cases, is vitamin C. Much of this new information is still in the theoretical stage, but it is intriguing. Here's a wrap-up of recent developments. (See the table, Best Food Sources of Vitamin C, on page 130, for additional sources of vitamin C in the diet.)

Vitamin C May Keep Cervical Dysplasia in Check

A low dietary intake of vitamin C is related to cervical abnormalities. That's what Seymour Romney, M.D., found when he tallied up the results of tests comparing women with normal Pap smears and those with cervical cancer or dysplasia—abnormal cell growth that may or may not lead to cancer.

Of the 80 women at the Bronx Municipal Hospital Center who had Pap smears taken, 34 had normal results. Their dietary intake of vitamin C was relatively high. The remaining 46 women took in considerably less vitamin C in the diet, and their diagnoses ranged from mild cervical inflammation to cancer (*American Journal of Obstetrics and Gynecology*).

Women with normal Pap smears had higher intakes of vitamin C.

Just a coincidence—or a connection? While there's still a lot of work to be done, Dr. Romney believes there is a definite relationship between cervical cancer and low vitamin C in the diet.

"A lot of people have been intrigued by the prospect that vitamin C may have antitumor properties, and there are reasonable scientific studies that support that idea," explains Dr. Romney.

Vitamin C may fight tumors.

How and why vitamin C may prevent tumors from forming isn't well understood, however. In fact, says Dr. Romney, vitamin C is probably just one part of the picture.

"Cancer is a terribly complicated disease," he says. "With regard to the role of any nutrients, their actions surely involve interactions with other chemicals in the body, which need to be looked into. It's not likely that a single nutrient, per se, is the cause and effect of a disease as complex as cancer."

The preliminary research suggests that women may not be getting enough vitamin C to prevent cervical cancer. Why? Because, says Dr. Romney, "If there's a disorder in the cervix, that increases the demand for ascorbic acid."

Can vitamin C prevent cervical cancer?

Whether you need more than the Recommended Dietary Allowance (RDA) of 60 milligrams of vitamin

C daily just isn't clear. However, Dr. Romney and his research staff would like to find out. "We're going to try to get some solid information on dosage and the effects of that dosage, whether there are side effects and how well it works."

Vitamin C versus Nitrosamines

Of course, cervical cancer is just one of many cancers, and research continues to determine how vitamin C affects other types of cancer, too.

You might have heard about the link between vitamin C and nitrosamines, cancer-causing substances formed by the interaction of nitrite—a common food additive—and chemicals in your body.

Vitamin C has long been believed to prevent nitrosamines from forming. A study reported in the journal *Carcinogenesis* lends strong support to that theory.

Vitamin C may break up cancer-causing agents in the stomach.

Researchers in Britain asked eight volunteers to take a gram (1,000 milligrams) of vitamin C every day for a week. Before and after the experiment, researchers siphoned off gastric juice from the volunteers' stomachs. In all but one of the volunteers, the levels of nitrosamines in the gastric juice were significantly lower at the end of the test.

Does this mean vitamin C prevents gastric cancer? No, but it may reduce the risk. Are the results definitive—that is, is this the last word? No. Further studies, and on a wider scale, should be done before coming to any definite conclusions. But the results of this study do give reason for optimism.

Relief for Arthritis— without Side Effects

Picture the body at war with itself. That's what happens in rheumatoid arthritis. The body's own cells mistake body tissues for foreign substances. To repel the "invaders," the cells manufacture antibodies to attack the tissue.

There is no cure for rheumatoid arthritis. Treatment often involves using steroids to reduce the pain and tissue swelling brought about by this disfiguring disease. But these anti-inflammatory drugs in themselves can cause side effects.

That's why Robert H. Davis, Ph.D., a professor in the Department of Physiology at the Pennsylvania College of Podiatric Medicine, has been exploring the use of vitamin C and aloe, two natural substances that cause few if any known side effects.

Vitamin C and aloe were teamed up to fight rheumatoid arthritis.

"It's an idea that goes back, for me, almost 30 years," says Dr. Davis. "Steroids and synthetic drugs have their place in the treatment of arthritis, but the side effects can sometimes be worse than the cure."

Why vitamin C? Simply this, says Dr. Davis: Vitamin C is an essential building block in the manufacture of the connective tissue called collagen. In rheumatoid arthritis, this connective tissue breaks down. But Dr. Davis believes that vitamin C, applied to the skin, may prevent or slow this tissue breakdown, reducing inflammation. And aloe also is believed to have healing properties.

One scientist says vitamin C may reduce the inflammation of rheumatoid arthritis.

In a prize-winning study that put his theory to the test, Dr. Davis and two students combined vitamin C, aloe and ribonucleic acid—a cellular building block also thought to reduce inflammation—in a cream ointment. Then they applied the cream to the arthritic hind paws of laboratory rats. The results were surprising. Joint-tissue swelling was reduced dramatically, both in the early stages of arthritis and later on, after the disease had progressed for several days (*Journal of the American Podiatric Medical Association*). "I honestly didn't think it would work," says Dr. Davis. "But I was able to repeat the results."

Of course, it is too soon to say what impact these studies will have on humans. Furthermore, it's important to understand that this report doesn't suggest that vitamin C is a cure for rheumatoid arthritis. But it offers some hope for an effective treatment that doesn't rely on steroids.

"I wouldn't recommend this kind of treatment to anyone until we get some real statistical data," says Dr. Davis. "I would like to say yes because rheumatoid arthritis is one of the tough ones. But I think it first has to go into a clinical trial and be evaluated. If some-

A Little Vitamin C May Go a Long Way

Elderly people with low vitamin C levels in their blood are usually given heavy doses of the vitamin to bring their plasma levels up to normal. Now a group of researchers in England says that may be overkill. A little vitamin C may go a long way.

Researchers at the University of Leeds and High Royds Hospital found that low blood levels usually meant low intake of foods rich in vitamin C—in part because of food preparation procedures in institutions and dental problems that made eating fruit impossible for the older people.

But by simply adding fresh orange juice or a vitamin C tablet to the diet—no more than the Recommended Dietary Allowance of 60 milligrams a day—the scientists found that they could bring those elderly with marginal deficiencies up to normal. Those who had deficiencies in the scurvy range, the researchers said, obviously need a larger dose. However, they added, the evidence indicates that there are far more elderly at risk of marginal deficiencies, which have their own potential health consequences, such as the delayed healing of injuries.

body has a real bad case of arthritis, they should be treated by a doctor."

Vitamin C Up, Heart Disease Down

Most animals make their own vitamin C. In fact, there are only a few species—humans, guinea pigs, monkeys and certain fruit bats—that have to get their vitamin C from what they eat.

Members of the one civilized, self-aware species in that group appear to suffer a chronic dietary shortage of vitamin C, says Anthony Verlangieri, Ph.D., of the University of Mississippi. And because of that deficiency, he says, "they may be more susceptible to heart disease."

Dr. Verlangieri theorizes that vitamin C deficiency causes atherosclerosis. True, cholesterol does clog arteries. But in Dr. Verlangieri's view, cholesterol is really a Johnny-come-lately, a cardiovascular bad guy who takes advantage of an already bad situation caused by a vitamin C deficiency.

One startling theory: Low vitamin C may cause heart disease.

One study by Dr. Verlangieri and colleagues at the University of Mississippi lends support to his controversial theory of vitamin C's role. Dr. Verlangieri and his staff reviewed health statistics from the period between 1964 and 1978. During that time, he noticed, Americans increased their intake of fruits and vegetables rich in vitamin C. Deaths from cardiovascular disease during that period declined.

When Americans ate more foods containing vitamin C, heart disease deaths decreased.

Other experts also have noted the decline in cardiovascular deaths and have attributed the slide to a number of factors, including a reduction in smoking, better eating habits and an increase in physical activity. But in his study, Dr. Verlangieri credited the increased intake of foods rich in vitamin C for the decline in heart deaths (*Medical Hypotheses*).

According to Dr. Verlangieri's research, vitamin C turns off an enzyme that attacks what are called endothelial cells in blood vessel walls. If you are vitamin C deficient—that is, if your cells aren't saturated with vitamin C—the enzyme is free to do its dirty work.

"The cells of blood vessels can be compared to bricks in a wall," explains Dr. Verlangieri. "Mortar holds the bricks in the wall together, but in blood vessels, a cement called the extracellular matrix holds the cells together. If the cement becomes defective, the cells loosen up. That leaves some bare spots. Normally, the cells provide a barrier to keep cholesterol off the blood vessel walls. But when the cholesterol gets into those bare spots, it causes inflammation. Vitamin C actually works at the level of the cell to inhibit an enzyme that chews up that cement."

Vitamin C may help keep cholesterol off the walls of your arteries.

If the body is low in vitamin C, the blood vessel walls become denuded in spots, says Dr. Verlangieri, leaving convenient places for cholesterol to take root. So cholesterol is an important part of the process once the disease begins, but it isn't how the disease begins.

Is the Recommended Dietary Allowance for vitamin C too low?

If the theory is true, how much vitamin C would people need to prevent cardiovascular disease? According to Dr. Verlangieri, the Recommended Dietary Allowance (RDA) of 60 milligrams isn't enough. "I think the evidence suggests that from 1,000 to 2,000 milligrams is probably what we need," he says.

Not a Do-It-Yourself Treatment

Before you consider increasing your intake of C, bear in mind that in many quarters this theory is still controversial. Many scientists do not think vitamin C is involved in coronary artery disease. Others do believe vitamin C appears to reduce coronary risks, but for altogether different reasons.

One study, for instance, suggests vitamin C in 1,000-milligram doses prevents blood platelets from clumping together and adhering to blood vessel walls. To find out whether this is true, researchers at

Tagore Medical College and Hospital in India gave volunteers 1,000 milligrams of vitamin C every eight hours for ten days. At the end of that period, they drew blood samples and found a significant drop in the rate at which blood platelets clumped together and adhered.

Vitamin C stopped the clumping that can lead to artery-clogging blood clots.

But at the same time, researchers noted that they were administering vitamin C in "pharmacologic doses"—doses so high they should be taken only under a doctor's supervision. They concluded that further studies needed to be done to confirm their findings (*Clinical Cardiology*). But whatever the connection, research at least suggests there might be one.

Chapter 20

Vitamin D:
How to Avoid a
"Hidden Epidemic"

A startling case of vitamin D deficiency.

He was certain he was about to die. At 82, the infirmities of old age had been limited to a mild case of diabetes and a hip fracture, from which he had recently recovered. Now he found himself back in the hospital, his bones weak and aching from what he was sure was an insidious cancer eating him alive.

Fortunately, his doctor's diagnosis wasn't made in such terrified haste. In fact, this physician even refused to jump to an easy conclusion when the X-rays showed the classic symptoms of osteoporosis: a wasting of bone mass and many collapsed vertebrae. His decision to prescribe vitamin D and calcium was based in part on something his frightened elderly patient told him in conversation: that he avoided sunlight and didn't drink milk or take vitamins.

Uriel A. Barzel, M.D., of New York City's Montefiore Medical Group and Albert Einstein School of Medicine, suspected that what he was seeing, X-rays and patient's fears aside, was osteomalacia, an adult version of a now rare childhood vitamin D deficiency disease called rickets. Both conditions are characterized by painful, thinning bones that, left untreated, can lead to deformities.

Until recent years, vitamin D deficiency was thought to be almost as rare as the bubonic plague, eradicated by D-fortified foods such as milk. But in the past few years, researchers and clinicians alike have become concerned that it may be a serious

Four New Healing Possibilities for Vitamin D

Vitamin D is converted by the liver and kidneys into its active form, a hormone called calcitriol that regulates the calcium balance in the body. Research in Japan has found that the hormone suppresses leukemia cells by causing them to be turned into noncancerous cells.

"Where this will go therapeutically isn't clear at this stage," says Hector DeLuca, Ph.D., professor of biochemistry at the University of Wisconsin, Madison. "In the long run, someday we may be able to control some types of leukemia. This may also have applications for controlling other types of malignancies."

Dr. DeLuca's own research also suggests that a vitamin D deficiency may lead to problems with glucose metabolism and, ultimately, insulin secretion. "Part of the falloff in glucose tolerance that occurs in many older people could be due to a lack of vitamin D, so if we can prevent the deficiency of calcitriol, perhaps we can control some cases of diabetes."

There's also a chance that a form of hearing loss associated with the cochlea, a tube shaped like a snail shell that forms a crucial part of the inner ear, can be prevented. Apparently, the cochlea needs vitamin D and calcium just as much as the skeleton and teeth do. When a deficiency occurs, minerals and hearing slowly fade. So far, hearing has been restored in some cases with daily supplements of calcium and vitamin D. (Refer your physician to the *Journal of Laryngology and Otology*, May 1983, pages 405–420.)

Preventing the hearing condition or catching it in the early phase is essential, since the deafness may be reversible. Just as important is the fact that early detection could point to the onset of osteomalacia, a bone-degenerating condition, before more serious skeletal problems occur.

As if the case for getting out in the sunshine weren't strong enough, a study spanning almost two decades found that men who developed colorectal cancer had lower intakes of vitamin D and calcium. A research team of scientists from across the country discovered that those men who developed cancer also weighed more and got less exercise than those who remained free of the disease, which, according to the researchers, "supports the suggestion that physical activity is inversely associated with the risk of colon cancer" (*Lancet*).

A lack of vitamin D may be rampant among elderly people.

hidden problem among the nation's elderly. One researcher calls it "an unrecognized epidemic," and it may be implicated as a factor in that scourge of old age, hip fracture. What's more, it's often difficult to diagnose, frequently masquerading as that other bone-thinning condition, osteoporosis.

Dr. Barzel took an educated guess with his patient and was proved correct in the best possible way—the man got well in three weeks of treatment with supplements. But, Dr. Barzel acknowledges, osteomalacia is a diagnosis that's easy to miss.

A Disease in Disguise

Doctors may overlook even obvious signs of a deficiency.

"Because vitamin D deficiency is uncommon in the general population, the family physician or internist may fail to consider vitamin D and may miss this diagnosis in the elderly," the physician says. "The symptoms and signs of early vitamin D deficiency may be difficult to recognize. The patient may have weakness, which may be attributed to coexisting disease. Although bone pain is quite specific, it may be mistaken for metastatic disease [cancer] or osteoporosis not only by the patient but also by the physician."

Though a bone biopsy may tell the most accurate story, Dr. Barzel has advised other physicians to first ask the right questions to pinpoint whether a patient is getting an adequate amount of D. If not, a short therapeutic trial with moderate amounts of vitamin D and calcium can be diagnosis and cure in one. "The response of the patient is both quick and dramatic and confirms the diagnosis," Dr. Barzel says.

One out of every two older people may get too little vitamin D.

Better diagnostic techniques are imperative because a number of studies give every indication that vitamin D deficiency is not rare. In fact, there may be cause for alarm. Studies of health-conscious and apparently healthy elderly participants showed that at least half got less than the minimum daily requirement of vitamin D—200 international units. A third were getting less than 100 international units. In a study of

142 elderly hip fracture patients at Massachusetts General Hospital in Boston, 40 percent were D deficient and three-quarters of them had osteomalacia. "As many as 30 to 40 percent of all hip fracture patients in the United States have osteomalacia," says researcher Samuel H. Doppelt, M.D., assistant professor of orthopaedic surgery and medicine at Harvard Medical School.

How Vitamin D Works

To understand these figures, it's first necessary to understand how vitamin D works. In the body, the raw vitamin is changed into its active form, a hormone known as calcitriol, by the kidneys and the liver. This active form enhances the absorption of calcium to nourish the nerves, muscles and skeleton. Without D, the body begins to strip-mine the bones for calcium to meet the needs of the nerves and muscles, leaving the bones thin, brittle and breakable.

In its advanced stages, osteomalacia can be extremely painful and may be accompanied by tetany, muscle spasms that are caused by a calcium imbalance. But even before pain starts, a D deficiency can do enough damage to cripple. It is a hidden epidemic in many ways. "A D deficiency of less severity can cause an accumulated bone loss with age and can be painless until a bone break occurs," says A. Michael Parfitt, M.D., director of the Bone and Mineral Research Laboratory at Henry Ford Hospital in Detroit. "And I'm afraid this is rather common among elderly people."

A severe lack of D can be crippling.

The reason? Although it is difficult for most of us to avoid getting enough vitamin D, it's even more difficult for elderly people to get enough. It's abundant only in foods that are hardly a staple of the American menu: fatty fish such as mackerel and swordfish. (See the table, Best Food Sources of Vitamin D, on page 147.) In the United States, vitamin D is added to milk, which many elderly people use simply

Older people often skimp on vitamin D-rich foods like milk.

to color tea or coffee. But it's most abundantly supplied when the sun's ultraviolet rays strike the skin, activating a vitamin D precursor. About 90 percent of the major circulating form of D comes from our skin supply. In fact, basking in the sun for about 30 minutes a day is enough to eliminate the need for any dietary D at all in healthy adults.

But, like Dr. Barzel's patient, many elderly people don't get enough sun. They may be housebound by

---

Older Skin Needs Its Day in the Sun

Researchers aren't sure why, but the skin of young people appears to be a more efficient vitamin D factory than the skin of older adults. As skin ages and becomes thinner, it becomes less productive at turning out vitamin D from sunlight, according to one study.

To prove the point, scientists took skin samples from a number of surgical patients. The patients ranged in age from 8 to 92. Each sample was bathed in ultraviolet light—similar to the ultraviolet light in sunlight. When they checked the samples, they found that young skin produced the most vitamin D. In the older, thinner skin samples, vitamin D production decreased in proportion to the age of the individual. The skin of one 82-year-old produced less than half the amount of vitamin D churned out by the 8-year-old skin (*Journal of Clinical Investigation*).

How much sunlight does older skin need to make enough vitamin D?

"That is almost impossible to say precisely," says Michael F. Holick, M.D., Ph.D., director of the Vitamin D and Bone Metabolism Laboratory at Tufts University in Massachusetts. Dr. Holick was one of the researchers in this study. "It depends on so many things—skin pigmentation, time of year, location and so on. But we can say this: If, say, you're in Boston in June at noontime, you should expose your hands, face and arms, 15 minutes at a time, two or three times a week. In the winter, you'd probably have to expose a much larger area of the skin for a much longer period of time because the sun's rays are much weaker [and even that may be insufficient]. In this case, vitamin D supplements are a desirable alternative," he says.

illness or disability, or simply less physically active and less likely to spend time outdoors. But, for whatever reason, they simply don't tap into the most available supply of D there is.

Sunshine is a primary source of vitamin D.

A Place in the Sun

Theoretically, doctors could solve the problem by prescribing cruises to warm, sunny islands or, at the very least, daily strolls in the afternoon sun. A group of British doctors stopped just short of recommending that when they assessed the vitamin D status of 110 men and women nearing retirement age. They extolled the virtues of "a sunny holiday" when they saw what it did to the vitamin D levels of their subjects. Almost all of those who had the highest concentrations of circulating D had been on vacation in sunnier climates, some as long as four months previously. One woman, whose diet was relatively poor in D, nevertheless had the highest concentration of D in her bloodstream. The reason? She had just gotten a two-week dose of sunshine on Malta (*Human Nutrition: Clinical Nutrition*).

But for many, a vacation in the sun simply isn't possible. And the sun isn't always an entirely reliable source of the sunshine vitamin either. During the winter months, the sun slants its rays through the ozone layer of the atmosphere, which filters out much of the ultraviolet light the skin needs to manufacture D. Studies show that blood levels of the vitamin tend to drop in the winter, especially among elderly women. Urban dwellers may see the sun even less than the housebound, especially if they live and work in the shadows of tall buildings. Pollution may also be a factor. A progressive increase in atmospheric ozone and pollutants between 1951 and 1972 produced a 20 percent decrease in the amount of ultraviolet radiation reaching the earth. Some researchers believe the decrease in ultraviolet light parallels a progressive increase in hip fracture mortality.

Pollution can block the production of vitamin D.

Vegetarians Need Vitamin D, Too

The elderly aren't the only people who need vitamin D. Everyone needs vitamin D for strong bones, but not everyone gets enough. Among the most vulnerable are vegetarians, whose diets don't always provide sufficient vitamin D. Additionally, the high percentage of roughage in a vegetarian's diet may interfere with the absorption of this important vitamin.

Consider, for example, the severe deficiencies reported by researchers in Norway among vegetarian children. Several children in that country were hospitalized for rickets, or osteomalacia, a disease characterized by progressive bone softening.

These children also may have been predisposed to rickets because of the vitamin D-deficient diets of their vegetarian mothers, according to researchers.

After they were diagnosed, the children were given vitamin D supplements, and the painful symptoms of rickets disappeared altogether (*Acta Paediatrica Scandinavica*).

Older people's metabolism may have trouble putting vitamin D to work.

There is another confounding factor. Elderly people also may have faulty vitamin D metabolism—an inability to convert vitamin D into its active form in adequate amounts. Hector DeLuca, Ph.D., professor of biochemistry at the University of Wisconsin, Madison, with his colleagues, was the first to demonstrate that D has to be changed into an active hormonal form before it can function. Since isolating the hormone, Dr. DeLuca and others have been experimenting with ways to use it pharmacologically to treat postmenopausal and old-age osteoporosis.

Faulty Metabolism Can Cause Trouble

"In both old age and the postmenopausal state, the vitamin D hormone doesn't respond as it should," says Dr. DeLuca. "Calcium absorption is low; bone turnover—the tearing down of old bone and the re-

building of new bone—is low. If you have low calcium absorption, the body continues to draw on bone
calcium to meet nerve and muscle needs. This contributes to the thinning of bones. When they become
thin enough, they fracture."

Several clinical tests have been "promising," says
Dr. DeLuca. Postmenopausal women given small
doses of the vitamin D hormone had increased calcium retention in the bones, increased bone mass and
a decrease in bone-fracture rates. The hormone
works, apparently, because it circumvents the metabolism problem. Giving D alone is ineffective, says Dr.
DeLuca.

But if your metabolism is working up to par and
you're in the high-risk category, a supplement may be
needed. "Without D, you can't make the hormonal
form," says the researcher. "I personally think the
best way to get D is by sunlight. But, unlike some

**A special form of vita-
min D helped prevent
broken bones.**

Best Food Sources of Vitamin D

Food	Portion	Vitamin D (I.U.)
Halibut-liver oil	2 tsp.	9,636
Herring, grilled	3 oz.	850
Mackerel, fried	3 oz.	717
Cod-liver oil	2 tsp.	675
Mackerel, raw	3 oz.	595
Salmon, Pacific, steamed	3 oz.	425
Sardines, canned in oil, drained	3 oz.	255
Tuna, canned in oil, drained	3 oz.	197
Milk, 1% fat	1 cup	102

SOURCES: Adapted from

McCance and Widdowson's The Composition of Foods, by A. A. Paul and
D. A. T. Southgate (New York: Elsevier/North-Holland Biomedical, 1978).

Bowes and Church's Food Values of Portions Commonly Used, by Jean A. T.
Pennington and Helen Nichols Church (New York: Harper & Row, 1980).

Handbook of Lipid Research: The Fat-Soluble Vitamins, by Hector F. DeLuca
(New York: Plenum Press, 1978).

other nutrition people, I recommend a multivitamin so you can get all the basic nutrients you need, including D."

One doctor's Rx: 400 international units of vitamin D daily.

If you are taking a D supplement, make sure it's no more than 400 international units a day. Vitamin D in larger amounts can be toxic. "Taking 400 international units once a day will keep you well below the level that can cause any harm," says Dr. Parfitt.

Vitamin E:
Protector of Cells

Vitamin E has been promoted as nothing short of a magical potion that restores everything from sexual potency to youth. Its widespread use led one wag at the *Harvard Medical School Health Letter* to suggest that vitamin E be classified as a "recreational drug."

All of this unfortunate ballyhoo has nearly obscured the facts about vitamin E, which in this case are proving to be far more remarkable than fiction. Vitamin E is being tested not only as a potential wound healer but as an anticancer agent and as a biochemical, not magical, antidote to aging. And there is some evidence that it may do all of these things because of its ability to protect healthy cells from damage.

In wound healing, scientists believe that vitamin E protects the lymphocytes, cells that produce antibodies against disease-causing organisms.

An aid to wound healing.

In cancer, some scientists believe E may diligently defend cell membranes against the assault of cancer-causing substances, notably the free radicals, highly unstable molecules that can scramble the genetic information the cells contain.

Those damaged cells can become, literally, an accident looking for a place to happen, starting a chain reaction that can lead to cancer.

Free radicals may play a role in aging, too. One theory—highly controversial—says that aging is not simply the inevitable ticking away of a programmed

E may be a cellular shield against cancer-causing substances.

(continued on page 152)

Using Vitamin E Externally

Vitamin E has a long history of being used topically by the public to soothe and heal everything from burns to warts. Researchers, though, are just beginning to examine vitamin E's topical use. There are some indications it can penetrate easily to the growing layers of the skin, work to reduce inflammation and heat in sunburned skin and protect tissues from the damage of cancer drugs.

The "Cell-Saver" Vitamin

Most of these benefits come from vitamin E's role as an antioxidant. It can neutralize harmful particles called free radicals formed by inflammation, ultraviolet light or chemotherapy, saving the cells from damage.

"Much more research must be done, but right now it appears that vitamin E has much more of a biological effect than any of us ever dreamed of," says Peter T. Pugliese, M.D., vice-president of research and development at the Xienta Institute for Skin Research in Bernville, Pennsylvania. There's good evidence, for instance, that vitamin E works as an anti-inflammatory when applied to the skin, he says.

Dr. Pugliese used vitamin E to reduce the amount of inflammation produced in the skin of mice by a mild "sunburn." Mice were irradiated with just enough ultraviolet light to produce a mild inflammatory response. Thirty minutes before the exposure, they had vitamin E rubbed into their skin. (The vitamin needs this time to penetrate to the growing layers of the skin, Dr. Pugliese says.)

The mice treated with a 5 percent solution of vitamin E were later found to have about a third less of a chemical secreted by the cells to initiate the inflammatory response. The mice treated with a 100 percent solution of vitamin E had a 93 percent reduction in this chemical.

"Vitamin E on the surface of the skin acts as a filter for ultraviolet light," Dr. Pugliese says. "But more important, it has a biochemical ability to short-circuit ultraviolet light's damaging effects by acting as an antioxidant."

According to Dr. Pugliese, vitamin E also affects the tiny blood vessels in the lower layers of the skin. These capillaries tend to leak excessively when they are stressed.

Researchers at Sapporo Medical College in Japan found that vitamin E applied to the skin constricts the capillaries and reduces their permeability, so less fluid leaks into surrounding tissues and less swelling occurs. This action also cuts down on surface skin temperatures by up to two degrees, creating a slight cooling effect, Dr. Pugliese says.

Reducing Side Effects of Chemotherapy

Researchers have noted that vitamin E used orally seems to help people better withstand cancer drug therapy. They think vitamin E acts to protect the body's healthy cells from these powerful free-radical-producing drugs.

Could vitamin E work to clean up a "spill" of chemotherapy drugs into the skin? Spills sometimes happen when these drugs are administered intravenously, and they can cause skin ulcers, says Ronald Barr, M.D., professor of pediatrics, McMaster University, Hamilton, Ontario.

Dr. Barr injected either low or high doses of the chemotherapy drug Adriamycin just below the skin layers of guinea pigs, then coated the site with either an organic solvent alone or in combination with a 10 or 50 percent solution of vitamin E. He continued coating the skin every three days.

The difference was dramatic between those guinea pigs receiving either concentration of vitamin E and those receiving none. Every one of the guinea pigs that received no vitamin E had complete ulceration of the skin by the ninth day after the injection of high doses of Adriamycin. And most were still completely ulcerated when the experiment ended 21 days later.

Skin ulceration was present in all animals receiving high doses of Adriamycin, but in the groups also receiving vitamin E, some of the animals showed evidence of healing. In animals receiving low doses of the chemotherapy drug (doses equivalent to accidental leakage during treatment), vitamin E not only diminished the amount of skin damage but also promoted more rapid healing.

"Vitamin E may help to reduce soft tissue damage by scavenging the free radicals produced by chemotherapy," Dr. Barr says. "We recommend that a solution of 50 percent vitamin E in an organic solvent be readily available at all times in locations in which patients are receiving intravenous chemotherapy drugs, so that it may be applied promptly to any site of a suspected spill into the tissue, with the view of preventing or at least diminishing the consequent tissue damage" (*British Journal of Cancer*).

biological clock but the result of a lifetime of avoidable damage caused by these molecules running amok.

Consider the Rotifer

"What E probably does is maintain the integrity of individual cell membranes," says James R. Litton, Jr., Ph.D., former assistant professor of biology at St. Mary's College, University of Notre Dame, South Bend, Indiana. "If we relate aging to the degradation of cell membranes, then, the theory is, if we maintain their integrity, we live longer."

Is vitamin E an anti-aging factor?

That theory is based on research such as studies conducted by Dr. Litton on very small animals called rotifers. The rotifer is a tiny aquatic creature that has a head that seems to spin like an outboard motor and also has a peculiar appetite for vitamin E. When the vitamin is added to a watery colony of rotifers, more of them live to a ripe old age. "We never increase their average life span," Dr. Litton stresses. "But we allow more of them to live a full life, which in the case of rotifers is 20-some days. They also have more offspring. Of course, if you live longer, chances are you produce more."

The rotifer is a minute, often microscopic, invertebrate that has just a little more in common with man than bacteria have. Is it possible that its reaction to vitamin E could have any human implications? "I'd be very hesitant to say that," says Dr. Litton. "But I would like to hope so."

The Anticancer Connection

Vitamin E may have the power to fight pain.

One area of research in which the human implications have extended beyond mere hope is in vitamin E's effect on cancer. A synthetic version of the vitamin is being used with cancer patients who have failed to respond to other therapies. Researchers report "some antitumor and analgesic effects." Though hardly a major breakthrough, they admit, "even a partial response by the infusion of vitamin E alone can be considered encouraging" (*Proceedings of the Society for Experimental Biology and Medicine*).

Animal studies suggest that the effects of E on one particular kind of cancer—breast cancer—are particularly encouraging, although the studies are limited to animals. In fact, even when E has no effect on other cancers, as in a British study on rats, it still lowers the incidence of breast tumors (*International Journal for Vitamin and Nutrition Research*).

The connection may be dietary fat. Some epidemiological studies show a correlation between breast cancer and high-fat intake. One of the end results of fat breakdown is the cell-damaging free radicals so strongly implicated in cancer. And, as we've noted, many scientists believe that vitamin E can protect the cells from free-radical assault.

Why does E have an effect on breast cancer? Theoretically, it could be E's stimulatory effect on the immune system—protecting the disease-fighting cells so they can do their work.

The Team Approach

That possibility was considered by Clement Ip, Ph.D., associate research scientist in the Department of Breast Surgery and the Breast Cancer Research Unit of Roswell Park Memorial Institute in Buffalo, New York. Dr. Ip used vitamin E as part of a one-two punch, along with the trace mineral selenium, on breast tumors in rats.

Vitamin E and selenium are both antioxidants, substances that protect cells from the damage caused during fat breakdown. Both have been shown in laboratory experiments to halt tumor growth.

In Dr. Ip's studies involving rats fed a high-fat diet, the vitamin E alone had no effect on chemically induced breast tumors. But when he paired vitamin E with selenium, there was a lower incidence of cancer.

In the laboratory, E and selenium paired up to fight cancer.

Why? Dr. Ip has two theories. One is that the vitamin E, a more powerful antioxidant than selenium, protected the cells from damage caused during the breakdown of fats and created a more favorable climate for selenium to inhibit tumor growth "via some other mechanism" as yet unknown.

Can Vitamin E
Help Prevent Heart Attacks and Strokes?

Vitamin E helps to prevent platelet aggregation—the "clumping" that occurs when red blood cells stick together like stacked poker chips, according to research by R. V. Panganamala, Ph.D., of the Department of Physiological Chemistry at Ohio State University School of Medicine. While such clumping is essential in the event of a cut, if it occurs in an intact blood vessel, it can trigger a heart attack or stroke.

Dr. Panganamala found that vitamin E maintains a healthy balance between two chemicals involved in platelet clumping. "Vitamin E works by blocking the production of a fatty acid that is used in the formation of a compound called thromboxane," he explains. "Thromboxane makes the cells stick together."

Vitamin E also stimulates the production of prostacyclin, a chemical secreted by the blood vessel wall, which helps keep the platelets "slippery."

To test vitamin E's effects on these two chemicals, Dr. Panganamala used two groups of rabbits. One group got a diet high in vitamin E; the other, no vitamin E at all. After 10 to 12 weeks, those animals deficient in vitamin E had significantly higher amounts of thromboxane, and their blood vessels had lost the capacity to produce prostacyclin. Giving vitamin E returned these animals to normal.

"There must be a proper ratio of thromboxane to prostacyclin for blood to flow without clumping," Dr. Panganamala says. "When the ratio gets out of balance, clumping is much more likely to occur. Vitamin E keeps these two substances in optimum balance."

Other work he's done with animals and humans makes Dr. Panganamala hopeful that vitamin E will alleviate some of the circulatory problems facing people with this illness.

Dr. Ip's second theory is that vitamin E and selenium stimulated the immune system, allowing the
body's own disease-battling cells to rid it of the cancer. In at least one experimental model, a deficiency
of antioxidants stimulates tumor growth. More important, when vitamin E and selenium are added to the
diet in quantities in excess of the recommended daily
requirement, the immune system seems to be stimulated. (Caution: Very high amounts of selenium are
toxic. The suggested range is 50 to 200 milligrams a
day.)

These nutrients may help your immune system fight cancer.

Vitamin E's stimulatory effect on the immune
system may have been responsible for the remarkable
recovery rate of laboratory rats from both gum
wounds and oral cancer in tests by researcher Gerald
Shklar, D.D.S., of the department of oral medicine
and oral pathology of the Harvard School of Dental
Medicine in Boston.

In the gum-wound study, the rats given daily
doses of vitamin E began to heal within two days of
their injury. The results of the cancer study were even
more astounding. "There," says Dr. Shklar, "vitamin E
very significantly delayed oral cancer formation and
in some cases even prevented it."

Vitamin E was used against gum wounds and oral cancer.

Alcohol Antidote?

Existing evidence hints that vitamin E may be
able to protect the heart from alcohol damage. Studies show too much alcohol can damage your heart,
leading to circulatory problems or cardiac failure.
Helmut Redetzki, Ph.D., a professor of pharmacology
at Louisiana State University School of Medicine, and
his co-workers found that in rats even a single intoxi-
cating dose of alcohol hurts heart muscle cells. "Alcohol generates free radicals that cause heart cells to
malfunction or die," he says.

But giving rats vitamin E first significantly reduced signs of cellular damage. Although the rats
received much larger doses than would be currently

Buffering the effects of alcohol on the heart.

considered appropriate in humans, normal amounts of vitamin E provide some protection from alcohol's effects, too, Dr. Redetzki says.

"We know that E-deficient animals suffer more heart damage from drinking than animals fed adequate E. Alcoholics often have lower blood levels of vitamin E, so they may be particularly prone to this kind of heart damage. And we know that in animals receiving adequate E in their diets, additional E boosted their protection from alcohol."

Heavy drinkers may benefit from E.

In humans, Dr. Redetzki theorizes, it may be that the more you drink, the more vitamin E you need. (See the table, Best Food Sources of Vitamin E, on page 158, for a list of vitamin E-rich foods.)

E-zier Breathing?

Air pollutants and cigarette smoke both generate plenty of free radicals that line up for a direct assault on the cells lining the lungs. A microscopic view of the lung cells of rats after 24 hours of exposure to a laboratory-concocted concentration of smog—the equivalent of a day in downtown Los Angeles—creates as much damage to the lungs as you'd see in a chronic cigarette smoker, says James Mead, Ph.D., professor emeritus of biological chemistry and nutrition at the University of California's Laboratory of Biomedical and Environmental Sciences. "It's horrifying to see the damage that takes place with smog or cigarette smoke," he says. "And even oxygen is somewhat toxic because it is the basis of free-radical formation."

Dr. Mead found that rats given vitamin E before exposure to pollutants had much less cell damage. The problem, though, was that massive doses were required to get the vitamin to the lungs in amounts large enough to provide optimum protection.

The solution, discovered by one of Dr. Mead's colleagues, was to put the vitamin into an aerosol spray that could be delivered directly to the lungs. He

uses a water-based spray with a water-soluble vitamin
E derivative. Rats that inhale this solution for half an
hour and are then exposed to a typical day's smog
show almost no lung damage, Dr. Mead says. "Vitamin E spray appears to work very well against air
pollutants. We know the protection we give the rats
lasts at least four days, and it may last considerably
longer." He hopes next to try aerosol E on people in
smog-heavy areas, smokers and those with lung diseases. "I'm already convinced of its safety and benefits, and I'd be happy to be the first volunteer," Dr.
Mead says.

A vitamin E aerosol spray protected against air pollution.

Good News—Maybe

A group of researchers in Minnesota, interested
in vitamin E's relationship to aging, did do their studies with humans. Because of suggestions that E could
retard the aging process, they tested the blood levels
of the vitamin in older people to determine if the
concentrations declined with age.

What they discovered was that total vitamin E
levels in the plasma, the fluid portion of the blood,
remained stable, although one form of the vitamin,
called gamma-tocopherol, declined significantly.
However, there were sharp declines of vitamin E in
the platelets, small disk-shaped components of blood
that assist in blood clotting (*Journal of the American
College of Nutrition*).

Levels of vitamin E drop with aging.

Their findings raise a question with serious implications for the elderly: Are the platelets harmed by
this loss of vitamin E in aging? The researchers don't
know. But they say "it is of crucial importance" to find
out.

One of them cautions against jumping to conclusions. "It may be that there is no added requirement
of vitamin E in the aging," suggests Govind Vatassery,
Ph.D., research chemist at the Geriatric Research,
Education and Clinical Center of the Veterans Administration Medical Center in Minneapolis.

Best Food Sources of Vitamin E

Food	Portion	Vitamin E (I.U.)
Wheat germ oil	1 tbsp.	36.3
Sunflower seeds	¼ cup	26.8
Almonds, whole, dried, unblanched	¼ cup	15.2
Wheat germ, raw	½ cup	12.8
Sunflower oil	1 tbsp.	10.9
Hazelnuts, dried, unblanched, chopped	¼ cup	10.2
Safflower oil	1 tbsp.	8.2
Peanuts, shelled, dried	¼ cup	6.0
Cod-liver oil	1 tbsp.	3.9
Peanut butter	2 tbsp.	3.8
Corn oil	1 tbsp.	2.9
Peanut oil	1 tbsp.	2.9
Corn oil margarine	1 tbsp.	2.7
Lobster, boiled	3 oz.	2.3
Salmon steak, broiled	3 oz.	2.0
Soybean oil, hydrogenated	1 tbsp.	2.0
Pecans, halves, dried	¼ cup	1.3

SOURCES: Adapted from

Composition of Foods: Fats and Oils, Agriculture Handbook No. 8–4, by Consumer and Food Economics Institute (Washington, D.C.: Science and Education Administration, U.S. Department of Agriculture, 1979).

Composition of Foods: Nut and Seed Products, Agriculture Handbook No. 8–12, by Nutrition Monitoring Division (Washington, D.C.: Human Nutrition Information Service, U.S. Department of Agriculture, 1984).

"Vitamin E Content of Foods," by P. J. McLaughlin and John L. Weihrauch, *Journal of the American Dietetic Association,* December, 1979.

Nutritive Value of American Foods in Common Units, Agriculture Handbook No. 456, by Catherine F. Adams (Washington, D.C.: Agricultural Research Service, U.S. Department of Agriculture, 1975).

McCance and Widdowson's The Composition of Foods, by A. A. Paul and D. A. T. Southgate (New York: Elsevier/North-Holland Biomedical, 1978).

Or, he speculates, it may be that enough E is stored in the liver and fat tissue that it can be mobilized to the bloodstream when it's needed. "You store it over the years, a little at a time. Vitamin E concentrations in the liver and fat tissues do go up with aging in experimental animals. It's as if you're writing a nutritional history of vitamin E in these tissues," he explains. "Whether that amount is rapidly and readily available in times of need is still controversial. Further study is absolutely essential."

Further study needed—these are the key words when it comes to vitamin E. Ultimate understanding of the health benefits of the much-hyped vitamin may be countless experiments away. But we have only to look at the direction research is taking to realize that all of the hullabaloo may not be wrong after all—just premature.

Chapter 22

Calcium: A New Look at an Old Friend

The milk mineral, the builder of bones, the maker of molars, is fast losing its ho-hum image bred in high school health classes of yesteryear.

For example: Just a couple of years ago, a panel of experts decided to rethink women's calcium Recommended Dietary Allowance (RDA) set by the National Research Council. The panelists, deliberating for the National Institutes of Health, proposed that the current RDA of 800 milligrams per day be bumped to a daily 1,000 milligrams before menopause and 1,500 milligrams after menopause.

Experts say the RDA for calcium may be too low.

Why all the fuss about more calcium for women? Osteoporosis. It's the bone-thinning, bone-fracturing disease that some experts say is virtually epidemic among older American women. For years medical people have suspected that calcium could prevent or impede the malady, and now the case for calcium therapy seems stronger than ever.

Why Many People May Need More Calcium

"It is by no means certain that lack of calcium causes osteoporosis," says Robert P. Heaney, M.D., an expert in bone physiology at Creighton University in Omaha. "But available evidence suggests that dietary calcium may have a positive effect on the dis-

Calcium may slow down or stop osteoporosis.

ease, which is a gradual loss of bone mass. We now know that bone loss happens to everyone after 35 or 45, but it's greatly accelerated in women past menopause. Osteoporosis is frequently the result, and calcium may counteract it."

So say several studies, including one from Australia. There, researchers selected 14 postmenopausal women with osteoporosis, gave them 1,000 milligrams of calcium daily for eight days, then measured the impact of the supplements on bone resorption, or degeneration. The effect was dramatic—the women showed "significant reduction in bone resorption" (*American Journal of Clinical Nutrition*).

Such data may be slowly changing the way doctors treat their osteoporotic patients. Most physicians now view calcium intake as an adjunct to estrogen therapy, a standard treatment for the disease. And some suggest trying calcium before resorting to estrogen, an agent whose long-term use is linked to an increased risk of uterine cancer.

An alternative to estrogen.

"Certainly the case for calcium as osteoporosis therapy isn't yet proved," Dr. Heaney says. "But I think it's best to take the course of least risk. If we say that increased calcium is ineffective, the damage can be great if we're wrong. If we recommend increased calcium and it does nothing, no one is harmed." (To help plan a calcium-rich diet, see the table, Best Food Sources of Calcium, on pages 164–65.)

Calcium and High Blood Pressure

But what of the case for calcium as a treatment for hypertension, the biological accomplice in thousands of American deaths?

More than a decade has come and gone since researchers first suggested that calcium in drinking water was related to lower blood pressure. And over

Scientists want to know if calcium can lower high blood pressure.

the years the calcium/hypertension link has grown stronger in surprising ways.

One of the biggest studies of the connection comes from a group of researchers at Oregon Health Sciences University in Portland and Temple University in Philadelphia. They borrowed data from a massive government study of the American population and analyzed the information for correlations between nutrient intake and high blood pressure. In over 10,000 men and women claiming they never had hypertension, the investigators assessed blood pressure and consumption of 17 nutrients, including vitamins A and C, iron, potassium and calcium.

As it turned out, about 9 percent had hypertension, which was more consistently associated with low-calcium intakes than deficits of any other nutrient. In fact, say the researchers, "none of the hypertensive subgroups had a mean intake of calcium equal to the current recommendation" of 800 milligrams per day.

More dairy products, less risk of high blood pressure.

And, not surprisingly, the consumption of dairy products—rich sources of calcium and potassium—was a strong indicator of whether someone over age 34 had high blood pressure. "The greater an individual's consumption of dairy products," say the investigators, "the less likely it was that he or she was hypertensive" (*Science*).

But an even more intriguing look at calcium's influence on errant blood pressure comes from a team of researchers at Cornell University Medical School, located in New York City. In one of the first research studies to actually test the power of calcium supplements against hypertension in humans, the researchers gave 26 mildly hypertensive patients 2,000 milligrams of oral calcium for six months. The result was a "modest but consistent" drop in pressure—from an average of 161/94 at the start of the study to 154/89 six months later.

For some of the subjects, the change was even

more dramatic. "The patients who started with lower levels of calcium in their blood showed the greatest decrease in pressures," says Lawrence M. Resnick, M.D., head of the research team. "In some cases, diastolic pressures dropped 10 to 20 percent. Patients with higher calcium levels, however, weren't helped at all by the calcium supplements. So the nutrient can benefit some, but not all, hypertensives."

A 20 percent reduction in pressure levels.

But how? "No one knows for sure," says Dr. Resnick. "My theory is that supplemental calcium alters the hormones that help regulate blood pressure. But a lot more research needs to be done before we figure out what's going on."

Moderate Amounts May Work Well

And more work *is* being done. In fact, Dr. Resnick's results have been corroborated by the investigators from Oregon Health Sciences University. They, too, found that oral calcium could lower blood pressure, but at a much lower dose.

For eight weeks they gave 1,000 milligrams of calcium or a placebo (dummy pill) to 70 patients, some with high blood pressure and some without. As expected, the nutrient pulled pressures down—in 42 percent of the hypertensives and 13 percent of those with normal pressures. And what's just as significant, none of the patients had to stop the calcium supplements because of side effects (*Clinical Research*).

1,000 milligrams of calcium daily pulled blood pressure down.

"These results," the researchers say, "suggest that long-term oral calcium may be effective nonpharmacologic [nondrug] therapy for reducing a subset of hypertensives' blood pressure and may also reduce blood pressure in selected normals [nonhypertensives]."

Is calcium just as effective as blood pressure medication?

And judging from the ongoing boom in calcium research, the calcium lessons in high school health class may never be the same.

Best Food Sources of Calcium

Food	Portion	Calcium (mg.)
Tofu, raw, firm, coagulated with calcium sulfate	3 oz.	581
Swiss cheese	2 oz.	544
Provolone cheese	2 oz.	428
Monterey Jack cheese	2 oz.	424
Yogurt, low-fat	1 cup	415
Cheddar cheese	2 oz.	408
Muenster cheese	2 oz.	406
Colby cheese	2 oz.	388
Brick cheese	2 oz.	382
Sardines, Atlantic, drained solids	3 oz.	372
American cheese	2 oz.	348
Ricotta cheese, part-skim	½ cup	337
Milk, skim	1 cup	302
Mozzarella cheese	2 oz.	294
Milk, whole	1 cup	291
Buttermilk	1 cup	285
Limburger cheese	2 oz.	282
Ice milk, soft-serve	1 cup	274
Salmon, sockeye, drained solids	3 oz.	271

SOURCES: Adapted from

Composition of Foods, Agriculture Handbook No. 8, by Bernice K. Watt and Annabel L. Merrill (Washington, D.C.: Agricultural Research Service, U.S. Department of Agriculture, 1975).

Composition of Foods: Dairy and Egg Products, Agriculture Handbook No. 8–1, by Consumer and Food Economics Institute (Washington, D.C.: Agricultural Research Service, U.S. Department of Agriculture, 1976).

Food	Portion	Calcium (mg.)
Ice cream	1 cup	176
Ice milk	1 cup	176
Tofu, raw, firm, coagulated with nigari	3 oz.	174
Pizza, cheese	⅛ of 14″ pie	144
Blackstrap molasses	1 tbsp.	137
Almonds	¼ cup	100
Scallops, steamed	3 oz.	98
Broccoli, cooked	½ cup	89
Soybeans, cooked	½ cup	88
Parmesan cheese	1 tbsp.	86
Collards, cooked	½ cup	74
Dandelion greens, cooked	½ cup	74
Navy beans, cooked	½ cup	64
Soy flour, defatted	¼ cup	60
Shrimp, raw	3 oz.	54
Mustard greens, cooked	½ cup	52
Kale, cooked	½ cup	47
Broccoli, raw	1 cup	42

Nutritive Value of American Foods in Common Units, Agriculture Handbook No. 456, by Catherine F. Adams (Washington, D.C.: Agricultural Research Service, U.S. Department of Agriculture, 1975).

Nutrient Data Research Branch, U.S. Department of Agriculture, Washington, D.C.

Chapter 23

Copper: Essential to Life and Health

W hen you think of copper, do you picture a roll of shiny new pennies? How about the pipes that bring water into your home? Or the gleaming pots and pans hanging in the kitchen? How about a healthy heart and a sound mind?

Probably not the latter. Even though it's absolutely vital to our good health, copper is just not a member of the nutrition Hall of Fame. Yet having the correct amount of this trace mineral (one we need in only tiny amounts) is indispensable to the development and maintenance of our nerves, blood vessels and bones. And although most of us have no difficulty keeping the amount of copper in our bodies at the proper level, for the few who encounter too little or too much, the results can be devastating.

That's because copper is both essential to human health and, like other heavy metals such as lead, cadmium and mercury, potentially toxic. Luckily, our bodies have mechanisms that control the amount of copper we retain. When there's a temporary deficiency of copper in our diet, we absorb more from the food we eat and excrete less. When there's an excess, we absorb less and excrete more.

A trace of copper is all we need.

What We Know about Copper

The copper that we do retain performs its functions as an integral part of more than a dozen proteins called enzymes. Cloaking the copper in these large protein molecules protects us from the toxic effects it would have if allowed to roam free.

Because we're so well protected from copper feast or famine, significant deficiency and poisoning are both uncommon. For that reason, much of what we know about those conditions comes from experiments with animals. Direct knowledge of their effects in humans comes from a few special cases.

Copper deficiency is uncommon.

"Our best evidence for copper's role in humans comes from children who have Menkes' disease," explains Joseph R. Prohaska, Ph.D., associate professor of biochemistry at the University of Minnesota School of Medicine in Duluth. "Menkes' is a fatal genetic disease of abnormal copper metabolism, in which the children die at two or three years of age." It's sometimes called kinky-hair syndrome because affected infants have peculiar kinky, white hair. Their symptoms are thought to reflect deficiencies of the copper enzymes.

"What happens to children with Menkes' disease is almost exactly what we see in copper-deficient experimental animals," Dr. Prohaska says. "Some of their brain cells die, some degenerate and in some there is a delay in the process of myelination, the formation of an insulating sheath around the neurons (the characteristic cells of the brain).

With too little copper, laboratory animals experience brain damage.

"These children also have abnormal blood vessels," he says. "They're twisted and have a tendency to rupture if blood pressure gets too high. The children's bones are weakened, too."

In children, a copper abnormality may result in fragile blood vessels.

Those abnormalities are thought to be a consequence of a low concentration of a copper enzyme involved in the cross-linking of collagen and elastin, connective tissue proteins. When strands of those molecules are properly cross-linked, the arteries are strong, elastic and capable of stretching as blood pulses through them, and the bones are formed with a solid matrix.

Unfortunately, there's no cure yet for Menkes' disease. Merely giving the children copper doesn't improve their condition or keep them from dying. The condition is still not completely understood.

A Kind of Nutritional Chore Boy

As you can see from the lethal effects of Menkes' disease, copper performs a number of crucial tasks. It's needed for the proper development of the brain, the cardiovascular system and the skeletal system.

Copper: essential for healthy blood vessels, brain cells and bones.

"The reason it affects so many different things," says Dr. Prohaska, "is that copper enzymes are ubiquitous in nature. Almost all cells in the body contain them. So when you start changing the copper nutriture, you're going to be changing the biological system in many different kinds of cells."

For instance, copper is part of a cell enzyme that is required for the release of energy. It's also part of an enzyme that is needed for the production of melanin, the dark pigment in hair and skin. The absence of this enzyme results in albinism.

Copper and iron keep anemia at bay.

Copper is involved in iron metabolism, too. Without it, iron cannot be properly incorporated into hemoglobin, the oxygen-carrying protein in the blood, and anemia ensues. Someone who has anemia caused by copper deficiency can't be cured by taking extra iron.

Copper-Clad Defense

Research suggests that copper may even have a role in immunity. "I knew that almost all of the infants with Menkes' disease die of some sort of an infection," says Dr. Prohaska. "That may or may not be due to an alteration in the immune system. But it was enough of a reason for me to suspect that might be the case."

In one study, Dr. Prohaska found that mice deficient in copper could not produce enough antibodies to a particular antigen (foreign protein) that they were given (*Science*). The mouse immune system is similar to our own.

"The number of cells that were able to make antibodies against that particular antigen was decreased in these mice roughly in proportion to how deficient they were," Dr. Prohaska reports.

"Some of the mice had only a marginal deficiency. Probably if they had checked into a mouse clinic, they'd have come out with a clean bill of health. Yet we were still able to detect a small change in the immune system.

"The ability to form antibodies is called the humoral immune response," he explains. "Another arm of the immune system, the cell-mediated immune response, relies not primarily on the production of antibodies but on cells in the immune system called T-cells. Subsequently we've shown that this arm of the immune system is also impaired in copper-deficient animals.

Is copper a vital factor in our immunity?

"We don't know yet exactly how copper is affecting these things," says Dr. Prohaska. "My research now is trying to elucidate whether there is a specific role for copper in the process or whether it's a secondary effect on something we already know about."

A Role in Heart Disease?

One of the most intriguing areas of copper research revolves around the theory that copper deficiency, or a relative copper deficiency, may be related to heart disease.

"The theory is based on the observation that there are a large number of similarities between animals that are deficient in copper and people with coronary heart disease," explains Leslie M. Klevay, M.D., research medical officer at the Human Nutrition Research Center in Grand Forks, North Dakota. "They both have abnormal electrocardiograms, abnormal connective tissue in the arteries and heart, death of some areas of the arteries, enlarged heart, a low copper level in the heart muscle and sometimes a ruptured heart.

Copper-deficient animals have heart disease symptoms. Is this a clue to preventing the disorder in humans?

"There are also biochemical similarities. The most important are glucose intolerance, hypercholesterolemia [high levels of cholesterol in the blood] and hyperuricemia [high levels of uric acid in the blood]. Glucose intolerance and hypercholesterolemia are two of the major risk factors for heart disease. And we know from the Framingham study that people with gout, who have high levels of uric acid, have twice the heart disease risk of people without gout. And the higher the uric acid, the higher the heart disease risk.

"I want to emphasize that we don't know whether these characteristics in humans are really due to copper deficiency," stresses Dr. Klevay. At this point it's still a theory.

An interesting corollary to that theory is that it's not only a deficiency of copper that might be related to heart disease but a relative deficiency of copper with respect to zinc. "In one of my earlier experiments, rats that were fed a diet with a high zinc-to-copper ratio had raised cholesterol levels," says Dr. Klevay.

How zinc and copper co-operate for health.

"And it's been shown in humans that too much zinc drives down HDL [high-density lipoprotein] cholesterol, the kind that is thought to be protective against heart disease. There's a lot of evidence that too much zinc can interfere with copper. That's how I explain those results."

One way zinc takes copper out of the picture is by blocking its absorption. "Metallothionein is a protein in the intestines that binds both zinc and copper and keeps them from being absorbed into the body," says Dr. Prohaska. "Normally, there's a very small amount of this protein. It can be induced to rather high levels, though, if presented with a large amount of zinc. But the protein tends to bind copper even tighter than zinc. Even in the face of a lot of zinc, this protein will preferentially bind to copper. Therefore you decrease the absorption of copper by giving large doses of zinc."

"From our animal studies, the ideal zinc-to-copper ratio seems to be four to one," says Dr. Klevay.

"Meddling" with Your Copper Supply

Just how much copper should we try to get? Because of insufficient information, the National Research Council hasn't set a Recommended Dietary Allowance. But based on all of the information they do have, they have estimated that a safe and adequate daily intake of copper for adults is two to three milligrams.

If that estimate is correct, there may be some cause for concern. Several studies have shown that we don't get that much copper.

"Considering several dietary studies, we found that 75 percent of the diets we checked contain less than two milligrams [2,000 micrograms] of copper," says Dr. Klevay. "Only 25 percent contained two or more milligrams.

A safe daily ration of copper: two to three milligrams.

"The best way to ensure you're getting enough copper is to eat foods that provide it in ample amounts," he recommends. Liver, shellfish, nuts and seeds, dried beans, wheat, barley and chicken are some of the best sources. (For others, see the table, Best Food Sources of Copper, on pages 174–75.)

"My feeling is that it's most important to get enough copper during growth and development," says Dr. Prohaska. "It's critical from pregnancy through the child's adolescence. It's especially important in adolescent pregnancies, where the growth of the mother as well as the baby adds to the requirements. In adults, especially the elderly, we just don't know yet. There's been very little research into their particular needs."

A critical nutrient for children and young mothers.

But there are some special situations to look out for. Some infants fed a diet of cow's milk have developed copper deficiency. That's because cow's milk contains almost no copper. People on total parenteral nutrition (intravenous feeding) may also be at risk of copper deficiency. So may those taking excessive quantities of antacids, those who've had intestinal bypass surgery and those on liquid protein diets.

In addition, there is evidence, based on animal studies, that large doses of vitamin C can interfere with copper absorption. To maximize vitamin C's benefits while minimizing its adverse effect on copper, it may help to divide the day's allowance into several smaller doses taken at intervals. Of course, it's equally important that the diet doesn't fall short of copper.

Too much vitamin C can meddle with copper absorption.

Copper's Tarnished Reputation

But what about the other side of the coin? Too much copper is just as dangerous as too little. "Because our bodies have mechanisms to detoxify copper and get rid of it, it's hard to get copper poisoning," says I. Herbert Scheinberg, M.D., professor of medicine and head of the division of genetic medicine at Albert Einstein College of Medicine in New York City. "You'd really have to work at it."

Chronic occupational exposure to copper in a form that could have toxic effects is relatively rare. Acute poisoning is also uncommon but can occur when too much copper is ingested by mistake. That can happen when acidic food or drinks, such as vinegar, carbonated beverages or citrus juices have prolonged contact with a copper container. It can also happen when water stands in copper pipes for a long period of time, only if the water is acidic. However, the problem is self-limiting. The vomiting and diarrhea caused by ingesting too much copper generally protect us from its more serious toxic effects.

Too much copper in the body is rare but dangerous.

But people with Wilson's disease are not protected. Wilson's disease results from a genetic defect in the mechanism that excretes copper, causing copper to accumulate in the liver, where it does great harm. Eventually it circulates out of the liver as free copper, causing damage to the brain, nervous system and kidneys, too. The disease first appears between the ages of 5 and 50, but most commonly around the age of 17.

Too Much Copper Can Be Hazardous

"In about one-third of patients, the first symptoms are signs of copper poisoning in the liver, such as jaundice, swelling of the abdomen and other signs similar to those found in hepatitis," Dr. Scheinberg explains. "In the other patients, psychiatric and neurologic symptoms may appear first. The psychiatric symptoms include behavioral disturbances, neurosis and psychosis. The neurological signs look like a combination of Parkinson's disease and multiple sclerosis. They include tremors, stiffness and difficulty speaking, walking, swallowing and writing. These eventually progress to the point of total incapacity.

The signs of copper poisoning.

"The disease is always fatal unless it's treated. The treatment is a drug called penicillamine, a derivative of penicillin. It combines with the excess copper so it can be excreted in the urine. If patients are treated before there is any irreversible damage, they can be brought back to normal health.

"There are an estimated 8,000 people with Wilson's disease in the United States," Dr. Scheinberg says. "Seven thousand of them will die because they are not properly diagnosed. Because the symptoms mimic hepatitis, neurological and psychiatric disorders, most of these people will get wrong treatment."

There are tests, however, that can diagnose Wilson's disease. One is a blood test for the copper protein ceruloplasmin. This protein, which normally protects us from copper poisoning, is deficient or absent in patients with the disease. If it's low, a liver biopsy can confirm the diagnosis.

"If someone in the family had Wilson's disease, it's important that a child be tested for it before the age of five," says Dr. Scheinberg. "And anyone who has unexplained symptoms of neurologic or psychiatric disorders, hepatitis or cirrhosis, especially if they're under 30, should be tested."

An alert for families of people with Wilson's disease.

Best Food Sources of Copper

Food	Portion	Copper (mcg.)
Crab, boiled	3 oz.	4,080
Liver, beef, braised	4 oz.	3,161
Cashews, dry-roasted	¼ cup	760
Sunflower seeds, dry-roasted	¼ cup	586
Sesame seeds, whole, dried	1 tbsp.	367
Peanuts, dried	¼ cup	366
Almonds, dried, unblanched, whole	¼ cup	335
Pecans, dried	¼ cup	320
Walnuts, black, dried	¼ cup	320
Whole wheat flour	½ cup	300
Prunes, dried, uncooked	¼ cup	173
Apricots, dried, sulfured, uncooked	¼ cup	140

SOURCES: Adapted from

Composition of Foods: Beef Products, Agriculture Handbook No. 8–13, by Nutrition Monitoring Division (Washington, D.C.: Human Nutrition Information Service, U.S. Department of Agriculture, 1986).

Composition of Foods: Breakfast Cereals, Agriculture Handbook No. 8–8, by Consumer Nutrition Center (Washington, D.C.: Human Nutrition Information Service, U.S. Department of Agriculture, 1982).

Composition of Foods: Fruits and Fruit Juices, Agriculture Handbook No. 8–9, by Consumer Nutrition Center (Washington, D.C.: Human Nutrition Information Service, U.S. Department of Agriculture, 1982).

Composition of Foods: Legumes and Legume Products, Agriculture Handbook No. 8–16, by Nutrition Monitoring Division (Washington, D.C.: Human Nutrition Information Service, U.S. Department of Agriculture, 1986).

Composition of Foods: Nut and Seed Products, Agriculture Handbook No. 8–12, by Nutrition Monitoring Division (Washington, D.C.: Human Nutrition Information Service, U.S. Department of Agriculture, 1984).

Food	Portion	Copper (mcg.)
Navy beans, cooked, boiled	¼ cup	134
Banana	1 medium	124
Raisins, seedless, not packed	¼ cup	112
Chicken, dark meat, cooked, without skin	4 oz.	91
Barley, raw	¼ cup	60
Halibut, steamed	3 oz.	60
Chicken, light meat, cooked, without skin	4 oz.	57
Wheat germ, plain, toasted	1 tbsp.	44
Mushrooms, raw, pieces	½ cup	39

Composition of Foods: Poultry Products, Agriculture Handbook No. 8–5, by Consumer and Food Economics Institute (Washington, D.C.: Science and Education Administration, U.S. Department of Agriculture, 1979).

Composition of Foods: Vegetables and Vegetable Products, Agriculture Handbook No. 8–11, by Nutrition Monitoring Division (Washington, D.C: Human Nutrition Information Service, U.S. Department of Agriculture, 1984).

"Copper Content of Foods," by Jean T. Pennington and Doris Howes Calloway, *Research,* August, 1973.

McCance and Widdowson's The Composition of Foods, by A. A. Paul and D. A. T. Southgate (New York: Elsevier/North-Holland Biomedical, 1978).

Chapter 24

What You Should Know about Iron

W hen it comes to iron, some of us may fool ourselves into thinking we know it all. Iron is certainly something we've heard enough about, thanks to advertising. It doesn't take a Ph.D. in biochemistry to understand that iron-packed red blood cells carry energy-giving oxygen to every part of our bodies, nor to realize that the end result of an iron-poor diet can be a foot-dragging weariness that leaves hardly enough pep to push a dustcloth, much less conduct an executive board meeting.

You don't have to be anemic to show signs of iron deficiency.

Further research, though, is taking iron beyond common knowledge and advertising clichés. With newer ways to assess how our bodies absorb, transport and store iron, doctors can now pinpoint body iron levels. They are finding that what once might have been considered an adequate amount of iron may not always be optimal, that the body can show symptoms even in mild iron deficiency, not just outright anemia. They are beginning to view iron deficiency as a "whole-body disease," one that affects immune response, body temperature and even learning and concentration.

Iron for Immunity

Researchers have known for a long time that iron is important to our ability to ward off infections in some way, says José I. Santos, M.D., an assistant professor of pediatrics and pathology at Boston University School of Medicine.

It's known that phagocytes, white blood cells that serve as the body's primary defense mechanism against bacterial infections, depend on iron-containing enzymes to do their job, Dr. Santos says. These cells engulf bacteria and secrete a variety of corrosive substances known as oxidants, which digest the invading microbe once it is engulfed. Phagocytes need plenty of oxygen to produce peroxides, and iron brings it to them. "Certainly iron deficiency is going to directly impede this process," Dr. Santos says.

Without enough iron, our body's defenses against infection start to break down.

Other white blood cells, known as lymphocytes, function even less well with inadequate iron. "Lymphocytes need iron for energy metabolism and for the production of enzymes important to their very specialized roles in the immune response," Dr. Santos says. The production of antibodies also requires iron-dependent enzymes, he adds.

But germs, especially bacteria, also need iron to survive and multiply, once they have invaded the body. That's why, when faced with some infections—malaria, for instance, or tuberculosis—the body begins to take iron out of circulation and store it in the bone marrow, liver and other areas where bacteria can't reach it. As if to counter this, bacteria produce chemical chelators (derived from the Greek word for *claw*), which grab iron away from the bloodstream or body tissues. So, paradoxically, low blood levels of iron are beneficial in resisting infection.

But the exact opposite is true where viral infections are concerned, Dr. Santos says. "Most viral diseases, including genital herpes, may become worse with iron deficiency." This is not surprising, since lymphocytes, the major defense against viral infections, also need iron for optimal activity.

Low iron levels leave you more vulnerable to viral attack.

Viruses also need iron to multiply, but they cannot garner it the way bacteria can. "Faced with a viral infection, the best thing we can do is to keep our iron levels up," Dr. Santos says.

Chill Resistance

Faced with a chilly winter, we may consider iron as essential as long johns. The ability to stay warm when it's cold out is affected by iron deficiency, according to researchers at the University of Washington Medical School, Seattle.

They found that after being exposed to 39°F temperatures for 24 hours, anemic rats became ill, whereas normal animals tolerated exposure. The anemic rats had lowered body temperatures, reduced oxygen consumption, and a less active thyroid, and one of their major heat-producing tissues, brown fat, showed markedly less metabolic activity than that of nonanemic control rats.

Does the cold really get to you? Maybe you need more iron.

"Abnormalities similar to those found in the rat seem to exist in iron-deficient humans," says Clement Finch, M.D., professor of medicine at the University of Washington Medical School. "We have found that people with iron-deficiency anemia aren't able to maintain their body temperature well when exposed to mild hypothermia."

The rats also showed a buildup of chemicals called catecholamines, which are secreted by the brain. Synthetic forms of these chemicals are used to treat shock, hypoglycemia and cardiac arrest. Along with thyroid hormone, catecholamines drive metabolic processes. But in this case, Dr. Finch says, they do double duty, acting as a reserve mechanism to try to keep the body generating enough energy to maintain its temperature.

Iron deficiencies may affect the way you think and behave.

In fact, some researchers believe that an imbalance in neurotransmitting chemicals, which require iron-containing enzymes, may be associated with the behavior and learning abnormalities seen in iron deficiencies. Infants and children with iron deficiencies often display symptoms of learning disability. They have been described as "solemn, irritable and inattentive." Teenagers with iron deficiencies have been described as restless, disruptive and inattentive.

But, at least with the children, only a few days of supplemental iron reversed this behavior. In Chile, researchers found that both anemic and nonanemic (but iron-deficient) 15-month-old youngsters showed a significant improvement in attention span and co-operativeness and did better in a psychological test ten days after starting iron supplementation.

Giving iron to iron-deficient kids can improve their dispositions.

Ernesto Pollitt, Ph.D., professor of human development in the Department of Applied Behavioral Sciences at the University of California at Davis, found that abnormalities in the ability to "receive" information in both mildly and severely iron-deficient children could be reversed with iron therapy.

"The findings suggest that the motivation to persist in intellectually challenging tasks may be lowered, attention span shortened, and overall intellectual performance diminished in iron-deficient children," Dr. Pollitt says.

Low Iron Leads
Nutritional Deficiencies

These findings are particularly worrisome when we consider the following: Although severe anemia is now becoming uncommon in the United States, iron deficiency is a leading nutritional deficiency problem, with infants, teenagers, women and the elderly its main victims.

Iron depletion may be the nation's number one nutritional deficiency problem.

A child from the age of nine months to two years is at high risk because the infant has used up its body stores of iron and may be weaned from iron-rich breast milk or iron-fortified formula to iron-poor cow's milk during this time, says Frank Oski, M.D., a pediatrician at Johns Hopkins Hospital and a professor of pediatrics at Johns Hopkins University School of Medicine in Baltimore, Maryland. Dr. Oski has found that iron deficiencies range from 10 to 25 percent in affluent suburban infants to as high as 50 percent in infants of lower socioeconomic classes.

Up to one-half of American women of childbearing age are iron deficient.

Iron deficiencies affect about 5 percent of all five- to eight-year-olds, 2.6 percent of all adolescents and 25 percent of pregnant teenagers. A screening of Yale University undergraduate women under age 21 found 18 percent mildly iron deficient. Surprising? "Maybe it is," says Dr. Oski, "when you think that here is a group of presumably very high socioeconomic status, yet they show this degree of anemia. But it's not surprising when you know that anywhere from 25 to 50 percent of American women in their childbearing years are iron deficient."

Older people, especially if they have low income and are over 60, are also vulnerable to iron deficiencies, studies have shown. Twenty-three percent of a group of low-income, older black residents of Washington, D.C., were found to be iron deficient by Allan Johnson, Ph.D., associate professor in the Department of Human Nutrition and Food at the School of Human Ecology, Howard University. Forty-one percent consumed less than the Recommended Dietary Allowance (RDA) of iron.

Absorption Factors

Is your body absorbing all the iron it needs?

Poor diet is certainly one cause of iron deficiency, but it's not the only cause. We may be eating enough iron but not absorbing enough of it to stay healthy, especially as we get older.

"Lack of iron could be the result of poor bioavailability rather than inadequate iron intake," says James D. Cook, M.D., director of the Division of Hematology of the University of Kansas Medical Center in Kansas City. He and colleague Sean Lynch, M.D., have tagged iron with radioactive particles to determine how well it is absorbed by the body in different situations.

Normally, we absorb only about 10 percent of all the iron we eat. And that's figured into the RDA. A young woman's RDA is 18 milligrams, but her body requires only 1.8 milligrams. (The RDA for men and for women 23 to 50 is 10 milligrams.)

There are two kinds of iron. Found only in beef, chicken, fish and other animal meats, "heme" iron is the easiest for our bodies to absorb.

Two kinds of iron—and the best sources of both.

"Heme iron makes up only about 5 percent of the iron we eat, but we can absorb about 25 percent of it," Dr. Cook says. And contrary to what you tried to make your mother believe, liver is definitely the best food source of iron. A 3-ounce serving of chicken liver has 7.2 milligrams of iron; sirloin, 2.9 milligrams and dark meat chicken, 1.1 milligrams.

But 95 percent of our iron comes from what are known as nonheme sources, iron compounds that are found in vegetables and grains and in meats. Liver is also the best source of nonheme iron, Dr. Cook says. Normally, only about 5 percent of the nonheme iron in foods is absorbed. (For a more complete list of sources of dietary iron, see the table, Best Food Sources of Iron, on pages 182–83.)

Boosting Iron Absorption

Unlike heme iron, the availability of nonheme iron is greatly influenced by what we eat along with it. It all has to do with about three feet of small intestine.

In the acid environment of the stomach, the iron molecule is free, but as soon as food moves into the small intestine and acidity drops, iron scrambles for a partner. How bioavailable the iron remains to us depends on how willing its partner is to give it up to the intestinal mucosa.

Amino acids in meats and vitamin C (ascorbic acid) are proving to be nonheme iron's indispensable escorts. Both can more than double the amount of iron absorbed, Dr. Cook says.

Meat and vitamin C can double iron absorption.

The addition of just 60 milligrams of vitamin C to a meal of rice will more than triple iron absorption. Adding papaya juice containing 66 milligrams of vitamin C to a meal of corn will boost iron absorption by 500 percent.

(continued on page 184)

Best Food Sources of Iron

Food	Portion	Iron (mg.)
Chicken liver, cooked	3 oz.	7.2
Crab, pieces, steamed	½ cup	6.0
Beef liver, fried	3 oz.	5.3
Soybeans, boiled	½ cup	4.4
Blackstrap molasses	1 tbsp.	3.2
Spinach, cooked	½ cup	3.2
Beef, rump roast, lean, cooked	3 oz.	3.1
Beef, sirloin, broiled	3 oz.	2.9
Potato, baked	1	2.8
Scallops, steamed	3 oz.	2.5
Sunflower seeds, dried	¼ cup	2.4
Pistachios, dried	¼ cup	2.2
Broccoli, cooked	1 spear	2.1
Cashews, dry-roasted	¼ cup	2.1
Lima beans, large, boiled	½ cup	2.1
Beef, ground, extra lean, broiled, medium	3 oz.	2.0
Swiss chard, cooked	½ cup	2.0
Turkey, dark-meat, cooked, without skin	3 oz.	2.0
Soybeans, dry-roasted	¼ cup	1.7
Lobster, broiled	½ cup	1.5

SOURCES: Adapted from

Composition of Foods, Agriculture Handbook No. 8, by Bernice K. Watt and Annabel L. Merrill (Washington, D.C.: Agricultural Research Service, U.S. Department of Agriculture, 1975).

Composition of Foods: Beef Products, Agriculture Handbook No. 8–13, by Nutrition Monitoring Division (Washington, D.C.: Human Nutrition Information Service, U.S. Department of Agriculture, 1986).

Composition of Foods: Fruits and Fruit Juices, Agriculture Handbook No. 8–9, by Consumer Nutrition Center (Washington, D.C.: Human Nutrition Information Service, U.S. Department of Agriculture, 1982).

Composition of Foods: Legumes and Legume Products, Agriculture Handbook No. 8–16, by Nutrition Monitoring Division (Washington, D.C.: Human Nutrition Information Service, U.S. Department of Agriculture, 1986).

Food	Portion	Iron (mg.)
Beet greens, cooked	½ cup	1.4
Tuna, canned in water	3 oz.	1.4
Almonds, dried, unblanched	¼ cup	1.3
Broccoli, raw	1 spear	1.3
Sesame seeds, whole, dried	1 tbsp.	1.3
Peanuts, dried	¼ cup	1.2
Peas, cooked	½ cup	1.2
Prunes, dried, cooked	½ cup	1.2
Chicken, dark-meat, cooked, without skin	3 oz.	1.1
Turkey, light-meat, cooked, without skin	3 oz.	1.1
Apricots, dried, sulfured, cooked	¼ cup	1.0
Brussels sprouts, cooked	½ cup	0.9
Chicken, light-meat, cooked, without skin	3 oz.	0.9
Cod, cooked	3 oz.	0.9
Raisins, seedless, packed	¼ cup	0.8
Spinach, raw, chopped	½ cup	0.8
Haddock, raw	3 oz.	0.6
Endive, raw	½ cup	0.2

Composition of Foods: Nut and Seed Products, Agriculture Handbook No. 8–12, by Nutrition Monitoring Division (Washington, D.C.: Human Nutrition Information Service, U.S. Department of Agriculture, 1984).

Composition of Foods: Poultry Products, Agriculture Handbook No. 8–5, by Consumer and Food Economics Institute (Washington, D.C.: Science and Education Administration, U.S. Department of Agriculture, 1979).

Composition of Foods: Vegetables and Vegetable Products, Agriculture Handbook No. 8–11, by Nutrition Monitoring Division (Washington, D.C.: Human Nutrition Information Service, U.S. Department of Agriculture, 1984).

Nutritive Value of American Foods in Common Units, Agriculture Handbook No. 456, by Catherine F. Adams (Washington, D.C.: Agricultural Research Service, U.S. Department of Agriculture, 1975).

Some escorts are notoriously unwilling to relinquish the iron they're teamed up with. In laboratory studies, Dr. Cook has found that the tannic acid in tea inhibits absorption by 64 percent and that in coffee by about 40 percent.

"Soy protein *does* inhibit iron absorption by 70 to 80 percent," Dr. Cook says. "But if you're adding it to a meal rather than using it to replace meat proteins, it has more than enough of its own iron to offset the inhibiting effect."

A phosphate compound found in egg yolks strongly binds the iron plentiful in the yolks and makes eggs a poor source of iron. The availability of iron in dairy products is also very low, but Dr. Cook is not sure why.

Eggs are a poor source of iron.

Calcium tablets should not be taken with iron, Dr. Cook says, since inorganic calcium compounds are potent iron blockers. And taking iron as part of a multivitamin may not be a good idea because iron will bind with many of the ingredients. The absorbed fraction of a 65-milligram iron supplement may drop from 8.1 milligrams when taken alone to 1.8 milligrams when part of a multivitamin that contains calcium, reports Gabe Mirkin, M.D., associate professor of pediatrics at Georgetown University School of Medicine, Washington, D.C.

Simply eating food at the same time you take your iron supplement can cut the amount of iron absorbed in half, Dr. Cook says. For maximum absorption, take iron tablets between meals, with vitamin C.

More Tips

You can rearrange your diet to take full advantage of the iron you do eat. Here are some dietary considerations for better iron absorption.

• Get some vitamin C with every meal. Drink orange or tomato juice, eat half a grapefruit or some strawberries. Include vegetables rich in C—tomatoes, green peppers, broccoli, radishes and green leafy vegetables like kale and turnip and collard greens. Season dishes with lemon or lime juice or parsley.

• Without necessarily increasing the amount of meat you eat, you may want to spread your meat protein out over more meals. Chicken and fish work as well as red meat. Serve smaller portions combined with whole grains and fresh vegetables.

Don't eat more meat, but eat it more often.

• Imitate the Italians. Long-simmering tomato sauces bring out the iron in any food. Or make like the Mexicans, whose ingenious use of a little beef with plenty of beans, rice and red chilies makes the most of each bit of iron.

• Use iron cookware. Simply cooking spaghetti sauce for three hours in an iron utensil increases its iron content to almost 30 times what it would be if prepared in glassware.

Cooking in iron cookware can boost the iron content of your food.

Eating right will help keep you rich in iron—and all the other vitamins and minerals you need for maximum performance.

Chapter 25

Give Yourself the Iron Test (and Rate Your Energy Reserves)

When it comes to your health, iron is a metal more precious than gold.

Though you may hoard it like a miser—banking the iron from a weekly serving of liver, a daily iron supplement and plates full of spinach and broccoli—your account may be regularly depleted by the iron robbers. If you are a menstruating woman, a dieter, a vegetarian, even a heavy tea drinker, you can find yourself overdrawn at the iron bank despite all your good intentions. In fact, you could be making withdrawals as fast as you're making deposits.

When that happens, your energy stores go bankrupt. Even before you're in the throes of full-blown anemia, you may experience fatigue, dizziness, nausea, loss of appetite and a shortened attention span.

Your body may be losing iron as fast as it's taking it in.

Are You Food Rich but Iron Poor?

How do you rate your iron levels? It's much like auditing any other account. First, you start by looking in the deposit column.

Part I of this quick and easy quiz will let you know roughly whether your weekly menu is iron rich or iron poor. It won't tell you if you're meeting the Recommended Dietary Allowance (10 milligrams daily for men, 18 milligrams for women). It's not that precise. But it will give you some idea of what kind of an iron-saver you are.

How to audit your body's iron account.

But the total of your deposits means nothing until you fill in the withdrawal column, part II of the quiz. These are the risk factors, each one a Willie Sutton eager to pocket your savings of this most precious metal. Needless to say, if your part II total equals or exceeds the total from part I (+16, –19, for example), you may have to make some dietary or lifestyle changes to avoid the penalties of iron deficiency. If your part I score is low, yet still higher than your score for part II (+9, –7, for example), you are probably not getting many iron-rich foods in your diet and, consequently, you may not be getting enough iron despite your low risk-factor score. If the scores are close (+15, –14, for example), you may still want to make some lifestyle or dietary changes that will shrink your withdrawals and boost your deposits.

What your score may mean.

Now take the following quiz, calculate *two* totals (don't add them), and compare. Then read the explanation of what it all means to your health.

Test Your Iron Level

Part I: Deposits

1. Do you eat beef liver at least once a week? (+3 points) ___

2. Do you eat a portion of beef, turkey, chicken, fish or shellfish at least once a day? (+3 points) ___

3. If you answered "no" to question 2, do you eat a portion of beef, turkey, chicken, fish or shellfish two to four times a week? (+1 point) ___

Bonus: Give yourself +3 points if you eat meat for three meals a day. ___

4. Does your diet include a serving of blackstrap molasses, almonds, lima beans, peas, sunflower seeds, prunes, dried apricots or broccoli at least twice a week? (+2 points) ___

Answer the next five questions and bonus questions only if you answered "yes" to any of the previous questions.

5. Does your diet include a serving of orange juice, green peppers, grapefruit juice, papaya, brussels sprouts, oranges, turnip greens, cantaloupe, cauliflower, strawberries, tomato juice, grapefruit, potatoes, raw tomatoes, cabbage, blackberries, blueberries or cherries at least twice a week?
(+2 points) ___

6. Does your diet include a serving of organ meats, yogurt, almonds, wild rice, ricotta cheese, Swiss cheese, Camembert cheese or Roquefort cheese at least twice a week?
(+2 points) ___

7. Does your diet include a serving of cashews, mushrooms, pecans, bananas, walnuts, peanuts, wheat germ, prunes or sesame seeds at least twice a week?
(+2 points) ___

Bonus: Give yourself +1 point each if your diet frequently includes broccoli, dried apricots or almonds. ___ Give yourself +½ point each if your diet frequently includes brussels sprouts, cauliflower, peas, bananas, strawberries, cashews, sunflower seeds, chicken, chicken livers or brewer's yeast. ___

8. Do you take a B-complex or riboflavin supplement (no score for multivitamins)?
(+2 points) ___

9. Do you take vitamin C supplements?
(+2 points) ___

10. Do you take an iron supplement?
(+3 points) ___

11. Does your typical meal include meat, a vegetable and one of the following: orange juice, green peppers, grapefruit juice, papaya, brussels sprouts, broccoli, oranges, turnip greens, cantaloupe, cauliflower, strawberries, tomato juice, grapefruit, pota-

toes, tomatoes, cabbage, blackberries, blueberries or cherries?
(+3 points) ___
    12. Do you frequently cook in iron pots?
(+3 points) ___

    Part I Total _____

Part II: Withdrawals

    1. Are you a menstruating woman?
(–3 points) ___
    2. Do you have heavy menstrual flow?
(–3 points) ___
    3. If you are a woman, do you give blood twice or more a year?
(–2 points) ___
    4. Have you recently had surgery?
(–3 points) ___
    5. Do you have a peptic ulcer, colitis or hemorrhoids?
(–3 points) ___
    6. Do you take aspirin often?
(–2 points) ___
    7. Are you on a low-calorie diet?
(–3 points) ___
    8. Are you over 65?
(–3 points) ___
    9. Do you drink a lot of tea, especially during or after meals?
(–3 points) ___
    10. Do you eat a lot of foods containing the preservative EDTA and phosphate additives?
(–3 points) ___
    11. Do you drink a lot of coffee, especially during and after meals?
(–2 points) ___
    12. Do you eat a high-fiber diet?
(–½ point) ___

13. Are you a vegetarian?
(–2 points) ___

14. Do you take calcium supplements?
(–½ point) ___

15. Do you frequently take antacids?
(–½ point) ___

16. Do you live in an area exposed to industrial pollution, particularly cadmium and lead?
(–1 point) ___

17. Are you involved in strenuous activity, such as long-distance running?
(–1 point) ___

18. Do you feel you are under a great deal of stress?
(–2 points) ___

Part II Total _____

Explanation

Part I: Deposits

1. Beef liver is one of the best sources of dietary iron, containing 5.3 milligrams per three-ounce serving. That doesn't mean your body can absorb the total amount. Only about 25 percent of the iron from animal sources is bioavailable—that is, absorbed by the body. Some medical experts believe many iron deficiency problems are the result of poor bioavailability rather than low-iron intake. That's why beef liver is so important: It gets high scores not only for iron content but also for bioavailability.

Liver: high levels, well absorbed.

In fact, you'd have to eat about 14 pounds of broccoli to get the amount of iron absorbed from six to seven ounces of liver. And there's a bonus, too. Liver also contains three other important nutrients: vitamin C, riboflavin and copper, all of which enhance the absorption of iron.

2–3. Again, only meat and fish have that double whammy, high iron and high bioavailability. Though red meat is highest on both counts, both poultry and fish are good substitutes. Three ounces of dark-meat turkey contain 2 milligrams of iron; a three-ounce slice of light-meat chicken provides 0.9 milligrams, but it also contains the enhancer riboflavin, which increases iron bioavailability. And if you choose lean cuts of meat, you can keep calorie and cholesterol levels down near those of fish and poultry.

Poultry and fish are good choices.

Bonus: Not only do you get a hefty dose of iron from meat but its presence in a meal will help you absorb iron from other foods you're eating. You can increase your iron intake by spreading out your meat protein—not necessarily increasing the amount you eat—over three meals instead of one or two.

Don't eat a day's worth of meat at one meal.

4. If you don't eat meat, and even if you do, you might want to consider including as many of these foods in your diet as possible. They're all iron rich, but only about 5 percent of the iron they contain is bioavailable.

But there are ways to increase bioavailability. Take a look at the foods listed in questions 5, 6 and 7 and the bonus question. If you can design your menu around these foods, you can sometimes double or triple iron absorption from both animal and plant sources.

A method to triple absorption.

5. The foods listed in this question are high in vitamin C. In one study done at the University of Göteborg, in Sweden, a glass of orange juice served with a meal of hamburger, string beans and mashed potatoes increased iron absorption from the meal by 85 percent (*Human Nutrition: Applied Nutrition*). The same researchers were also able to significantly boost the iron absorption from a vegetarian meal by making sure it had a high C content (*American Journal of Clinical Nutrition*).

6–7. These are the high-riboflavin and high-copper foods, respectively. Again, they're the helper nutrients that make sure you get the most out of your iron deposits.

Bonus: Why extra points for these foods? Broccoli, dried apricots and almonds not only contain iron but they also contain at least two iron enhancers. The foods in the second bonus list contain iron and at least one enhancer nutrient.

Dried apricots and other iron enhancers.

8–10. Needless to say, taking supplements of iron and the enhancer nutrients can help if you can't eat enough to boost your iron savings.

11. You may recognize this food list. These are the vitamin C foods, and this is the ideal iron-rich meal: meat, iron-rich vegetable and vitamin C food.

12. Iron pans for iron nutrition? It sounds farfetched, but it really helps. The cooking process permits a considerable amount of iron to be absorbed by the food. In some cases, food cooked in iron cookware can have three or four times more iron than the same foods cooked in aluminum or glass. If you do a lot of wok cooking, you can bring up your deposit score.

Part II: Withdrawals

1–6. A government survey estimated that about 93 percent of all American women eat less than the Recommended Dietary Allowance of iron. That's the first strike against women. The second is blood loss from menstruation.

Why women need almost twice as much daily iron as men.

Iron is used by the body to form hemoglobin in the blood to help circulate oxygen and carbon dioxide. Because of its presence in the blood, any blood loss—from menstruation, surgery, ulcers, colitis, hemorrhoids, blood donations, even minor bleeding caused by aspirin—can leach iron from your system. Though men can certainly undergo surgery, have colitis or take aspirin, they're not as vulnerable as women. Why? Because menstruation, especially heavy menstruation (such as that caused by intrauterine devices), is a regular, monthly blood loss. It's an iron withdrawal women can, unfortunately, count on.

That's why the Recommended Dietary Allowance for women is almost twice that for men. And women also often face a third strike: a low-calorie (and often low-meat) diet.

7. Even when women aren't dieting, they simply do not eat as many calories as men, and their intake of red meat and liver is lower. Some researchers believe they would have to eat at least as much as men to get that precious 18 milligrams of iron a day.

8. Here's another rub for women. When menopause hits, it becomes much easier for a woman to get enough iron. But menopause means you're getting older, and studies have shown the risk of iron deficiency increases with age for both men and women.

9. Drinking a cup of tea with a meal, even a meal containing a large quantity of meat and vitamin C, can reduce your iron absorption by one-half to almost two-thirds, according to several studies. Why? Researchers believe it's the tannic acid in tea that binds to the iron in the meal and makes it impossible for the body to absorb it. There are a number of other iron inhibitors.

Tea with meals can cheat your body of iron.

10. The common additives EDTA and phosphates, which are added to soft drinks, baked goods and other foods, can prevent iron from being absorbed.

11. Though not as potent as tea, coffee taken during or after a meal can decrease iron absorption by about 39 percent.

Coffee, too, can block iron uptake.

12. Diets high in fiber can also inhibit iron absorption, so if you're taking an iron supplement, it would be best to take it well before meals.

13. Because the most bioavailable iron is in meat, vegetarians have a harder time getting the iron they need. More careful diet management—assembling a menu rich in iron-containing vegetables and nutrient enhancers—as well as supplementation might be in order for these individuals.

14. Inorganic calcium can be a potent iron blocker. Researchers have also looked at dairy prod-

Antacids, pollution and stress also take their toll.

ucts that are high in calcium, but there's no clear evidence available to include them in the risk-factor category.

15. Why antacids? They can decrease the ability of gastric juices in the body to dissolve dietary iron.

16. Cadmium and lead, common industrial pollutants, are known iron inhibitors.

17. Strenuous exercise can rob you of iron. So-called sports anemia is relatively rare and may, in fact, be more related to diet than to exercise. Unless you are a very active person eating a low-calorie, iron-poor diet, you probably do not have to worry about this risk factor.

18. Stress robs us of so many things that it should be no surprise that iron is among them.

The Health Power of Magnesium: A Medical Roundup

M rs. C. B. arrived in the hospital in really bad shape. The 82-year-old woman was so weak and unresponsive that the admitting doctors suspected that she had had a stroke or had low-grade spinal meningitis, but tests for those conditions proved negative.

John Sheehan, M.D., examined her. She had long-term but controlled congestive heart failure. For several years she had been taking both a diuretic and digitalis. She also took potassium chloride to counteract the potassium-draining effect of the diuretic. In the past year, she had become increasingly drowsy and weak and then completely bedridden.

Dr. Sheehan did two very simple things. He tested the woman's blood for its level of magnesium. Her level fell within what some doctors consider a low but normal range, but one that Dr. Sheehan considered too low. Then he started Mrs. C. B. on intravenous magnesium sulfate. Some 24 hours later, the treatment completed, Mrs. C. B. got out of bed and walked—for the first time in six months.

A dramatic case of too little magnesium.

The Secret of Her Success

Mrs. C. B.'s almost instant rejuvenation may seem miraculous, but it came as no surprise to Dr. Sheehan. First in Dublin, Ireland, then at the Cleveland Clinic Foundation's Department of Endocrinology, and now at University Hospital's Department of Medicine, also in Cleveland, he has been using different forms of magnesium for several years to treat patients like Mrs. C. B. for a variety of arrhythmias (heartbeat irregularities), all with success.

Over an 18-month period, for example, Dr. Sheehan examined 25 patients with uncontrolled atrial fibrillation—heartbeat irregularities—that were not responding to traditional treatment. He found that 20 of the patients were magnesium deficient. The fibrillation stabilized in every case when they were given magnesium by injection. And it remained stable as long as their magnesium levels remained normal and they avoided alcohol, which causes magnesium to be excreted in the urine. One man who had controlled his heart palpitations very nicely for three months by eating four magnesium-rich bananas a day and staying on the wagon found his heart arrythmia returned after a weekend of beer drinking. Magnesium corrected the problem promptly.

Alcohol can flush out magnesium.

Work by other researchers indicates that magnesium deficiencies may play a crucial role in many of the major diseases that plague us—congestive heart disease, heart attacks (particularly sudden attacks), angina, arrhythmia, strokes, high blood pressure and even epilepsy and migraine headaches.

Magnesium deficiencies may be involved in major circulatory diseases.

Burton M. Altura, Ph.D., of the Downstate Medical Center in Brooklyn, and his wife, Bella T. Altura, Ph.D., are probably the world's experts on magnesium. It is their belief that magnesium deficiencies are a likely factor in many diseases or conditions that involve constriction or spasm of the heart and circulatory system. Their findings also indicate that an optimum intake of magnesium can go a long way toward preventing those diseases and alleviating their symptoms.

In fact, the only really surprising thing about magnesium is that so few doctors outside the research field diagnose and treat its deficiency or use it to help maintain health.

Just what is magnesium and how does it work?

Magnesium Involved in Many Body Functions

Magnesium is one of the body's major electrolytes, along with potassium, calcium and sodium. When dissolved, these minerals form the salty, electricity-conducting soup that bathes and permeates the cells of our body —in blood serum, spinal fluid and intracellular liquid.

Magnesium is known to be involved in many functions, including enzyme and hormonal actions, the metabolism of carbohydrates and DNA production. But one of its more important and better-studied roles is in nerve and muscle tissue function. Magnesium seems to regulate the balance of calcium and sodium in our cells, particularly in our heart and blood vessels.

The Alturas, in a review article of 30 years of research, published in the journal *Magnesium*, say magnesium may control what they call the "sodium-calcium pump," which is essential for the maintenance of normal coronary artery muscle tone.

Too little magnesium allows calcium and sodium to flood the cells. And since those two minerals are constricting agents, the muscle tissue turns to knots.

All this means is that an adequate intake of magnesium helps our hearts to beat smoothly and regularly and withstand the stress and abuse of daily life. It also means magnesium helps our blood vessels remain open and relaxed, lowering our blood pressure.

A buffer against life's stresses and strains.

Hard Water Provides a Clue to Heart Health

Numerous studies done in England, Finland, Ireland, Canada and the United States show that people who live in areas with magnesium-rich "hard" water have a lower rate of cardiovascular disease and sudden-death heart attacks than people who live in areas with magnesium-poor "soft" water. People living in many soft-water regions are also found to have higher-than-normal blood pressure levels.

Researchers have known for years that inducing a magnesium deficiency in dogs raises their blood pressure and, conversely, that an infusion of magnesium lowers their blood pressure. It hasn't been until relatively recently, though, that magnesium has been tried in clinical experiments to reduce blood pressure in people.

In 1982, doctors at the Veterans Administration Medical Center in Oklahoma City found that patients with low serum magnesium required more drugs to control their high blood pressure than those with normal levels.

Magnesium can make it easier to control blood pressure with drugs.

They also noted that low magnesium levels may be caused by the diuretics given for high blood pressure, which in turn may interfere with the effectiveness of other blood pressure medications.

And at University Hospital in Umea, Sweden, 20 patients receiving long-term diuretics—18 for high blood pressure, 2 for congestive heart failure—were given 365 milligrams of magnesium supplements for six months. Nineteen of the 20 showed a drop in blood pressure. In 3 patients, blood pressure dropped so low that the amount of magnesium was reduced. In 3 others, the amount of diuretic being used to treat the hypertension was reduced (*British Medical Journal*).

Magnesium and Artery Health

According to Dr. Burton Altura, high magnesium levels correspond with lowered levels of cholesterol. He said that it is possible to prevent the formation of the plaque found in degenerated and thickened blood vessel tissue experimentally by increasing the dietary intake of magnesium.

An intriguing possibility: preventing life-threatening blood clots.

Magnesium deficiency is known to be accompanied by an increased tendency of blood to clot. Says Dr. Altura, "Since magnesium is also known to possess platelet-stabilizing action, one must consider the strong possibility that this mineral may either reduce the incidence of, or prevent, thrombosis [blood clotting] in the coronary, pulmonary and cerebral" blood vessels, which can be life-threatening.

The brain's blood vessel tissues have twice the concentration of magnesium of any other tissue in the body, and they seem particularly sensitive to changes in its concentration. A magnesium deficiency causes these vessels to clamp down just as surely as it does heart vessels.

Using dogs, the Alturas measured the degree of tension in cerebral arteries, first in a magnesium-free solution, then in a magnesium-rich one. Without magnesium, the arteries showed a rapid increase in tension, the Alturas report. In contrast, a sudden increase in magnesium resulted in a rapid relaxation of tension in the cerebral arteries.

Can magnesium reduce the risk of stroke?

The Alturas also found that potent brain blood vessel spasms brought on by other substances such as serotonin and prostaglandins were relaxed "rather easily and dramatically" by the addition of magnesium.

The Alturas suggest that magnesium therapy may be beneficial in brain ischemia (blood deficiency) and blood vessel spasm of unknown origin, and for the prevention of strokes and the blockage of the brain's blood vessels.

Magnesium May Relieve Migraines

Migraine headaches are also known to be caused by blood vessel spasm. In fact, migraines are common in early and late pregnancy, a time when women are often magnesium deficient. They can also suffer from another deadly disease, preeclampsia, which current research shows is related to magnesium deficiency.

Migraines respond to magnesium.

Migraines are particularly responsive to magnesium therapy, says Kenneth Weaver, M.D., of East Tennessee State University. He studied 500 women:

300 were pregnant, and about 60 were taking oral contraceptives, which often induce migraine. All 500 suffered from migraine headaches. Each began taking 200 milligrams a day of magnesium. Eighty percent soon found their migraines were completely gone. In fact, relief was so quick that a woman feeling a migraine headache coming on could take magnesium, and within half an hour, the symptoms would disappear.

A dietary approach to epilepsy.

Researchers at the International Center for the Disabled (ICD) in New York City have found magnesium deficiencies in the red blood cells of a number of epileptics whose seizures were not being controlled by medication. Robert Fried, Ph.D., director of research, and Richard Carlton, M.D., have reported that by using biofeedback, controlled breathing exercises and a diet free of excess dairy products, sugar, coffee and alcohol, they were able to cut the number of seizures from up to five a week to one or less a month. Some of the patients have been seizure free for months at a time for the first time in many years.

The researchers said they plan to add magnesium supplements to their patients' diets. They expect this will lead to even fewer seizures for their epileptic patients.

A True Deficiency

Fifteen or 20 years ago, magnesium deficiencies were considered rare. Now, those in the forefront of magnesium research say this mineral deficiency is much more widespread than most doctors realize and that it is rapidly becoming more common.

Are doctors overlooking magnesium deficiencies?

"Nutritional statistics, especially in the Western world, indicate that our dietary intake of magnesium has been steadily declining since the turn of the century, to where many of us now border on a 'true' deficiency," say the Alturas. A study done at the University of Tennessee at Knoxville found that most of the pregnant women questioned got 60 percent or less of the Recommended Dietary Allowance (RDA) of magnesium. Dr. Weaver estimates that "at least" 50 percent of the young women he sees are magnesium deficient. Dr. Sheehan believes that about one-half of the older adults he treats suffer from magnesium deficiency.

Many doctors rarely think of the possibility of a magnesium deficiency, Dr. Sheehan says. In the patients he sees, for instance, the attending doctor often assumes symptoms of weakness, heart irregularities and depression are the untreatable result of the underlying disease, which is often congestive heart failure. In the patients whose heart arrhythmias he successfully treated with magnesium, none of the physicians taking care of the patients acknowledged the low-magnesium laboratory report or treated the patient with magnesium.

Dr. Sheehan also says the lower limit of what is considered a "normal" serum magnesium level keeps dropping, which it shouldn't. "If I had accepted what some doctors say is a normal serum blood level of magnesium, I would have had to drop half of the patients in my study, all of whom benefited greatly from magnesium treatment."

Certainly one of the reasons for an increase in magnesium deficiencies is that people are living longer and surviving chronic diseases with treatments—diuretics, digitalis, antibiotics, chemotherapy—that are all magnesium depleting.

Poor diet is a major cause, and one we can do something about. The RDA for magnesium is 350 to 400 milligrams a day, and many researchers say that amount is too low. Nuts, beans, whole grains and green leafy vegetables are good sources of magnesium. (For others, see the table, Best Food Sources of Magnesium, on pages 202–3.) Alcohol, fats and too much protein deplete magnesium. And magnesium works in close balance with calcium. You should be getting about 1½ times more calcium than magnesium. You can enhance magnesium's healing properties by getting adequate amounts of vitamin B_6.

Balancing magnesium with other nutrients.

Best Food Sources of Magnesium

Food	Portion	Magnesium (mg.)
Soy flour, full fat, raw	½ cup	180
Tofu, regular, raw	½ cup	127
Almonds, dried, unblanched	¼ cup	105
Black-eyed peas, dried	¼ cup	98
Soybeans, dry-roasted	¼ cup	98
Wheat germ, toasted	¼ cup	91
Cashews, dry-roasted	¼ cup	89
Brazil nuts, dried, unblanched	¼ cup	79
Spinach, cooked	½ cup	79
Swiss chard, cooked, chopped	½ cup	75
Rye flour, light	½ cup	74
Soybeans, boiled	½ cup	74
Whole wheat flour	½ cup	68
Peanuts, all types, dry-roasted	¼ cup	64
Walnuts, black, dried	¼ cup	63
Oatmeal, regular, quick	1 cup	56
Peanut flour, defatted	¼ cup	56
Potato, baked	1 medium	55

SOURCES: Adapted from

Composition of Foods, Agriculture Handbook No. 8, by Bernice K. Watt and Annabel L. Merrill (Washington, D.C: Agricultural Research Service, U.S. Department of Agriculture, 1975).

Composition of Foods: Beef Products, Agriculture Handbook No. 8–13, by Nutrition Monitoring Division (Washington, D.C.: Human Nutrition Research Service, U.S. Department of Agriculture, 1986).

Composition of Foods: Breakfast Cereals, Agriculture Handbook No. 8–8, by Consumer Nutrition Center (Washington, D.C.: Human Nutrition Information Service, U.S. Department of Agriculture, 1982).

Composition of Foods: Dairy and Egg Products, Agriculture Handbook No. 8–1, by Consumer and Food Economics Institute (Washington, D.C.: Agricultural Research Service, U.S. Department of Agriculture, 1976).

Composition of Foods: Fruits and Fruit Juices, Agriculture Handbook No. 8–9, by Consumer Nutrition Center (Washington, D.C.: Human Nutrition Information Service, U.S. Department of Agriculture, 1982).

Food	Portion	Magnesium (mg.)
Shredded wheat, small biscuit	1 cup	55
Blackstrap molasses	1 tbsp.	52
Beet greens, cooked	½ cup	49
Lima beans, baby, boiled	½ cup	49
Avocado	½	40
Kidney beans, all types, boiled	½ cup	40
Banana	1	35
Pecans, halves, dried	¼ cup	35
Salmon, sockeye, canned	4 oz.	33
Brown rice, cooked	½ cup	28
Milk, skim	1 cup	28
Peanut butter, smooth	1 tbsp.	25
Beef, round, full cut, separable lean only, broiled	3 oz.	24
Buckwheat flour, light	½ cup	24
Chestnuts, European, roasted	½ cup	24
Spinach, raw, chopped	½ cup	22
Collards, cooked, chopped	½ cup	11

Composition of Foods: Legumes and Legume Products, Agriculture Handbook No. 8–16, by Nutrition Monitoring Division (Washington, D.C.: Human Nutrition Information Service, U.S. Department of Agriculture, 1986).

Composition of Foods: Nut and Seed Products, Agriculture Handbook No. 8–12, by Nutrition Monitoring Division (Washington, D.C.: Human Nutrition Information Service, U.S. Department of Agriculture, 1984).

Composition of Foods: Vegetables and Vegetable Products, Agriculture Handbook No. 8–11, by Nutrition Monitoring Division (Washington, D.C.: Human Nutrition Information Service, U.S. Department of Agriculture, 1984).

Nutrient Data Research Branch, U.S. Department of Agriculture, Washington, D.C.

Chapter 27

More Health Power from Magnesium

Everybody needs it, some owe their lives to it and doctors are starting to give it serious attention—magnesium is a little mineral with a big future. And the main reason is that scientific evidence on the health benefits of this mineral is coming in too fast to ignore.

Here's a rundown on further developments in this research.

Angina Attacks Stopped Cold

Following in the footsteps of other scientists, researchers in Israel have successfully treated 15 people afflicted with recurring spasm angina. At each bout of chest pains, the doctors injected the patients with magnesium. And 30 seconds to 5 minutes later, the attacks ceased. Ordinarily such attacks would last 5 to 15 minutes.

After these scientists demonstrated that they could use magnesium in angina treatment, they set out to test the mineral in angina prevention. They found that in several patients they could consistently provoke an angina attack by immersing the patients' hands in cold water. But if they injected the patients with magnesium before immersion, no attacks occurred. Magnesium apparently stopped the chest pains before they got started.

The results of these and other studies suggest that magnesium may one day replace or complement drugs as therapy for angina.

Magnesium stopped angina attacks before they got started.

Diabetic Seizures Vanish

It's well established that intravenous magnesium is an anticonvulsant (agent for preventing or relieving convulsions) and that people with magnesium deficiencies sometimes suffer convulsions and tremors.

Doctors at the Bronx-Lebanon Hospital Center in the Bronx, New York, have used magnesium to stop seizures in people who have uncontrolled diabetes mellitus.

The seizures—marked by convulsive muscle contractions and jerky movements—afflicted three women with the disease. When the women were admitted to the hospital, their seizures were lasting from 30 seconds to three minutes, occurring every five to ten minutes. The doctors treated the patients' diabetes, but the seizures wouldn't stop. Since the physicians knew that magnesium deficiency is common in people with severe diabetes mellitus, they decided to inject the women with the mineral—and the injections worked. The seizures vanished within 24 hours after starting magnesium therapy.

Magnesium relieved seizures in diabetic women.

"It therefore appears," the doctors report, "that magnesium deficiency was the main cause of the neuromuscular abnormality."

These results will have to be confirmed by additional research. But they do suggest an intriguing question: Can magnesium quell other kinds of seizures, including epileptic ones? Scientists surely will try to find out.

Heart Attack Damage Reduced

Research in both animals and people has hinted that magnesium may do "damage control" work during a heart attack, lessening the destruction of vital heart tissue.

Magnesium may reduce damage from heart attacks.

Sherman Bloom, M.D., of George Washington University School of Medicine in Washington, D.C., has confirmed the earlier investigations. In a study focusing on heart attacks in dogs, he discovered that the animals on a low-magnesium diet suffered twice as much heart damage after an attack as animals on diets with adequate magnesium.

"When people have heart attacks—and they can have them without even knowing it—the critical consideration is how much damage is done to the heart muscle," Dr. Bloom says. "Every increase in infarcted area [destroyed tissue] increases your chances of dying in the aftermath of an attack. My study and research done by others indicate that magnesium is one very important determinant of how much damage a heart attack does."

"The data suggest," says Dr. Bloom, "that dietary magnesium intake is an important determining factor in your ability to withstand a heart attack. You should ensure that you're getting adequate amounts of magnesium in your diet."

Type-A Behavior and High Blood Pressure

The available evidence has suggested a compelling hypothesis: Type-A people (those who are hard-driving, impatient and excitable) react to stress by developing magnesium deficiencies, which in turn exaggerate the ill effects of stress and lead to high blood pressure.

Stress depletes the body of magnesium.

Not too long ago, investigators in Paris reinforced the hypothesis when they studied 20 Type-A young men under stress.

When they gave those Type-A young men a stress-producing task to perform and monitored the magnesium in their bodies, the researchers uncovered an odd biochemical routine. Magnesium leached out of red blood cells and was shunted out of the body via the urine. This magnesium depletion happened in almost twice as many of the Type-A people as in a comparable group of more relaxed Type-B subjects.

"Type-A behavior personalities," says head researcher Jean-Georges Henrotte, M.D., "would be involved in a vicious circle in which their tendency to chronic self-induced stress would lead them to a progressively increasing state of magnesium deficiency."

And a lack of magnesium, as other research indicates, is probably a contributor to high blood pressure. Conversely, magnesium supplementation has actually been used to lower blood pressure.

Magnesium has been used to lower high blood pressure.

"These results," says Dr. Henrotte, "should be, of course, confirmed on a larger group of individuals."

The Unhealthful Impact of Stress

Researchers have concluded that Type-A people may not be the only ones caught in a cycle of stress and magnesium deficiency. Studies have suggested that stress in almost anyone can deplete magnesium and that such depletion can magnify stress-induced ills.

Scientists at the University of Hohenheim in West Germany uncovered evidence that this stress/depletion cycle may be halted with magnesium supplements.

In studies of thousands of pigs subjected to the typical stresses of confinement, the researchers found that they could reduce the death rate of the animals by giving them extra magnesium. In fact, the death rates of supplemented pigs were one-seventh to one-half as high as the death rates of pigs getting normal levels of magnesium.

Magnesium supplements reduced the death rate.

"These studies and others like them," says chief investigator Hans G. Classen, Ph.D., "indicate that with adequate magnesium stores, people may be better able to withstand the ravages of stress in their daily lives."

Irregular Heartbeat Normalized

Doctors have shown that magnesium may play a key role in the treatment of the potentially dangerous condition of arrhythmia, or irregular heartbeat.

**Magnesium halted ar-
rhythmias.**

Investigators at the University of California-Irvine College of Medicine corroborated the earlier evidence by using magnesium successfully to treat arrhythmia patients after standard therapies had failed.

"We've studied several patients with acute, life-threatening arrhythmias that wouldn't respond to either drugs or shock therapy," says chief researcher Lloyd T. Iseri, M.D. "But when the patients received magnesium, their heartbeats reverted to normal rhythm. The magnesium had an almost instant effect, whereas some drugs may take minutes to influence the arrhythmias."

It remains to be seen whether magnesium will become the therapy of choice in the treatment of arrhythmia.

Better Brain Function

Medical people have firmly documented the harm done to muscles and nerves by magnesium deficiency, but they know much less about what a lack of the mineral can do to the brain.

**Magnesium brought pa-
tients out of comas.**

Paul G. Cohen, M.D., of Atlanta, reports that he's treated three adults suffering from brain disease and low magnesium levels. All three eventually lapsed into a coma. But when he gave them magnesium, they responded immediately. There was, Dr. Cohen says, "prompt reversal of encephalopathy [brain dysfunction] and coma."

Just how common are such symptoms in people lacking magnesium? How often is the magnesium connection overlooked? Future research and clinical experience will have to supply the answers.

Toxic Shock Syndrome Responds to Mineral Replacement

In toxic shock syndrome (TSS), the rare but sometimes fatal disorder found predominantly but not exclusively in menstruating women, doctors know that calcium deficiency is common. What they don't know is what role magnesium plays in this disease.

J. H. Rudick, M.D., of Case Western Reserve University in Cleveland, and a colleague discovered that magnesium depletion may be a little-known finding in

Is magnesium deficiency a key to toxic shock syndrome?

Dossier on Magnesium

Here's an abbreviated report on magnesium: how much you need, who may be deficient, and why it's necessary.

Recommended Dietary Allowance (RDA)
> 300 milligrams daily for nonpregnant women.
> 450 milligrams daily for pregnant women.
> 350 milligrams daily for men.

Maximum Recommended Dosage
> 400 milligrams for nonpregnant women. (Although dosages slightly above this are considered safe, medical supervision is recommended when this limit is exceeded.)

Possible Deficiency Symptoms
> Irritability, nervousness, muscle weakness, high blood pressure, convulsions, tremors, arrhythmia.

Prevalence of Deficiencies
> Surveys indicate that average daily diets contain only 200 to 250 milligrams of magnesium. Deficiencies may be especially widespread in pregnant women. One study of expectant mothers revealed that most got only 60 percent or less of the RDA of magnesium.

TSS—a feature that could contribute to the severity of hypocalcemia (low levels of calcium in the blood) found in TSS patients.

The doctors examined two women with TSS and found low magnesium levels and functional hypoparathyroidism—two conditions known to sometimes accompany one another. "We conclude," Dr. Rudick says, "that life-threatening hypocalcemia in certain magnesium-depleted TSS patients may be averted by magnesium replacement therapy. And it seems reasonable that physicians should consider testing magnesium levels in TSS cases."

Selenium:
The Great Protector

Selenium is best known as a cancer fighter. That exciting news was first heralded a decade or so ago when selenium—initially thought to cause cancer—was found in low levels in the soil in areas where cancer incidence was high. And a lot has been happening in selenium research ever since. Positive—but preliminary—anticancer results have been found in people as well as in animals for skin, lung, mouth and throat cancers. Let's take a look at some of the evidence of that research.

A Roundup
of Encouraging Studies

At the University of North Carolina in Chapel Hill, 240 people with skin cancer were compared with people who were similar in all respects except they had no cancer. Patients with low selenium levels had a consistent increase in the risk of skin cancer (*Dietary Aspects of Carcinogenesis*).

At the University of Miami, researchers tested the theory that people who live in geographical areas where the soil and crops contain higher levels of selenium are less likely to get head and neck cancer. (In Florida, selenium levels are among the lowest in the nation.) They found that the 52 cancer victims in their study had depressed levels of selenium in their red blood cells as well as low levels of the important

Evidence shows selenium is an anticancer agent.

enzyme GSH-Px. However, selenium levels in their blood plasma were high compared to the control group, indicating to the scientists that the cancer patients had a blunted ability to transport selenium into their cells (*Cancer*). These results, say the researchers, suggest that selenium supplements might help correct this problem.

Then there's a lung cancer study published in China. "There was an area of China that had a very high incidence of lung cancer, and the researchers wanted to find out why," says Gerhard N. Schrauzer, Ph.D., a pioneer in selenium research who is familiar with the Chinese study. "When the subjects were analyzed, it turned out they had very low selenium levels. The soil in the area in which they lived had very low selenium levels also. So they went to an area where the selenium in the soil was very rich. The people there had a very low lung cancer rate."

People living in areas with selenium-rich soil had less lung cancer.

Finally, there are animal studies: At Baylor College of Medicine in Houston, researchers found that selenium supplementation reduced the incidence of breast tumors from 80 percent to 18 percent in mice. Selenium also reduced the incidence of other cancer-induced tumors from 40 percent to 6 percent (*Dietary Aspects of Carcinogenesis*).

At the Eppley Institute for Research in Cancer, at the University of Nebraska Medical Center, Omaha, both very high (toxic) and very low doses of selenium were fed to male and female rats. Colon cancer was found in only 16 out of 30 male rats fed very high doses of selenium but in 28 out of 29 of the male rats on the low-selenium diet. Lung cancer was found in none of the 30 male rats fed the high-selenium diet, while the incidence of cancer for those on the low-selenium diet was 14 percent. None of the female rats developed cancer at either selenium dosage (*Cancer Research*).

In animals, high doses of selenium meant a low incidence of cancer.

In Germany, animals were fed selenium to test its cancer-preventive ability. Of 50 mice not treated with selenium, 31 developed tumors. Of the 50 animals treated with selenium, only 14 developed tumors. And these tumors were less than half the size of the tumors that developed in the nontreated animals (*Journal of Cancer Research and Clinical Oncology*). "We must infer that selenium must be one of the few chemical elements to which a tumor-preventive effect can be attributed," noted the researchers. "The results of our own investigations enhance and amplify present knowledge of this anticarcinogenic action of selenium."

How Selenium Battles Disease

Why does selenium work so well against cancer? "Selenium stimulates the immune system," says Dr. Schrauzer. "It also alters the metabolism of carcinogenic substances, thus preventing an accumulation of free radicals."

One of the biggest mysteries in selenium research is still in the investigative stage: How much selenium do we actually metabolize from the foods we eat? Ara Nahapetian, Ph.D., was among a group of researchers at the Massachusetts Institute of Technology (MIT) who tried to answer just that question.

How much selenium can our bodies derive from food?

"Selenium is an essential micronutrient," he says. "Without it, we will die. But we also know that taking too much can have harmful effects. What we're trying to find out is how much is absorbed and how much is excreted." Using a state-of-the-art technique, the MIT researchers measured small amounts of the trace mineral as it goes through the human system. But a full understanding of how efficiently our bodies use the nutrient is still up in the air, says Dr. Nahapetian.

Where to Find Selenium?
Think "Protein"

But until we find out, it's good to know that there are plenty of foods that contain selenium. Fish is by

Selenium and Vitamin E versus Aging

Large doses of vitamin E and the trace mineral selenium significantly improved the overall well-being of a group of elderly nursing-home residents, Finnish researchers reported in *Biological Trace Element Research*.

The researchers gave daily doses of 400 milligrams of vitamin E, 8 milligrams of sodium selenate and 50 micrograms of organic selenium to 15 residents (average age 76) for a year. Compared with a similar, untreated control group, the vitamin-treated subjects showed significant improvement in mental alertness, emotional stability, depression, anxiety, fatigue and other measures of overall health. "A distinct improvement of the general condition was noticed after only two months, and the improvement continued up to the end of the one-year study period," the researchers noted. "There were no side effects whatsoever," they added.

Warning: In large doses, selenium can be toxic. *Moral:* Let the dust settle on this exciting new discovery until safe guidelines can be established.

The best sources of selenium.

far the richest source of selenium, and tuna fish is one of the best. Whole wheat bread, liver, kidneys, Brazil nuts and rice are other rich sources of selenium. The mineral can also be found in many protein-rich foods.

While the Recommended Dietary Allowance (RDA) for selenium is 50 to 200 micrograms per day, Americans get, on average, only 85 micrograms a day. Dr. Schrauzer thinks that just isn't enough. "I feel 200 micrograms is the minimum and from 250 to 350 micrograms is the optimal total intake for preventive measures," he says.

Too much selenium can be toxic; in *supplement form,* probably no more than about 100 micrograms a day should be taken.

"Selenium is probably one of the least-thought-about trace minerals there is. But the evidence keeps piling up that selenium is important in preventing a whole list of conditions, and at the top of the list is cancer," says Dr. Schrauzer.

"A lot of people worry about their intakes of calcium and iron," he continues. "I predict in a few years selenium will also be a common concern. When it comes to trace minerals, don't forget selenium!"

Chapter 29

Zinc:
The Whole-Body
Mineral

I t has only been since 1974 that zinc was recognized as essential and given a Recommended Dietary Allowance (RDA) of 15 milligrams daily. But in that short time, this trace mineral has been shown to have a profound influence on the body's ability to grow and to resist disease. Male sexual maturity and fertility depend on adequate zinc. And some researchers think our declining ability to absorb zinc, along with other nutrients, as we age is one reason we become more vulnerable to disease.

So far, researchers have found more than 90 zinc-dependent enzymes in the body—more than those of all the other minerals combined, including iron. Each is involved in a different biochemical reaction. But we need to know only two closely related facts about zinc to understand a good part of its importance.

Over 90 enzymes in your body need zinc to do their job.

The Facts about Zinc and Basic Good Health

First, zinc is needed for the body to make protein. Zinc-containing enzymes help to string together the long chains of amino acids that make up each molecule of protein.

Second, every cell's genetic material, its DNA and RNA, is derived from protein.

What this means is that your body needs zinc to make every one of its cells—from the hair on your head to the soles of your feet. Severe deficiencies mean that needed cells may not get made. They also mean that it is more difficult to repair damaged genetic material.

Because cell growth is so dependent on zinc, it's first missed when or where rapid cell growth occurs—in pregnancy, childhood, wound healing and any other situation involving rapidly dividing cells. One of these areas is the immune response.

Rapid cell growth—in wound healing, for example—demands zinc.

"Severe zinc deficiency has been shown to cause major abnormalities in the body's immune defense," says Susanna Cunningham-Rundles, Ph.D., at the New York Hospital, Cornell Medical Center in New York City.

One reason for this impact is that any effective immune response involves a massive buildup of the white blood cells that fight bacteria, viruses and cancer. For instance, one type of white blood cell, called a neutrophil, can multiply five times within a few hours after infection sets in. And another kind of white blood cell, called a lymphocyte, can divide and form up to 500 new cells in four days.

Immunity lags without enough zinc.

"Studies show that if zinc is not present in the quantities needed, this sort of cell proliferation is reduced, and the immune response will be lessened," Dr. Cunningham-Rundles says.

And there are other roles zinc plays in the immune response.

"Zinc is probably essential for the work of thymic hormones," Dr. Cunningham-Rundles says. These hormones, secreted by the thymus gland, are responsible for the development of T-cells, types of lymphocytes central to the fight against viral and bacterial infections.

Zinc will also increase the activity of lymphocytes called natural killer cells, even when there is not an apparent zinc deficiency. Because these cells are able to destroy a virus- or bacteria-invaded cell without the prior sensitization that all other lymphocytes require, they are considered part of the body's first line of defense against disease.

Your body needs zinc to fight off bacteria and viruses.

Zinc teams up with A to protect skin cells.

Zinc also seems to interact with vitamin A, a nutrient that seems to have a protective effect against cancer. Certain cells, called epithelial cells, may be particularly dependent on both A and zinc. These cells cover a surface, like the skin, or line a cavity, like the bladder. It's not incidental that these cells also have the most rapid turnover of any in the body. Or that throat cancers have been linked with both vitamin A and zinc deficiencies.

One area where epithelial cells are found is in the mammary gland. Michael Bunk, Ph.D., a research scientist at Memorial Sloan-Kettering Cancer Center in New York City, found that mice made zinc deficient also became deficient in vitamin A.

Zinc, the Thymus and Immunity

We all know that it's our immune system that comes between us and disease. But for some (especially older people and children with Down's syndrome), the system all too often fails. In the past, doctors usually placed the blame on a faulty thymus gland.

Italian researchers have found that a deficiency of zinc (and not the thymus) may be directly responsible for at least part of that failure in these two groups of people. Here's how.

The thymus puts out a hormone called FTS, which is needed for immunity. But this hormone's activity is dependent on zinc. When the researchers measured FTS and zinc levels in these patients, they found both a zinc deficiency and diminished FTS activity.

The researchers think that even marginal zinc deficiencies (which are widespread) may impair FTS activity. Therefore, "careful zinc monitoring should be applied to all patients who show low FTS activity" (*Lancet*).

"It's pretty well known that zinc deficiency affects the release of stored vitamin A from the liver," Dr. Bunk says. He thinks there may be a second connection, that a zinc deficiency impairs the uptake of vitamin A by the epithelial cells, putting them at risk for developing cancer or other diseases.

Zinc and vitamin A work hand in hand.

Links with Eating Disorders

Doctors have known for some time that too little zinc can alter the senses of taste and smell. A lack of zinc changes the chemistry of saliva, which directly affects the way things taste in the mouth. Zinc-poor people have trouble tasting sweets, for instance.

But zinc may also affect areas of the brain that receive and process information from taste and smell sensors. And that, in part, has led some researchers to speculate that zinc could influence areas of the brain that control eating and drinking behavior.

"Animal studies seem to indicate that zinc deficiencies could play a role in eating disorders like anorexia and bulimia," says Craig McClain, M.D., associate professor of medicine and director of the Division of Gastroenterology at the University of Kentucky School of Medicine, Lexington. Studies he and his colleagues have done indicate that zinc-deprived rats develop the same bizarre eating habits as teenage girls diagnosed as anorexic, bulimic or bulimirexic, a combination of both disorders. Like the girls, the zinc-deprived rats ate less and less until they were consuming only about a third the normal amount. When they did eat, they tended to pig out, and they also tended to easily regurgitate their food. What's more, when they were subjected to stress (mildly pinched tails), they headed straight for the rat chow! When adequate zinc was added to their diet, the rats' eating behavior returned to normal (*Physiology and Behavior*).

In another study, Dr. McClain found that nine bulimirexic women were extremely low in zinc, even when they were within normal weight ranges, and other nutritional signs were normal. "Many of these

Animals without zinc act like people with bulimia or anorexia.

women's habits—laxative abuse, vomiting, dieting—would definitely put them at risk for a zinc deficiency," Dr. McClain says (*Clinical Research*).

One question is, which comes first: the zinc deficiency or the eating problem? "It's possible that a zinc-poor diet, which wouldn't be all that unusual in teenage girls, could trigger eating problems," Dr. McClain says. "Or the eating problem could be triggered by psychological or social problems."

Can zinc supplements help anorexics break the habit? Perhaps, Dr. McClain says. "That's what we intend to study next. Until results are in with humans, though, about the only recommendation I can give people with eating disorders is to make sure they're getting the RDA of zinc."

Advice for people with eating disorders: Get your daily ration of zinc.

Zinc, Alcohol and Obesity

Surprising connections also seem to exist between zinc deficiencies, alcohol abuse and obesity, says Platon Collipp, M.D., former professor of pediatrics at State University of New York, Stony Brook.

He found that rats fed zinc-deficient diets voluntarily drank much more alcohol than rats fed adequate zinc. (The rats could choose between water and alcohol in their cages.) When they were then given enough zinc, their drinking declined to normal (*Alcoholism: Clinical and Experimental Research*).

Can zinc help solve drinking problems?

"People have been speculating for some time now that food intake can influence drinking behavior. I think zinc is one nutrient that could have a possible effect," says Dr. Collipp. "It would be very interesting to see how or if zinc reduces the craving for alcohol in alcoholics. I haven't been able to do that study, but it should be done. So should a study to see whether zinc supplementation in the children of alcoholics, who may be genetically zinc deficient, reduces their five-times-greater-than-normal chances of becoming alcoholics themselves."

Dr. Collipp also made an interesting discovery that may help some heavyweights. He found that a zinc deficiency is associated with the way the body handles glucose (blood sugar).

A zinc-dependent enzyme in the liver acts as a kind of railroad switch in glucose metabolism. Called a branch-point enzyme, it's located right at the spot in glucose metabolism where one reaction leads to energy burning and the other to fat storage.

The zinc/blood sugar link.

"Studies of rat livers show that when there's not enough zinc to go around, this enzyme becomes inactive," Dr. Collipp says. "The result is that glucose is shunted toward making triglycerides [blood fats] that can be stored in the fatty tissues rather than being burned for energy (*Pediatrics Annals*).

"There are some people who say that everything they eat turns to fat," he says. "Well, those people may be zinc deficient."

A Satiation Link?

Dr. Collipp also thinks there may be psychological connections in zinc's effect on eating and drinking. Zinc-deficient children don't seem to rely on "internal cues" for their behavior, he says. Such children might not be able to discern the difference between feeling hungry and feeling full, for instance.

"Quite a few studies link zinc deficiencies with brain disorders, like learning problems," Dr. Collipp says. "I think a zinc deficiency may also affect some part of the brain involved in the self-monitoring of the body, a kind of satiation center that lets you know when you've had enough to eat or drink."

Healthy Gums Need Zinc

Zinc deficiency is especially detrimental to the gums. The tissue is loaded with fibrous protein strands, and the thin layer of cells right next to the tooth's root is epithelium, says Henry Mallek, D.M.D., Ph.D., professor at the Georgetown University School of Dentistry in Washington, D.C.

You need zinc to keep your gums in the pink.

A zinc deficiency doesn't actually *cause* gum disease. Plaque does. But a deficiency makes the gums much less likely to be able to withstand the bacterial assault of plaque that inflames gums and loosens teeth.

"There are many reasons to think that people with gum disease may have zinc deficiencies," Dr. Mallek says. "I've seen people with long-term gum problems who had conventional treatment. Although it helped, the gums were not completely healthy. But when the zinc deficiency was corrected, the gum problems were resolved."

Zinc for Herpes?

Zinc helped cold sores heal rapidly.

Herpes infections—both the cold-sore and the genital kind—have been found to respond to applications of zinc in experimental treatment. Doctors at Hadassah University Hospital in Jerusalem found that herpes simplex sores treated with zinc healed in about 9½ days, compared with an average of 16 days with other forms of treatment (*Acta Dermato-Venereologica*). In Swedish studies, continued use of zinc solution after the sores healed prevented a recurrence (*British Journal of Dermatology*).

Zinc may offer hope for genital herpes.

Could zinc someday offer hope to genital herpes victims? An animal study by Patrick Tennican, M.D., director of internal medicine, Spokane, and a clinical associate professor at the University of Washington, Seattle, indicates it might, but only if it's used very early in the course of the disease.

Female mice with genital herpes were treated with either a zinc-soaked sponge, a nonmedicated sponge or oral zinc, which was started two days before they were infected. The difference between the topically treated group and the other two groups was great. Thirty-two percent of the untreated group had moderate to severe herpes symptoms by the ninth day after treatment. Only one animal with topical zinc treatment had these symptoms, and for one day only. The mice receiving oral zinc actually had more symptoms than the control group.

Encephalitis, another sign of herpes infection (in mice *only*, not in humans) was greater in the oral zinc and untreated groups. Both had a 40 percent death rate by the 15th day of the experiment, while none of the topically treated mice died. Dr. Tennican thinks the zinc prevented the herpes virus from multiplying by interfering with essential enzyme systems necessary for its replication.

Topical zinc may prevent the herpes virus from multiplying.

"I'm afraid the problem with genital herpes is that the virus quickly moves away from the site of infection to where no topical agent is going to reach it," Dr. Tennican says. "The idea of using a zinc solu-

---

Zinc and Vaccinations

Keeping your body's immune function at its best does more than prevent disease from occurring. It's also what helps make you well again when a nasty germ does get in. Either way, it can't do the job alone. That's where zinc comes in.

In one study, scientists from Michigan State University in East Lansing found that without enough zinc, the body may lose its ability to remember what it's been immunized against. The zinc deficiency may actually destroy the so-called immune memory cells, making it virtually impossible to successfully vaccinate against common diseases.

The researchers point out that simply improving the diets of malnourished people may not be enough to restore their immune response to some diseases they've previously been exposed to or vaccinated for. These people may need to be vaccinated after their bodies' nutritional stores of zinc have once again been brought up to optimal levels (*Journal of Nutrition*).

tion as a kind of 'morning after' treatment is interesting, but the fact is that there is no known topical treatment that has prevented the recurrence of genital herpes."

Zinc and Fertility

There is probably more zinc in seminal fluid than in any other fluid in the body. That finding led urologist Joel L. Marmar, M.D., to wonder if certain male fertility problems might be caused by a zinc deficiency.

Zinc may be important to the motility of sperm.

He tested some patients in his Cherry Hill, New Jersey, practice. He reports, "Out of our infertile population, 10 to 15 percent have truly low zinc levels." Zinc, he says, has an apparent influence on the swimming ability of sperm, which must be strong enough to reach a woman's fallopian tubes and penetrate the egg for fertilization to take place.

Dr. Marmar isn't sure exactly why it works, but he has had some success using zinc supplements with that small, select group of infertile patients.

Of course, not every malfunction in our body is necessarily the result of a drop in a nutrient stockpile. But new technology, allowing scientists to examine functioning nutrients in living tissue, are helping pinpoint the ones that are.

Zinc for Osteoporosis?

Osteoporosis is a hot topic these days. Increased calcium intake and weight-bearing exercises can help head it off. And it seems zinc might help, too.

Bone metabolism is another area where zinc-dependent enzymes play a role, says Joseph Soares, Ph.D., a professor of nutrition at the University of Maryland, College Park.

In bone calcification in children, the role is clear, Dr. Soares says. Zinc is needed to produce a matrix of protein threads onto which the bone-forming calcium is laid. In older people, though, the process is much slower. "Calcium deposition and removal continues into old age, but if more calcium is lost than is deposited, osteoporosis will be the result," Dr. Soares says.

"We'd like to find out if zinc can help to boost calcium deposition in the elderly. It would seem to make sense, but it's a difficult question to answer." Dr. Soares's continuing work will determine the role of supplementation in bone calcification in quail and rats. If it does, he says, "an important new development in the study and control of osteoporosis may be available."

A promising prospect: Zinc may help weak bones attract calcium.

One study by researchers in Turkey showed that victims of osteoporosis had zinc levels 25 percent lower than those without the disease. "Many older people are getting too little zinc, just as they're getting too little calcium, because of overall poor nutrition," Dr. Soares says. In fact, there's evidence to indicate that zinc intake is below the RDA for other groups as well.

A survey by the Beltsville Human Nutrition Research Center in Maryland found that middle-class adults were getting only about three-fourths of the RDA for zinc, averaging 9.9 milligrams a day. Women fared worst. Their intake was only 57 percent of the 15-milligram requirement.

Many middle-class adults are not getting enough daily zinc.

Make your food choices zinc-wise. Oysters are the richest source of zinc. Organ meats and beef are the next-best source. Three ounces of lean beef has nearly four milligrams of zinc. Grains and nuts contain fairly good, but probably less absorbable, amounts. (For a list of other zinc-rich foods, see the table, Best Food Sources of Zinc, on pages 226–27.) In fact, a nutritional survey showed vegetarians on low-calorie diets to be at particular risk for zinc deficiencies. (If you feel you need supplemental zinc, be sure not to take more than 30 milligrams a day without medical supervision.)

Zinc research can only continue to confirm how important it is to get the right amount of this essential trace mineral.

Best Food Sources of Zinc

Food	Portion	Zinc (mg.)
Oysters, raw, meat only	⅓ cup	7.12
Chicken heart, cooked	3 oz.	6.00
Calves' liver, cooked	3 oz.	5.20
Beef liver, braised	3 oz.	5.16
Beef, ground, lean, broiled, medium	3 oz.	4.56
Lamb, lean, cooked	3 oz.	4.20
Pumpkin seeds, roasted	¼ cup	4.20
Tuna, canned in oil, drained	½ cup	4.01
Beef, round, full cut, separable lean only, broiled	3 oz.	3.98
Turkey, dark-meat, cooked	3 oz.	3.80
Chicken liver, cooked	3 oz.	3.70
Chicken, dark-meat, cooked	3 oz.	2.40
Swiss cheese	2 oz.	2.20
Cashews, dry-roasted	¼ cup	1.90

SOURCES: Adapted from

Composition of Foods: Beef Products, Agriculture Handbook No. 8–13, by Nutrition Monitoring Division (Washington, D.C.: Human Nutrition Information Service, U.S. Department of Agriculture, 1986).

Composition of Foods: Breakfast Cereals, Agriculture Handbook No. 8–8, by Consumer Nutrition Center (Washington, D.C.: Human Nutrition Information Service, U.S. Department of Agriculture, 1982).

Composition of Foods: Dairy and Egg Products, Agriculture Handbook No. 8–1, by Consumer and Food Economics Institute (Washington, D.C.: Agricultural Research Service, U.S. Department of Agriculture, 1976).

Composition of Foods: Legumes and Legume Products, Agriculture Handbook No. 8–16, by Nutrition Monitoring Division (Washington, D.C.: Human Nutrition Information Service, U.S. Department of Agriculture, 1986).

Food	Portion	Zinc (mg.)
Cheddar cheese	2 oz.	1.80
Sunflower seeds, dry-roasted	¼ cup	1.70
Turkey, light-meat, cooked	3 oz.	1.70
Brazil nuts, dried	¼ cup	1.60
Black-eyed peas, cooked	½ cup	1.50
Clams, raw, meat only	3 oz.	1.34
Chick-peas, boiled	½ cup	1.25
Lentils, boiled	½ cup	1.25
Peanuts, all types, dry-roasted	¼ cup	1.20
Chicken, light-meat, cooked	3 oz.	1.10
Peas, cooked	½ cup	1.00
Filberts, dried	¼ cup	0.70
Tuna, light, canned in water	½ cup	0.70
Oats, regular, cooked	½ cup	0.60

Composition of Foods: Nut and Seed Products, Agriculture Handbook No. 8–12, by Nutrition Monitoring Division (Washington, D.C.: Human Nutrition Information Service, U.S. Department of Agriculture, 1984).

Composition of Foods: Poultry Products, Agriculture Handbook No. 8–5, by Consumer and Food Economics Institute (Washington, D.C: Science and Education Administration, U.S. Department of Agriculture, 1979).

Composition of Foods: Vegetables and Vegetable Products, Agriculture Handbook No. 8–11, by Nutrition Monitoring Division (Washington, D.C.: Human Nutrition Information Service, U.S. Department of Agriculture, 1984).

Journal of the American Dietetic Association, April, 1975.

McCance and Widdowson's The Composition of Foods, by A. A. Paul and D. A. T. Southgate (New York: Elsevier/North-Holland Biomedical, 1978).

Part **IV**

SPECIAL NUTRITIONAL ALLIES FOR HEALTH

Amino Acids: Building Blocks of Well-Being

To make muscle, you need protein. To make protein, you need amino acids.

That's one side of the amino acid picture. Scientists believe there's another side, though, one in which amino acids are no longer confined to the limited role of microscopic puzzle pieces that fit together to make protein.

Amino acids may be more than just building blocks. These essential nutrients may help regulate our emotions, lower cholesterol and reduce the pain of serious injury. Science continues to methodically peel back the layers on many amino acids, learning more about how they work in our bodies.

Identifying new health roles for protein's building blocks.

Phenylalanine and Depression

A serious shortage of certain amino acids—including phenylalanine (PHE)—may account for some depressive disorders, according to the researchers at Rush-Presbyterian/St. Luke's Medical Center in Chicago.

The Chicago researchers supplemented the diet of depressed patients with phenylalanine and discovered that, in many cases, the depression eased. It didn't work for everybody, but for some people whose lives are devastated by black moods, phenylalanine can be a godsend.

When some seriously depressed people took PHE, their depression decreased.

"In general, phenylalanine is a useful alternative to antidepressant drugs in a limited number of cases involving depression of the bipolar type," says Hector C. Sabelli, M.D., Ph.D., a psychopharmacologist on the Chicago research team. " 'Bipolar' patients can be recognized by the fact that they have recurrent depressions, they tend to be impulsive rather than anxious and they sleep too much rather than too little."

The Chicago study evolved from years of study into the brain chemistry of depressive patients.

PHE can work like an amphetamine to elevate mood.

"In the body, phenylalanine turns into the active compound phenylethylamine (PEA), which functions something like an amphetamine," says Dr. Sabelli. "It's a natural amphetamine of the brain. The question is, why do some people not form enough phenylethylamine? Is it because they don't get enough phenylalanine in the diet or they don't absorb enough, or is it that they can't transform the phenylalanine into phenylethylamine? We don't really know yet."

Most people get all the phenylalanine they need in their diet—about two grams—says Dr. Sabelli. There's some phenylalanine in all protein foods, he adds. In treating depressives, the Chicago researchers usually give two to four grams a day.

Until more is known about phenylalanine, however, Dr. Sabelli says it would be wise for those who suffer from depression to consult their family doctors or psychiatrists. He says too much phenylalanine can function like a mild amphetamine. But for many depressed people, in a clinical setting, he adds, "Phenylalanine can help a lot."

PHE can ease aches and pains.

As useful as phenylalanine may be in treating the emotional pain of depression, it may also be helpful in easing some physical aches and pains. But, as with clinical depression, phenylalanine doesn't appear to help everyone.

British researchers tested phenylalanine on 22 volunteers who suffered from a wide variety of long-standing ills, from lower back pain to spinal fusion. In seven patients, the phenylalanine, given in 250-milligram daily doses, did ease the pain. But for all the rest of the patients, phenylalanine had no effect (*Advances in Pain Research and Therapy*).

Phenylalanine may be a boon for some people, but for a small minority born with a rare genetic disorder, the problem is not too little but too much phenylalanine. The disorder is called phenylketonuria, or PKU.

People with PKU have chronically elevated levels of phenylalanine. If left untreated, a child born with PKU could become mentally retarded. With treatment—that is, a diet in which the phenylalanine content is very closely regulated—normal mental development is all but assured. But there can be serious problems—hyperactivity, short attention span and impaired motor skills—for those who go off the prescribed low-protein diet.

A low-PHE diet to treat a rare genetic disorder.

The Recovery Team: Valine, Isoleucine, Leucine

One solution to the behavioral problems caused by PKU might be found in three other amino acids— valine, isoleucine and leucine. These aminos appear to compete with phenylalanine for transport into the brain, according to researchers at the College of Mount St. Joseph in Cincinnati. Tests on six PKU patients showed that with these three neutral amino acids, behavioral and motor problems improved (*Developmental Medicine & Child Neurology*).

These three—also known as branched-chain amino acids, or BCAAs—may also help alleviate the suffering of seriously injured patients.

Studies are under way at the University of Alabama in Birmingham to confirm the theory. Palmer Q. Bessey, M.D., assistant professor of surgery, believes this amino trio might change the way the body responds to trauma.

A way to protect trauma patients.

Studies have shown that when the body is seriously injured, muscle tissue is broken down rapidly as a source of protein which, in turn, is a source of BCAAs. It's also thought that injured people are more resistant to insulin than normal, healthy people. This may be partly responsible for the breakdown of muscle protein during trauma. BCAAs may prove useful in decreasing muscle breakdown in injured patients.

Arginine: Potential against Cancer

Cancer is a complex medical puzzle for which there is no miracle cure. Bearing that in mind, it's also fair to say that scientists are making some headway. One potential anticancer drug, in fact, is not really a drug at all, but the amino acid arginine.

Arginine as an anticancer drug.

Tests on laboratory rats have demonstrated that arginine discourages tumor growth, though the reasons for this aren't clear. Scientists suspect arginine boosts the cancer-fighting powers of the white blood cells (*Journal of Parenteral and Enteral Nutrition*).

Helping skin to heal faster after surgery.

Arginine may also help the skin heal after major surgery, according to Hans Fisher, Ph.D., professor and chairman of the Department of Nutrition at Rutgers University. "Healing involves the formation of scar tissue, and scar tissue is made up of collagen," he says. "And collagen contains a high percentage of arginine and another amino acid, glycine."

Sleeplessness and Tryptophan

Try to find something tryptophan *doesn't* do. It has been proposed in the past as a painkiller, a natural antidepressant and as a nondrug means of bringing the sandman.

Tryptophan is converted in the body to serotonin, a powerful neurotransmitter, a biochemical used to relay nerve impulses. That's the key to this amino acid's versatility.

Tryptophan has been used as an experimental treatment for the mental disorder called mania. Researchers suspect tryptophan stimulates the production of more serotonin, which reduces the symptoms of mania (*Biological Psychiatry*).

Tryptophan Better than Counting Sheep

For thousands of people who have trouble falling asleep, tryptophan (the amino acid commonly found in milk) has become as popular as counting sheep used to be. But does it *really* work—scientifically—to induce sleepiness? Yes, say a group of researchers from the Massachusetts Institute of Technology in Cambridge.

The researchers administered various tests to measure the mood state and performance of a group of men after they had taken tryptophan and after they had taken a placebo (dummy pill). After the tryptophan, the men reported increased drowsiness and decreased vigor, while their performance was not impaired on any of the tests given by the researchers.

Because of this, the researchers think tryptophan is a good choice for use in inducing sleepiness. Most prescription drugs currently used as hypnotics, they say, impair performance not only immediately after administration but also the next day. Tryptophan "may be preferable to such drugs, particularly if a less potent hypnotic would be sufficient," say the researchers (*American Journal of Clinical Nutrition*).

Investigators from the University of California at Los Angeles also got positive results with tryptophan. They tested it on elderly patients with persistent insomnia. Although it doesn't work for all types of insomnia, the doctors say that for those responsive to it (about 30 percent of those tested), there was a "dramatic and sustained relief of insomnia" (*Journal of the American Geriatric Society*). As for side effects, they seem to be virtually nonexistent. Even so, the researchers caution that there are some patients who should not take tryptophan—those with liver disease and those on certain medications. In fact, anyone who is undergoing any medical treatment should check with his doctor first before using the amino acid.

Tryptophan may help battle depression, insomnia and pain.

Earlier medical reports suggest the possibility of help for those who periodically become depressed, suffer from sleeplessness or require pain relief. Dr. Fisher points out that tryptophan supplements tend to work best when taken along with carbohydrates—starchy foods such as bread, cereal or potatoes—and not with proteins. Protein foods, says Dr. Fisher, tend to send other amino acids rushing to compete with tryptophan for delivery to the brain.

Note: Since relatively little is known about the safety of amino acids, be guided by your physician in the medical use of any of these substances.

Taurine for Gallstone Control?

Can taurine prevent formation of gallstones?

Gallstones are painful, but until recently science hasn't been able to come up with a way to control them. A Japanese study of the amino acid taurine, however, may provide hope for gallstone sufferers. Researchers fed mice a high-cholesterol diet supplemented with taurine. After a few weeks, cholesterol levels in the liver dropped significantly, despite the continuous influx of cholesterol. As a result, gallstones, which are formed from cholesterol-laden bile, weren't able to form.

If the relationship between taurine and gallstones can be confirmed, the implications for humans are obvious. But, the researchers stress, further studies should be done before drawing any firm conclusions (*Journal of Nutrition and Scientific Vitaminology*).

Tyrosine versus Stress

If we can call tryptophan the anti-insomnia amino acid, then we can call tyrosine the antistress amino acid.

When certain laboratory mice are placed under physical or emotional stress, they stop probing their environment, poking their way through mazes or sitting up on their haunches to look around. But if those mice are supplemented with tyrosine before being exposed to stress, they don't lose their natural inquisitiveness. Their bodies apparently convert tyrosine into norepinephrine, a brain neurotransmitter that is known to be depleted by stress.

Do these findings apply to people? Yes, says Richard Wurtman, Ph.D., of the Massachusetts Institute of Technology, the experiment's author. "Supplemental tyrosine may be useful therapeutically in people exposed chronically to stress," he says. The catch, however, is that only those people who are under stress would receive a boost from tyrosine. "We did not observe behavioral effects when unstressed rats were given tyrosine," Dr. Wurtman adds (*Brain Research*).

An antidote for unrelenting stress.

Tyrosine may also help fight depression, or at least magnify the effects of antidepressant medication. One of Dr. Wurtman's depressed patients "improved markedly" after two weeks of tyrosine therapy, and her symptoms returned within a week after she stopped taking the supplements.

One thing to keep in mind: Don't take a supplement of valine, another essential amino acid, when you take tyrosine. Valine may block tyrosine's entry to the brain.

Parkinson's disease may also respond to tyrosine supplementation, though the evidence is weak. By a series of biochemical reactions, the body can turn tyrosine into dopamine, a vital neurotransmitter that Parkinson's patients are usually low in. The tyrosine seems to work best when the disease is still in its mild, early stages (*Neurology*).

Tyrosine may help in the treatment of Parkinson's disease.

Lysine Reputed to Reduce Herpes Attacks

Few people had ever heard of this amino acid before it was publicized in the late 1970s as a natural remedy for cold sores, shingles and genital herpes.

Can lysine cure cold sores?

Lysine is now popular with those afflicted with herpes—especially those people who suffer frequent attacks.

The theory behind lysine supplementation is this: Researchers discovered in the 1950s that the herpes virus can't survive without a diet of arginine. Arginine, like lysine, is an amino acid, one that is plentiful in nuts, seeds and chocolate. Researchers also discovered that lysine competes with arginine, somehow

---

Fighting Cholesterol with Amino Acids

Eating a low-fat, high-fiber diet can help lower cholesterol levels in the blood, but it may also assure that we get the right balance of amino acids to maintain good health. And, in a roundabout fashion, a proper amino balance, too, may lower cholesterol.

The positive health benefits of a diet high in plant protein—fruit, whole grains, beans, vegetables, nuts—are well known. Still, researchers wondered, is there more to plant protein than high fiber and low fat? The answer isn't clear, but researchers at Loma Linda University in California believe that in addition to low fat and high fiber, plant protein offers a balance of amino acids that regulates cholesterol.

When you eat a diet that is high in plant protein, the lysine levels in your blood go down in relation to arginine levels. Scientists have observed that when this happens, blood cholesterol levels go down, too.

Additionally, Loma Linda researchers found out, many other amino acid levels change when diet is changed from high fat to high fiber. Glycine and serine, for example, increase; valine, leucine, histidine and tyrosine decrease. Is it a coincidence or is there a cause-and-effect relationship?

"We're still trying to find out. But anything that appears to regulate cholesterol is important," says Albert Sanchez, Dr.P.H., professor of nutrition at Loma Linda University School of Health. "Fats, carbohydrates, fiber and simple sugars—all these factors seem to regulate cholesterol. But we're looking at another aspect of diet that appears to be regulating cholesterol. And what this could mean is that we may have to go to a higher plant-food diet if we want to avoid cholesterol problems."

elbowing it out of the way and making it inaccessible to the herpes virus. If lysine could prevent arginine from reaching the virus, the theory went, it could prevent the viruses from multiplying and setting off an active infection.

In a study published in 1983, a group of researchers polled more than 1,500 people who had purchased lysine. Among those polled (whose average daily intake of lysine was over 900 milligrams), 88 percent said that the amino acid has indeed helped them. Lysine, they said, seemed to reduce the severity of their attacks and accelerated the healing time (*Journal of Antimicrobial Chemotherapy*).

Many say that 88 percent of those polled said lysine helped.

These results have been disputed, however, by scientists who attribute them to the placebo effect. University of Miami researchers found that when they gave sugar pills to herpes sufferers and told them it was lysine, most of the patients reported an improvement. The same researchers found that giving 1,200 milligrams of lysine a day failed to help those people with severe, frequent herpes episodes (*Archives of Dermatology*).

Glutamine of Interest to Alcoholics

Twenty-five years ago, nutritionist Roger J. Williams, Ph.D., wrote a book called *Alcoholism: The Nutritional Approach.* The regimen that he recommended for alcoholics included supplements of glutamine, one of the nonessential amino acids. Dr. Williams claimed that glutamine reduces the usually irresistible craving for alcohol that recovering drinkers almost inevitably encounter.

Glutamine may reduce the craving for alcohol.

Many authorities on alcoholism reject the very notion that a "sobriety nutrient" exists. But others say glutamine seems to help.

"I've been using a combination of glutamine, vitamin C and niacinamide, 500 milligrams of each,

A triple nutrient mixture for alcoholics.

one to three times a day," says Harry K. Panjwani, M.D., a Ridgewood, New Jersey, psychiatrist and a former member of the Advisory Committee of the National Council on Alcoholism. "We don't know how it works. We can only say that somehow the craving is gone. We've used it extensively, and the findings have been the same in every case."

Dr. Panjwani isn't alone. Jerzy Meduski, M.D., Ph.D., a professor at the University of Southern California and a member of the Task Force for Nutrition and Behavior in Los Angeles County, also reports that he has had success with glutamine. "The craving for alcohol seems to be the effect of an imbalance in nutrition," he says. "There is no doubt that there is a positive response to nutritional supplementation."

Safety Is the Bottom Line

When you think about amino acids, think safety.

Until more is known about the safety of amino acids, they shouldn't be used for the self-treatment of serious illnesses. At the same time, they shouldn't be taken in large amounts for long periods.

But many of those who are researching amino acids feel that it is only a matter of time before the benefits of these nutrients are fully appreciated. They believe that amino acids may eventually replace certain drugs in the treatment of diseases such as those mentioned here and potentially many others.

The Fish-Oil Factor:
Healthy-Heart
Gift from the Sea

Thou Shalt Not Eat Shellfish, for It Hath Cholesterol. Remember this dietary commandment legislated by science?

It may now be rescinded by something that has been changing minds and turning heads in scientific circles for over a decade—fish oil.

The news comes from William E. Connor, M.D., professor of medicine, and a colleague at Oregon Health Sciences University in Portland. There, they put a group of patients on control diets that were very low in cholesterol, then later on diets high in shellfish (and therefore high in cholesterol). To gauge the effects of the regimens, the researchers monitored the levels of cholesterol and triglycerides (circulating fats) in the patients' blood. And the results were just what shellfish lovers want to hear: Overall, the two kinds of diets had virtually the same impact on both blood factors (*Metabolism*).

Shellfish is not taboo.

Moderate Amounts of Shellfish Are Okay

"This means that eating moderate amounts of shellfish—three or four ounces a day—is perfectly acceptable," says Dr. Connor.

To some people that makes about as much sense as a flat earth. Research has shown time and again that cholesterol-rich foods drive up cholesterol in the blood, so what's so different about shrimp and lobster and scallops?

The big difference is a class of polyunsaturated fatty acids called omega-3, says Dr. Connor. They're the healthy-heart factors found mostly in fish oils, including the oil in shellfish. Among researchers they've earned a reputation as arch foes of elements that clog the circulation.

Introducing a true friend of the heart: omega-3 fatty acids.

"The implication of our findings," says Dr. Connor, "is that the omega-3 fatty acids helped neutralize the impact of the high-cholesterol shellfish diets."

And so it goes. Reports like this have been coming in for years, consistently defining certain elements of fish oils as potent forces for coronary health.

First came news that Greenland Eskimos were practically immune to heart disease despite diets loaded with fat, a known cause of heart trouble. The natives ate staggering amounts of whale blubber, seal and fatty fish but appeared to have some of the healthiest hearts in the world. Then there was word that scientists had found a clue: The Eskimos had high levels of omega-3 fatty acids in their blood—substances derived directly from their marine food. It soon became clear that the fatty acids might somehow be compensating for the fatty meals. Researchers had uncovered a dietary ally in the war on heart disease.

Omega-3 oils were the Eskimos' secret to healthy hearts.

It wasn't long after this first bit of detective work that investigators figured out which members of the omega-3 class were chalking up most of the good deeds. Scientists called them eicosapentanoic acid (EPA) and docosahexanoic acid (DHA). In patient after patient, researchers pitted these against high levels of cholesterol and triglycerides as well as excessive blood clotting, a process that can cause a heart attack or stroke. And EPA and DHA almost always came out ahead.

EPA and DHA decreased blood fats and excessive blood clotting.

Consequently, the questions surrounding omega-3 today are more intriguing than ever. Just how far can fish oil go toward the prevention of heart disease? Can omega-3 do any more for your heart than other poly-unsaturated fatty acids? Are omega-3 supplements just as good as a seafood diet? How much fish oil do you really need each day? Since there are now many omega-3 research projects going full tilt, the answers are getting better by the minute.

Omega-3, Gram for Gram

William S. Harris, Ph.D., formerly of Oregon Health Sciences University, can attest to that. He and his colleagues may have settled a scientific argument that's been around for years—whether polyunsaturated fish oil is better for your heart than polyunsaturated vegetable oils. Researchers have known for two decades that moderate intakes of such vegetable oils could push down cholesterol levels, but can fish oil do just as good a job—or better?

Which is better for your heart—polyunsaturated vegetable oils or fish oil?

To find out, Dr. Harris and his colleagues put seven people on three consecutive diets, each containing equal amounts of cholesterol and 40 percent of their calories in fat. A control diet imitated the American standard, making up its 40 percent in saturated fat. Another of the diets got its fat from polyunsaturated safflower and corn oil. And the third diet had its fat derived from salmon and salmon oil, both rich in EPA and DHA.

The researchers checked the subjects' levels of cholesterol and triglycerides each step of the way. And when all the data were in, there was plenty to think about. The salmon and the vegetable-oil diets reduced cholesterol by about the same margin—an average of 11 percent below control-diet levels. But the salmon regimen did something that its vegetable-oil counterpart couldn't: It forced down triglycerides. It reduced triglycerides an amazing 33 percent below control levels (*Metabolism*).

"No other polyunsaturated oils have been able to get triglyceride levels to drop in this way," says Dr. Harris. "So the impact of the fish-oil diet is really significant. For a person with high triglyceride levels, a 33 percent reduction would be an important change toward better cardiovascular health."

But there was more meaning embedded in the study than this. With the information the researchers had acquired, they were able to directly compare the effects of the two major classes of polyunsaturated fatty acids—omega-3 and omega-6 (the principal cholesterol-lowering agent in polyunsaturated vegetable oils).

"There's no question," says Dr. Harris. "Gram for gram, omega-3 fatty acids were far more potent than omega-6 fatty acids, not only in reducing triglycerides but in lowering cholesterol levels as well."

On Omega-3 Frontiers

A group of scientists in Munich would no doubt salute this kind of research, for they've been scrutinizing omega-3 themselves—but from a different angle. They've been looking at the effect that this class of fatty acids has on something called platelet function, that secretive process of the blood that can tilt the scales between coronary health or heart attack and stroke.

Platelets are those tiny blood elements so crucial to the clotting process. When you cut yourself, you need them there at the wound. Otherwise you want them to stay loose and out of mischief—to not aggregate, or clump up, choking off the flow of blood, begging for some coronary catastrophe.

But sometimes platelets become too "sticky" and start to aggregate at the wrong times. Or there's an overabundance of thromboxane in the bloodstream, a substance that sets platelets to clumping and causes vessels to constrict.

These are the problems that the West German researchers hoped omega-3 fatty acids could take on. And in a definitive study on the subject, they demonstrated that these simple derivatives of fish oil are up to the job.

The fish-oil diet reduced triglyceride levels by an amazing 33 percent.

A new way to cut the risk of heart attack and stroke.

For 25 days they supplemented the diets of a group of men with daily doses of nearly three table-spoons of cod-liver oil—rich in EPA and DHA. Then they ran a battery of tests to evaluate the men's cardiovascular systems, particularly the action of platelets. (For the sake of comparison, the men also took the tests either just before the 25-day trial or a month after.) And in factors measuring clotting activity, the men registered significant improvements because of their fish-oil intake. Platelet aggregation decreased, the production of thromboxane went down, the number of platelets diminished, even bleeding times increased, another indication that the risk of dangerous clotting had been reduced (*Circulation*).

Cod-liver oil reduced the risk of blood clots.

"The findings," say the investigators, "paralleled observations in active Eskimos, who have unique nutrition and low morbidity from atherothrombotic disease [heart trouble caused by fatty deposits and blood clots]."

But the biggest surprise of all was what the fish oil did for the men's blood pressure: It actually pulled it down. While they were taking the cod-liver oil, their systolic blood pressure dropped an average of nearly ten points.

A scientific surprise: Fish oil lowered blood pressure.

And, the researchers say, there were no side effects at all from the treatment, even though three tablespoons of cod-liver oil is normally an excessive dose, containing exceptionally large amounts of vitamins A and D. (*Caution:* These amounts were used under controlled medical conditions. Routine supplementation should never approach those levels.)

Omega-3 fatty acids, the researchers note, may be a new preventive for atherothrombotic disease—a preventive that should be stacked against the best conventional therapies currently available, including antiplatelet drugs and omega-6 fatty acid diets.

A Lack of Omega-3

All of which is worth taking to heart. But amid these signs that a little bit of fish oil goes a long way,

Most of the population is deficient in omega-3 fatty acids.

there are warnings from scientists that a little bit is far more than most people are getting.

Donald O. Rudin, M.D., former director of the Molecular Biology Department at Eastern Pennsylvania Psychiatric Institute in Philadelphia, thinks that the situation may be worse than expected.

"After years of research," he says, "we now know that omega-3 fatty acids are absolutely required by the human body. They're not optional nutrients. Yet most of the population is deficient in them. The consumption of cholesterol and fat is way up at a time when omega-3 consumption is way down.

"We obviously need these fatty acids more than ever. They're the last major nutrient family to be recognized. In more ways than one, they're our nutritional missing link," says Dr. Rudin.

More Good News about Omega-3

Heart disease, psoriasis, rheumatoid arthritis, breast cancer, migraine headaches. There's a common thread running through this rogues' gallery of modern ills: an unsaturated fat called omega-3. With this thread, scientists hope to unravel the mysteries of some of our most perplexing diseases.

Every new study demonstrates the heart-healing properties of this important group of fatty acids. Most medical experts now greet each new bit of information about omega-3 with enthusiasm.

"These highly unsaturated fats seem to give benefit in every study we've reviewed," says William Castelli, M.D., director of the Framingham Heart Study.

Reel in the Fish

Another prominent omega-3 researcher, William E. M. Lands, Ph.D., professor of biological chemistry at the University of Illinois at Chicago, also favors including more fish in the diet.

"The best way to obtain the beneficial omega-3 fatty acids is to eat more seafood," he says. "All the reasons for eating polyunsaturated oils from vegetables remain, certainly. But we need to balance them with omega-3 oils from fish. Omega-3 moderates the body's overutilization of chemicals called eicosanoids, formed from polyunsaturates."

Why doctors say, "Eat more seafood."

One of the prime beneficiaries of a diet high in omega-3 is your heart. That's where the most intensive research has been done. Studies cited in the preceding chapter show that omega-3 reduces harmful cholesterol and triglycerides and helps keep arteries clear of blood clots that can cause a heart attack or stroke. But more recently, scientists have been finding other uses for this highly unsaturated fat.

Fishing for Arthritis Relief

One of the most intriguing areas of research involves rheumatoid arthritis.

A reduction in arthritic pain and swelling.

There is no cure for this painful disease. But some researchers have found that omega-3 fatty acids might offer some relief from the pain and swelling. "We may be recommending omega-3 as an adjunct to traditional therapy in the future," says arthritis researcher Joel M. Kremer, M.D., of Albany Medical College.

A group of eicosanoids called leukotrienes, formed in the body, is thought to cause the characteristic pain and inflammation of rheumatoid arthritis. But omega-3 appears to change the chemical composition of the leukotrienes, making them less inflammatory.

In a study conducted by Dr. Kremer and associates, 23 arthritis patients each were given 1.8 grams of a concentrated fish-oil supplement every day for 12 weeks. Twenty-one other patients received placebos—capsules filled with nothing but wax. As the study progressed, the pain and swelling were reduced in the patients taking supplements. The patients taking placebos showed no improvement (*Lancet*). "The results are very encouraging," says Dr. Kremer.

Relief from the itching and scaling of psoriasis.

Patients with psoriasis may also benefit from omega-3, since leukotrienes are believed to trigger the characteristic inflammation and scaling of this skin disorder. In British and U.S. studies, omega-3 fatty acids appeared to render leukotrienes less active, resulting in some improvement—but not in all cases. In any event, omega-3 may give some relief from the itching and scaling of psoriasis (*Annals of Allergy*).

Omega-3 also appears to reduce the body's rejection of tissue grafts, though it isn't clear how or why. It's believed graft failure has something to do with the function of blood platelets, which are involved in blood clotting. Tests on laboratory animals show that a diet high in omega-3 reduces tissue-graft failure, presumably by changing the function of the blood platelets (*Journal of Surgical Research*).

Help for Migraines

One reason why migraine sufferers are predisposed to these unusually painful headaches might be a shortage of eicosapentanoic acid, or EPA, one of the omega-3 fatty acids found in fish. Without EPA, says Robert J. Hitzemann, Ph.D., associate professor of psychiatry and behavioral sciences at the State University of New York at Stony Brook, the body releases too much serotonin, a brain chemical that has the capability of either tightening or loosening blood vessel walls in the brain. All that excess serotonin appears to put the squeeze on blood vessels, resulting in pain.

Migraine sufferers may be deficient in omega-3.

To test the theory, Dr. Hitzemann and his colleagues gave omega-3 supplements to 15 migraine patients. For about half the test subjects, the supplements alleviated pain and resulted in fewer headaches. But all the news wasn't as good, says Dr. Hitzemann. Three of the migraine sufferers didn't notice any change and 4 actually became worse.

It's too soon to tell whether eating fish or taking fish-oil supplements can help relieve most migraines, says Dr. Hitzemann. But, he adds, if you've already sought conventional medical advice, it might be worth a try.

"I can't make sweeping recommendations on the basis of a 15-patient study," says Dr. Hitzemann.

"Nevertheless, I think we're all convinced this is a breakthrough." (Guidelines for the safe intake of fish-oil supplements conclude this chapter.)

Tumor Prevention?

Scientists studying omega-3 also appear to have taken a hopeful step in the battle against breast cancer. Studies linking omega-3 to prevention of breast tumors are still in a very early stage, but they seem to hold promise.

A group of eicosanoids known as prostaglandins lowers immunity and encourages tumor growth, says Rashida A. Karmali, Ph.D., associate professor of nutrition at Cook College, Rutgers University.

As a result of an overabundance of these chemicals, says Dr. Karmali, "tumors form faster, and the body can't fight them off."

Omega-3 appears to fight off the harmful effects of these overactive chemicals. Dr. Karmali fed fish oil to laboratory rats with breast tumors. The result was a reduction in the number of tumors. "Even when we transplanted tumors from one rat into another, the growth of those established tumors was much slower when we fed them fish oils," she says.

In laboratory animals, fish oil reduced the number of breast tumors.

It is one thing to prevent cancer in rats. It is quite another to prevent cancer in people, Dr. Karmali cautions. But the preliminary results of her studies offer some encouragement.

Other studies in the United States tend to support Dr. Karmali's theory. In one study, conducted at the University of Rochester School of Medicine, rats fed fish oil developed fewer tumors (*Journal of the National Cancer Institute*).

Researchers at Cornell University had encouraging results, too, when they fed fish oil to laboratory rats. There were fewer tumors, and the tumors that did develop were smaller (*Federation Proceedings*).

No one can guarantee that eating fish will definitely help prevent breast cancer. But if you want to hedge your bets, Dr. Karmali advises eating more fish.

Back to the Heart

Omega-3 may be very beneficial to people whose cholesterol levels are on the high side—between 230 and 260 milligrams per deciliter of blood. According to Dr. Castelli, people with cholesterol levels this high are particularly at risk for heart attack. Despite this, he says, many doctors don't express concern until the levels reach 300 or higher.

"Doctors are missing three-quarters of all the heart attacks in their town by overlooking all the lower numbers," Dr. Castelli says. "The bulk of all our heart attacks occur at cholesterol levels between 230 and 260. If you do not lower cholesterol, you will not have a favorable effect on heart disease."

One way to lower your cholesterol, says Dr. Castelli, is simply to eat more fish.

In one study at Vanderbilt University School of Medicine in Nashville, patients took about three tablespoons of an omega-3-rich fish-oil supplement every day. At the end of the four-week study, serum cholesterol was reduced by 15 percent (*Internal Medicine News*).

Three tablespoons of fish oil a day lowered cholesterol by 15 percent.

Adding Fish to Your Diet

You don't have to eat as much fish as the Eskimos do to decrease your risks of heart disease, cancer and other illnesses. Experts think we might prevent disease by eating comparatively little.

Most researchers believe as few as two to four fish meals a week might be sufficient. The more you eat, obviously, the better.

"The ideal amount to eat probably varies from person to person," says William E. Connor, M.D., professor of medicine at the Oregon Health Sciences University in Portland and one of the pioneers in omega-3 research. "A couple of six-ounce fish meals a week is probably the minimum. I certainly enjoy three or four servings of fish a week."

A prescription for heart health: at least two six-ounce fish meals a week.

Selected Food Sources of Omega-3

Seafood	Omega-3 (g.)
Mackerel, Atlantic	2.6
Mackerel, chub	2.2
Mackerel, king	2.2
Scad, muroaji	2.1
Dogfish, spiny	2.0
Trout, lake	2.0
Mackerel, Japanese horse	1.9
Herring, Pacific	1.8
Herring, Atlantic	1.7
Tuna, bluefin	1.6
Sablefish	1.5
Salmon, chinook	1.5
Sturgeon, Atlantic	1.5
Tuna, albacore	1.5
Whitefish, lake	1.5
Anchovy, European	1.4
Salmon, Atlantic	1.4
Saury	1.4
Herring, round	1.3
Salmon, sockeye	1.3
Sprat (small herring)	1.3
Bluefish	1.2
Capelin	1.2
Mullet	1.1
Salmon, chum	1.1
Conch	1.0
Salmon, coho	1.0
Salmon, pink	1.0
Eel, European	0.9
Halibut, Greenland	0.9
Bass, striped	0.8
Smelt, rainbow	0.8
Periwinkle, common	0.7
Rockfish, brown	0.7

SOURCE: Adapted from "Provisional Tables on the Content of Omega-3 Fatty Acids and Other Fat Components of Selected Foods," by Frank N. Hepburn, Jacob Exler, and John L. Weihrauch, *Journal of the American Dietetic Association*, June 1986.

NOTES:
All portions are raw. Cooking does *not* decrease the omega-3 content of fish. Figures are based on a 3½-oz. serving.

Of course, Dr. Connor adds, you ought to watch your weight, keep your blood pressure under control, avoid stress, eat fewer saturated fats and stop smoking. "The omega-3 theory is a tremendous advance," Dr. Connor told a symposium audience. "But there are other basic things to consider."

Most experts agree that fish should be substituted for red meat and poultry and not eaten in addition to what you normally consume. The meat we get from farm animals is low in omega-3.

Not all fish contain the same amount of omega-3. Generally, fattier fish—salmon and mackerel, for example—contain more. Ocean fish have more than freshwater fish. (See the table, Selected Food Sources of Omega-3, on page 252, for a more complete list.)

Fatty ocean fish are the richest sources of omega-3.

If you don't like fish, supplements may be an alternative. Ten capsules of concentrated marine lipids supply 1.8 grams of eicosapentanoic acid. A serving of salmon (about four ounces) contains about an average of 2 grams of EPA. Cod-liver oil also contains EPA, but the amount varies according to brand. Cod-liver oil usually contains high amounts of vitamins A and D, however, and in large amounts these can be toxic, so cod-liver oil should not be used for this purpose.

Supplements are an alternative.

Chapter 33

Chromium and Choline: Promising Possibilities for Health

The research into chromium and choline is in its infancy—tentative, preliminary, unconfirmed. But the little that is known about these two nutrients is encouraging.

Chromium, the Insulin Regulator

Our bodies require only the tiniest bit of the trace mineral chromium—50 to 200 micrograms a day—but many of us don't get enough of it, particularly as we get older. Chromium is a natural, and very effective, insulin regulator. It is essential for insulin to work efficiently in our bodies.

Older people may not get enough chromium.

"Insulin is required to remove glucose [sugars] from the blood," explains Richard A. Anderson, Ph.D., of the U.S. Department of Agriculture's Human Nutrition Research Center in Beltsville, Maryland. When blood glucose levels are high, as they are shortly after eating, the pancreas secretes insulin, which stimulates cells to take up the glucose and burn it for energy. "Chromium makes the insulin more efficient at stimulating the cells. The body needs less to do the job, and so blood insulin stays at a healthy lower level," Dr. Anderson says.

Supplements normalized blood sugar metabolism.

In one study, Dr. Anderson gave healthy volunteers 200 micrograms of chromium a day for three months. He reports that chromium supplements or brewer's yeast (which is rich in chromium) normalized glucose metabolism.

In the volunteers who had slightly elevated blood sugar levels before taking chromium, there was a significant drop of about 20 points in blood sugar level. And in those who started out with moderately *low* blood sugar (hypoglycemia), chromium supplementation was associated with about a 10-point increase in blood sugar levels.

"Chromium truly is a regulator of insulin," says Dr. Anderson, whose work suggests that chromium may alleviate many of the major symptoms of low blood sugar. "With chromium, you don't have insulin 'overshooting' its target," he says. "You don't get too much insulin in the blood, or too little. You avoid the seesaws in blood sugar that come as a result of fluctuating insulin levels."

Brewer's yeast containing chromium also may help to regulate fats in the blood. People who took about two tablespoons of chromium-rich brewer's yeast each day for eight weeks had significant drops in their cholesterol levels, according to research by J. Clint Elwood, Ph.D., professor of biochemistry at State University of New York and Health Science Center at Syracuse. The average decrease for all the subjects was 10 percent, but a few of the volunteers had dramatically larger drops. Their cholesterol levels went from over 300 to within a normal range of less than 250.

Brewer's yeast may help lower cholesterol.

"The higher the cholesterol level, the better the response was to the brewer's yeast," Dr. Elwood says. "But what interested us most was that what we consider to be normal cholesterol levels could also be lowered with brewer's yeast. We still don't know the best level of cholesterol for optimum health."

What Choline Can Do for the Brain

Many of the foods touted as "brain foods"—fish, for instance, and liver and eggs—contain choline, a substance researchers think may help preserve the brain's ability to reason, learn and remember.

Researchers at Ohio State University, for instance, found that mice fed a diet heavy in choline-rich lecithin, or one of lecithin's "brain active" ingredients, phosphatidylcholine, had much better memory retention than mice on regular diets. They took much longer to go into a back room in their cages where they had received a mild electric shock, meaning they hadn't forgotten their unpleasant experience.

Can choline improve your memory?

What's more, their brain cells, examined under a microscope, showed fewer of the expected signs of aging, says Ronald Mervis, Ph.D., of Ohio State University's Brain Aging and Neuronal Plasticity Research Group.

"Normally, as the brain ages, its cell membranes become more rigid with fatty deposits and lose their ability to take in and release brain chemicals and to relay messages," Dr. Mervis says. This can cause memory loss and confused thinking. But a lecithin-rich diet seems to repress or delay this membrane hardening.

As part of the deterioration process, aging brain cells also tend to lose dendritic spines, the chemical receptor areas that are vitally important in passing along information. Having too few dendritic spines is like having a bad phone connection. Messages get distorted and lost. But lecithin-fed older mice had the same number of dendritic spines as much younger mice.

Why lecithin is considered "brain food."

"Despite the differences between mice and men, there are, nevertheless, remarkable similarities in the structure of their nerve cells," says Dr. Mervis. "I believe lecithin could help to repress or delay similar problems in man, although we have yet to verify that."

Part V

SOLVING
HEALTH
PROBLEMS
WITH
NUTRITION

An Alternative Way to Fight Alcoholism

"I don't think I could have stayed sober this long if I hadn't found out about nutrition."—James A.

At the age of 29, James A. had been an alcoholic for 15 years. During that time, he was committed to hospitals and "dried out" twice. He was asked to dredge up memories of an alcoholic father who died when he was only 10. He listened to countless "drunkologues"—life stories of recovered alcoholics who "had been there"—and met doctors who tried to scare him with greenish dissected livers. But after both treatments, he returned to his job as a bartender in a Minneapolis singles club and to his habit of drinking a quart of vodka and 12 cans of beer a day. Sobriety just didn't work out for him.

"I stayed sober for a year the last time," he says, "but it wasn't a pleasant experience. I had problems with depression and anxiety. I'd be walking down the street and—whap—I'd have an anxiety attack. And I had a bad sweet tooth. I drank several quarts of pop a day. I remember thinking to myself, 'If this is what being sober is like, I don't want it.' "

The misery—and nutritional backlash—of one man's post-alcoholic sobriety.

Standard Treatment Often Fails

The treatment James received was typical of that given in many hospital-based rehabilitation centers and ARUs, or alcohol recovery units. The first stage is detoxification, when an alcoholic goes cold turkey for a week—sometimes with the help of tranquilizers. The next step includes encounter sessions and lectures in the hospital. The third step, when the patient goes home, calls for regular attendance at Alcoholics Anonymous meetings. The treatment's customary goal is to heal the alcoholic's psyche and spirit. It's hoped that he'll discover the emotional and psychological roots of his addiction and "talk them out."

Eighty-five percent of all dried-out alcoholics eventually go back to drinking.

Those methods have saved many alcoholics from a miserable life and a premature death. But, as valuable as such techniques may be in individual cases, their overall performance record has not been outstanding. They haven't put a dent in these vital statistics: An estimated 85 percent of all dried-out alcoholics eventually go back to drinking; half of all traffic fatalities are linked to alcohol; 20 percent of all hospital beds are filled by people with alcohol-related illnesses. In all, the public pays billions of dollars a year in terms of medical care and lost productivity as a result of alcoholism.

A Different Approach

An unusual kind of alcoholism treatment: nutrition.

That rate of failure has motivated a lot of people in the alcoholism treatment field to look for more effective therapies. Although they're still very much in the minority, there's a growing number of M.D.'s and others who say that more attention should be paid to the physical disease of alcoholism. They agree that emotional problems have to be faced. But they also argue that the alcoholic, in order to recover, must discover the underlying biochemical factors that created his disease and treat them. They say that the alcoholic who undergoes a radical nutritional overhaul—a switch from sugar, cigarettes and coffee to whole grains, fresh produce and vitamin supplements—has a much better chance of staying permanently dry than one who doesn't.

One member of this new and vocal minority is Joan Mathews-Larson, Ph.D., director of Health Recovery Center, a state-licensed clinic for alcoholics in

Minneapolis. Motivated by the suicide of her alcoholic son a few years ago, she decided to pursue a doctorate in nutrition and to open a treatment center where alcoholism would be treated by restoring the normal biochemical balance through diet and supplements as well as with psychological counseling. She knows she is a maverick, but she thinks her controversial program works.

According to one expert, the nutritional treatment of alcoholism works.

"Only a small percentage of the alcohol treatment centers in the United States use the nutritional approach," she says. Much of the field still treats alcoholism as a psychological disorder. And most members of Alcoholics Anonymous don't even know that there's a physical and nutritional approach.

"But people recover very nicely here without confessing their sins in group therapy sessions and without being made to feel ashamed of their disease. What we're doing is much more basic to their recovery. You wouldn't put a diabetic in group therapy and expect him to 'talk out' his disease. Yet this is what many people expect alcoholics to do."

Alcoholism, for Dr. Mathews-Larson (she is a certified chemical-dependency practitioner in Minnesota), is an inherited physical disorder that has severe psychological complications. She says that alcoholics have a peculiar genetic defect that causes their bodies to metabolize alcohol into a highly addictive, morphinelike substance called tetrahydro-isoquinoline, or THIQ. Most alcoholics also develop hypoglycemia, or low blood sugar, she says. They crave alcohol and sugar in any form, but both substances put them on a physical and emotional roller coaster that only more of the same can bring to a temporary halt. Certain food and chemical allergies, she says, can also cause a craving for alcohol.

Is alcoholism the result of a genetic defect?

Do Alcoholics Need Extra Vitamins?

This vicious cycle can be broken, she says. When alcoholics first enter her six-week program, she sends them through a battery of tests to check for hypoglycemia and nutrient deficiencies. She puts them on a fast to unmask potential food allergies and has a staff doctor check for hidden physical and psychiatric problems.

Then come the nutrients. Recovering alcoholics need replacement of the B vitamins, plus plenty of vitamin C and certain amino acids, she says. To stay in her program, they must also kick their coffee, tobacco, white flour and sugar habits. While most alcoholism counselors say that their patients need those crutches in order to cope with withdrawal, Dr. Mathews-Larson believes they just delay recovery.

No more coffee, tobacco, white flour or sugar.

Success Stories

James A. was one of Dr. Mathews-Larson's clients. With the aid of emotional counseling, he has been sober ever since going through her program in 1982. He has only good things to say about it. "I remember the first group meeting I went to there," he says. "I heard people saying that alcoholism was a biochemical problem, not a mental problem. And I thought, 'Maybe it's just a problem in my biochemistry. Maybe I'm not going crazy.' After the program, I felt like I was on a fairly even keel for the first time in my life. People who knew me couldn't believe it."

"I was on an even keel for the first time in my life."

Other patients at the Health Recovery Center have had similar success. Mary W., a 27-year-old mother of two boys, was one of them.

"Both of my parents were alcoholics, and I started drinking when I was 14," she says. "I was always very depressed, and when I started drinking, it made me feel good. I could hold my liquor better than anybody, but I was still always tired and unhappy."

Mary went to the Health Recovery Center when she was planning her second pregnancy. She had been drinking and using drugs during her first pregnancy, and her son grew more slowly than normal. He later became hyperactive and suffered from multiple allergies. With her second child, she wanted to avoid making that mistake again. Having known Dr. Mathews-Larson from a prior attempt to dry out, she went to see her. She found out that hidden food allergies may have made her depressed and added momentum to her alcohol abuse.

"I found out that I was allergic to beef, wheat and dairy products," she said. She also learned a lot about healthy food. "In group therapy, we didn't talk about what was wrong with our marriages. Instead, we talked about good places to buy wholesome food and ways to cook it. We found out what to have for breakfast and what to snack on during the day. And one of the workers took us on a tour of natural food co-ops."

Confession of an alcoholic: Food was part of the problem.

After going through the program, Mary said she was happier than she had ever been. "I wake up feeling good, and I feel good all day. And my second baby was much bigger and stronger than the first."

The Role of B Vitamins

One mainstay in the Health Recovery Center treatment regimen is glutamine, a little-known amino acid. More than 25 years ago, nutrition pioneer Roger J. Williams, Ph.D., professor emeritus in chemistry at the University of Texas, began recommending this amino acid to alcoholics. Glutamine, he said, could allay the unendurable craving that causes so many alcoholics to backslide. Dr. Mathews-Larson agrees. "We've found that glutamine does everything that Dr. Williams says it does," she says.

The B vitamins can also reduce the craving for alcohol, Dr. Williams believes. That alcoholism can cause B vitamin deficiencies, most experts in the field agree. But Dr. Williams reversed that formula and took the unorthodox position that a deficiency of the B's can cause excessive drinking. He may be right, though the case is far from proven. Some years ago, experiments in Finland showed that rats made deficient in B vitamins are more likely to choose alcohol

B vitamins may reduce the craving for alcohol, says one scientist.

than water when both are offered to them. But vitamin supplementation reversed their tastes (*British Journal of Addiction*).

Some M.D.'s share Dr. Mathews-Larson's views. One of them is Harry K. Panjwani, M.D., a Ridgewood, New Jersey, psychiatrist and former member of the Advisory Committee of the National Council on Alcoholism. He says that by mixing vitamins and psychotherapy he has helped many alcoholics turn their lives around within a few months.

Dr. Panjwani puts each new patient on a regimen of glutamine, niacinamide and vitamin C. He believes that alcoholics who regain their health via good nutrition are much better at working out the problems that gave rise to their addiction. Just taking the liquor away and leaving a person with addictions to cigarettes, coffee and sugar isn't enough, he says. "That's treating the disease, not the whole person."

A regimen of glutamine, niacinamide and vitamin C.

A New Regimen

Nutrition is also stressed at Brunswick House, an alcoholism treatment facility at the Brunswick Hospital Center in Amityville, New York. Joseph Beasley, M.D., who is the medical director of the 86-bed facility, says that his patients are asked to give up sugar, cut back on refined food, and begin a multivitamin program after rigorous individualized diagnoses. They're also encouraged to participate in the entire treatment program, including therapy, lectures and activities such as using the paddleball courts and Nautilus machines at the facility. "We feel that this, along with traditional therapies, is where alcoholism treatment is now," Dr. Beasley says.

In California, Jerzy Meduski, M.D., Ph.D., a professor at the University of Southern California and a member of the Task Force for Nutrition and Behavior in Los Angeles County, also believes in giving vitamins and glutamine to recovering alcoholics. In one study, he supplemented the diets of 100 alcoholic prison inmates for two years and achieved great results.

"The craving for alcohol seems to be the effect of an imbalance in nutrition. That is almost always the case," Dr. Meduski says. "There is no doubt that there is a positive response to nutritional supplementation."

A positive response to nutritional supplements.

Yet another nutrition-minded alcoholism counselor is Mark Worden, former editor of *Alcoholism: The National Magazine.*

"Does a poor diet increase the chances that an alcoholic will go back to drinking?" Worden asks rhetorically. "You can say that if an alcoholic's body is well prepared for stress by good nutrition and a healthy lifestyle, then the likelihood of his going back to his old way of dealing with stress—alcohol—is probably less."

Comparing Recovery Rates

Is the nutritional approach, then, the most effective form of treatment? The only way to find out would be to compare recovery rates. The program that kept the most alcoholics dry for the longest amount of time would emerge the winner. Such data are hard to come by. It's just too impractical to keep tabs on a large group of people for several months or years. But the few figures that are available on this subject lend credence to the nutritional approach.

Dr. Mathews-Larson claims, for instance, that one year after leaving her program, about 82 percent of her patients are still sober. Those results are far better, she says, than the numbers reported by other, more traditional, programs, which generally show that only one-third of their clients are alcohol free by the end of one year.

Still sober a year after trying the nutritional treatment.

A nutritionist at the Elmhurst Alcoholism Program in New York City also came up with pronutrition figures. Lillian Yung, Ed.D., studied a group of 64 alcoholics to see whether the ones who stayed sober the longest ate differently than those who quickly went back to the bottle.

The results surprised her. She found that 45 percent of the alcoholics who stayed sober for more than

Did supplements make the difference?

50 days after leaving treatment were using vitamin supplements. But only 19 percent of those who couldn't stay sober for 50 days used supplements.

"The failure rate for conventional alcoholism treatment is in the upper 80th or even 90th percentile," Dr. Yung says. "There have been reports that much of the counseling and group therapy that alcoholics get has no effect on how long they stay sober. That encouraged me to look at the problem from a nutritional standpoint."

A study in Texas adds more evidence to the nutrition theory. At a Veterans Hospital Medical Center in Waco, Ruth Guenther, Ph.D., looked at the effects of nutrition on a group of hard-core alcoholics. These were men who had been drinking, on the average, the equivalent of 13 ounces of alcohol a day for the previous 15 to 20 years. She discovered that alcoholics who ate well could stay sober longer.

Alcoholics who ate well stayed sober longer.

The men were studied in two groups. Dr. Guenther asked the first group to stay on the standard hospital diet and asked the second group to switch to a special diet plan that she had prepared. This experimental diet included foods like wheat germ, bran, decaffeinated coffee and unsweetened fruit in conjunction with the regular hospital diet. She also asked the second group to swear off all snacks except for the nuts, cheese, peanut butter and milk that she provided. Finally, she asked them each to keep taking a multivitamin supplement for six months after their release from the clinic.

The special diet made a difference in mood and sobriety.

The results were gratifying. When interviewed, the alcoholics on the special diet told Dr. Guenther that they felt "calmer and more relaxed." More important, their recovery rate was very high. Six months after they went home, 81 percent of the vitamin group was still sober. By comparison, only 38 percent of the control group had not taken a drink (*International Journal of Biosocial Research*).

Anemia:
Who Gets It and
What to Do about It

"I feel so much better—I never realized I haven't had the energy I should."

This is a common reaction from people who've bounced back from iron-deficiency anemia, a common blood disorder whose hallmark is feeling tired and washed out.

"Very often, we'll give an iron supplement to people who are only slightly anemic, and they'll report feeling more energetic," says Suzanne McClure, M.D., assistant professor of medicine in the Division of Hematology-Oncology at the University of Texas Medical Branch in Galveston.

Restoring energy with iron.

"We have seen reports," adds Annette Natow, R.D., Ph.D., professor of nutrition at Adelphi University in Garden City, New York, showing "that just having low-iron intake—without being full-blown anemic—might result in some people having concentration ability and immune-system responses that aren't up to par."

People who develop more pronounced iron deficiency may have fatigue compounded by depression, fainting spells, headaches, heartburn, irritability, itching, pale lips and skin, poor appetite or memory, a sore tongue or brittle nails. Also, people with angina may notice their condition getting worse.

The many symptoms of severe iron deficiency.

Supply Down, Demand Up

The body's energy levels are taxed when it doesn't get enough iron for one of the mineral's chief functions: producing hemoglobin. It's iron-based hemoglobin that carries oxygen to tissues and cells to energize them. If iron levels drop, then hemoglobin and energy fade, too.

Doctors first look at what factors in a person's lifestyle might be acting alone or in combination to deplete iron stores.

Iron deficiency and anemia often hit people who've set themselves up this way: Neglecting to put enough iron-rich foods in their diet, they don't have enough of the mineral packed away in their bone marrow for "emergencies" like they should. Then they start to lose blood for expected reasons (menstruation, pregnancy) or unexpected reasons (ulcers, hemorrhoids). The blood loss bills the body for extra iron to make up for what's lost—and the body can't pay the balance.

This is just one anemia scenario. Prolonged, paltry iron intake alone, without a blood loss condition, can make some people anemic. On the other hand, it's possible to not get enough iron and escape any adverse effects.

A doctor can do a full-scale blood chemistry test to analyze several factors, one being hemoglobin levels, and determine if iron is in short supply. He or she will also check to see if any of the following risk factors are coming into play.

Too many people are in "iron debt"—-and suffer the consequences.

Menstruation Puts You at Risk

If you're a menstruating female, you're the most likely candidate for anemia. "It's almost impossible for most women to get anywhere near the iron they need from their diets," says Dr. Natow. "If a woman's on a 1,000-calorie reducing diet, for example, she's probably only taking in 6 milligrams of iron—pitifully less than the Recommended Dietary Allowance (RDA) of 18 milligrams. Even if she eats 2,000 calories a day, which is generally way more than figure-conscious women will allow themselves, her iron intake will average only about 12 milligrams. Add to

The number one candidate for iron-deficiency anemia.

that the fact most women choose iron-poor 'diet foods' like cottage cheese, yogurt, lettuce and fruit juice for a good percentage of what calories they do consume, and iron deficiency becomes even more likely." (*Editor's note:* The RDA for women 11 to 22 is 18 milligrams; for women over 22, the RDA is 10 milligrams.)

Menstruation compounds the iron problem even more. Women with heavier flows face greater odds of being iron deficient; birth control pill users run a lessened risk due to usually lighter periods. Pregnancy especially takes its toll on iron by assigning the mother's iron supply to double-duty nourishing.

"A woman can suffer from somewhat of an iron deficit after years of simply being female," Dr. McClure notes. She once attended a health fair for hospital employees where all female nurses had their iron levels evaluated. "Over one-quarter of the women were iron deficient and a few were outright anemic. These were health-conscious people who knew all about, and cared about, eating well, but menstrual blood loss was still sapping their iron. This is why women should have their blood checked at regular intervals," says Dr. McClure.

Recommendation for women: Have your blood checked regularly for low iron.

Iron Losses in the GI Tract

Gastrointestinal disorders may contribute to anemia. This is the main thing that puts a man at risk for iron-deficiency anemia, because men easily consume their RDA of 10 milligrams of iron each day.

Many things might cause gastrointestinal bleeding. Some, like hemorrhoids, can obviously be noticed by a person. Other conditions—benign or malignant polyps, or bleeding ulcers, for example—may go undetected without an internal exam. Irritable bowel syndrome can sometimes cause blood loss, too. "When you hit 40 and older, you enter a higher risk group for GI conditions," Dr. McClure explains. "You can't always notice blood in your stool, either, because it may not be red. It's a good idea to do one

For unexpected reasons, some men are also at risk for iron deficiency.

of the home stool tests, or get one from your doctor, every year. This isn't on people's list of top ten things to do, but it's an important diagnostic test that shouldn't be avoided." The American Cancer Society's guidelines of having a thorough colon and rectal exam between ages 40 and 50, followed by another exam every three to five years, are also wise measures.

One additional stomach irritant: aspirin. It can cause bleeding in people who take large amounts. (It's not uncommon for arthritis sufferers to take four tablets every four hours, says Dr. Natow, to relieve pain.)

Children Need Plenty of Iron

"A growing child needs to get lots of iron to handle the job of building all the new red blood cells in the growing volume of blood," explains Myron Winick, M.D., a New York City pediatrician and director of the Institute of Human Nutrition at Columbia University College of Physicians and Surgeons. "His or her diet needs lots of iron-rich meats and vegetables, or iron-fortified cereals. If the child's a picky eater, iron supplements are in order to make sure the body can keep up with the increased iron need.

Good sources of iron for babies: breast milk or iron-fortified formula.

"Babies, until about their first birthday, should either keep receiving breast milk or iron-fortified formula," stresses Dr. Winick. "Starting a baby on whole milk earlier than this deprives him or her of iron. Not only because whole milk simply doesn't have any but also because it contains high amounts of protein which can cause microscopic bleeding in the gastrointestinal tract and cause blood to be lost in the stool. Breast milk's iron is very well absorbed, on the other hand."

Iron Blockers to Watch Out For

Certain dietary factors inhibit iron absorption. Coffee and tea contain tannin, a substance which, if the beverages are taken with meals, can cut the amount of iron absorbed by 40 to 95 percent. If these drinks are one of your favorite pleasures, try waiting until an hour or two after a meal to have them.

Iron is also blocked by the phosphates in ice cream, candy bars, baked goods, beer and soft drinks. EDTA, an additive in many canned and processed foods, has the same inhibiting trait. (Check labels for EDTA if you're concerned.)

Two additives that subtract iron.

Calcium, important for bones though it may be, may also be guilty of iron inhibition when it's taken as a supplement with meals. To avoid interfering with iron absorption, women seeking to guard against osteoporosis should not take their calcium supplements with foods serving as a primary source of iron.

Gatekeepers of Iron

In addition to being aware of iron sappers, you can make the most of iron enhancers. Beef, veal, fish, lamb, poultry and game all multiply iron absorption fourfold. These meats encourage your body to take in nonheme iron, a form of the mineral that isn't easy to absorb.

Vitamin C lends a hand in nonheme iron absorption, too. Dr. Natow suggests if you take an iron supplement, you drink vitamin C-rich orange juice at the same time. Good vitamin C bets are citrus fruits, cabbage, peppers, tomatoes, broccoli, cantaloupe and strawberries. Still another iron pick-up from vegetables and citrus fruits: lots of folate, a B vitamin that iron needs to pair up with for optimal performance. Folate is also abundant in liver and beans.

Vitamin C helps your body absorb iron.

The iron-pot trick can boost iron intake threefold. As your food simmers in the skillet, some of the pot's iron comes off into the food and strengthens its nutritional value.

Finally, these foods, and perhaps an iron supplement if needed, are the best at keeping your iron stores stocked:

Iron-boosting foods.

- Beef and chicken liver, roast beef, lean ground beef, chicken, dark-meat turkey.
- Prunes, dried apricots, blackstrap molasses, sunflower seeds.
- Lima beans, soybeans, broccoli, spinach, peas, beet greens or kidney beans.

Arrhythmias:
Heartthrobs You Can
Live Without

There you are, sitting down with a mug of coffee in the tranquillity of your own kitchen, when your heart races as if you'd just run up a flight of stairs. Or, while sleeping on your left side, you're suddenly awakened by the pounding of your heart. Or, for no reason at all, you feel as if butterflies are fluttering where your heart should be. When this happens, it's scary—scary enough to make you consider an immediate trip to the cardiologist.

Sometimes these arrhythmias, as they're called, do mean that something is wrong with the heart. Ventricular fibrillation, in which the heart beats randomly and recklessly, can lead to death. Certain kinds of bradycardia or tachycardia, which means the pulse is too slow or too fast, may mean that there is some underlying ailment.

But more often than not, temporary arrhythmias aren't cause for mental anguish. "Mild arrhythmias are the most common reason for referral to a cardiologist," says one doctor, and others say that occasional mild arrhythmias "no more augur sudden death than a sneeze portends pneumonia." In fact, healthy people whose hearts never miss a beat are very much in the minority.

When the beating of your heart is cause for concern.

Irregular but Not Abnormal

A significant advance in cardiology in recent years has been the discovery that arrhythmias are

Arrhythmias: worrisome, but not rare.

Some heartbeat irregularities are perfectly normal.

As we get older, erratic heartbeats become more common.

common among normal, healthy people. Irregularities once thought to be life-threatening—fast pulse, ventricular ectopic beats (irregular beats) and even some types of heart block (a failure in the flow of electric impulses across the heart muscle)—happen to, but seem not to bother, people who are otherwise in good health.

In England a few years ago, researchers set out to discover "the rhythm of the normal human heart," studying the electrocardiographs of 86 healthy people who had no trace of heart disease. To the scientists' surprise, most of the study group possessed a rhythm disturbance of some kind. The normal, in other words, was abnormal. To explain why these people seemed to do just fine even with arrhythmias, the researchers said, "Perhaps these disturbances may well be tolerated by a normal heart" (*Lancet*).

Others have agreed with them. "When ventricular ectopic beats occur in someone who has heart irregularities, they can generate a lethal disturbance," says Bart Gershen, M.D., "but in a healthy person, this arrhythmia might have no effects at all."

Indeed, even the healthiest people suffer arrhythmias. Dr. Gershen surveyed 50 healthy medical students at Holy Cross Hospital in Silver Spring, Maryland, and found that at least half showed skipped beats, palpitations or pounding in their chests, while their pulses at times soared as high as 180 and as low as 37 beats per minute. Other cardiologists have found that harmless arrhythmias commonly show up in superfit distance runners, even while they run (*American Heart Journal*).

It is also entirely normal, apparently, for arrhythmias to become more frequent as we get older. Even the elderly shouldn't become alarmed just because a few mild ventricular arrhythmias show up on their electrocardiograms. A survey of 106 active people over age 75 showed that most of them had signs such as irregular beats or racing pulse, but the symptoms didn't cramp their lifestyle. In fact, among those 106 relatively healthy elderly persons, only 24 (23 percent) could boast of a "normal" heart rate for 24 hours straight (*American Heart Journal*).

Causes of Arrhythmias

Of course, cardiac arrhythmias are sometimes an indication that something has gone awry with the heart. This "something" could be anything from advanced heart disease to nothing more serious than a reaction to strong coffee.

Heart Attack

Ventricular arrhythmias, for instance, often accompany a heart attack, appearing at the time of the attack and in the weeks that follow. It used to be gospel that post–heart-attack arrhythmias could trigger a second attack. For that reason, doctors often plied their heart patients with antiarrhythmia drugs. But studies have shown that those arrhythmias are an effect rather than a cause of heart attack and may not require medication (*British Medical Journal*).

Are arrhythmias that accompany heart attacks a cause for alarm?

Similarly, atrial fibrillation, in which the heart may have an irregular rhythm, is also associated with diabetes, and it greatly increases the chance of a fatal heart attack. But there's a more positive note: Atrial fibrillation is much less dangerous when it strikes someone with a fairly healthy heart (*New England Journal of Medicine*).

Lack of Magnesium

On the other hand, arrhythmias may not indicate a heart attack at all. They might be a symptom of magnesium deficiency.

Magnesium deficiency causes out-of-sync heartbeats.

Anyone who uses diuretic medication to control high blood pressure is a candidate for magnesium deficiency. Diuretics drain the body of magnesium, and they are among the most commonly prescribed types of drugs in America.

But those not on diuretics are also vulnerable. The average magnesium intake by Americans in 1900 was 475 milligrams a day. Today, however, the average intake is only 245 milligrams a day—well below the 300 to 350 milligrams a day recommended by the National Academy of Sciences.

"Any patient who is on diuretic therapy and has irregularities in the heart rhythm should be checked for serum magnesium levels," says Eugene Coodley, M.D., of the Veterans Administration Medical Center in Long Beach, California. "If they are low, they should be brought up with magnesium sulfate."

Diuretics can lead to a lack of magnesium— which may warp heart rhythm.

It should come as little surprise that magnesium is essential for a regular pulse. On a cellular level, a magnesium-dependent enzyme helps generate the energy that gives each heartbeat its oomph, and there have been cases in which people with life-threatening arrhythmias have recovered their natural rhythm with no other treatment than magnesium supplementation (*Acta Medica Scandinavica*).

Caffeine

Caffeine has been implicated as a dietary inducer of arrhythmia. Americans consume about 2.2 billion pounds of coffee a year, and the caffeine in that coffee disturbs the pulse possibly in the same way that it creates alertness and insomnia—by triggering the release of adrenaline. People with existing heart problems are especially vulnerable to caffeine, and for that reason most cardiac care units allow only decaffeinated beverages as a matter of policy (*New England Journal of Medicine*).

Palpitations after morning coffee.

Coffee-induced arrhythmias, in fact, can be frightening, and they send many anxious people in search of a cardiologist. "We see a number of people who developed palpitations after their morning coffee," says Carl V. Leier, M.D., of Ohio State University. "Some people are more sensitive than others, and the phenomenon isn't universal," he says, "but about half of the people we see with arrhythmias also are coffee drinkers. If you have an arrhythmia and drink a lot of coffee, our advice would be to cut down."

Stressful Lifestyle

Emotional stress can also raise the body's adrenaline levels and increase the likelihood of arrhythmias. The same high-stress life agenda that gives heart attacks to driven executives often gives them arrhythmias as well. Researchers at Harvard School of Public Health say that "psychological stress profoundly lowers the cardiac threshold for ventricular fibrillation"—the arrhythmia that causes sudden death.

Almost any kind of stress seems to do. Studies with animals have shown that such things as offering and denying food and mild physical restraint in unfamiliar surroundings may cause arrhythmia. In humans, feelings of abandonment, depression, alienation and even violent dreams are thought to cause arrhythmia.

Acute anger, researchers think, disrupts heart rhythms the most. Anger releases body chemicals that may constrict the arteries that supply the heart itself with blood (*Annual Reviews in Physiology*).

Is stress throwing your heartbeat off its pace?

Warning: Anger can be hazardous to your heartbeat.

Alcohol and Cigarettes

There is also a link between alcohol, cigarettes and cardiac arrhythmias, but doctors aren't sure how strong it is. In one of the studies mentioned here, British researchers found no obvious relationship between smoking and the type or number of arrhythmias in people over age 75. Another study has shown that, in a group of men and women of good health, smokers had faster but not less-regular heart rates.

But nicotine, like anger, unleashes adrenaline, and "cigarette smoking has been shown to lower the threshold for ventricular fibrillation during a heart attack." Dr. Coodley urges his heart patients to "reduce all coffee and alcohol and eliminate tobacco" because all "are capable of initiating arrhythmias."

As for alcohol, this oft-abused substance is known to be responsible for a syndrome called "holiday heart." Every year between Christmas Eve and

Alcohol: The cause of the frightening "holiday heart."

New Year's Day, apparently, hospital emergency rooms are frequented by people who develop severe arrhythmias as a result of alcoholic binges. In many cases, the specific arrhythmia is atrial fibrillation. It usually subsides when the alcohol wears off.

Many doctors believe that holiday heart occurs only among alcoholics or those with a long history of immoderate drinking. But Dr. Gershen says, "Any time someone overdrinks, there's the possibility of an irregular heartbeat. Alcohol is a potential toxin to the heart, and you don't have to be an alcoholic to be affected by it."

Drugs

Watch out for stimulants in over-the-counter medicine.

Almost any stimulant can adversely affect the heart, Dr. Gershen says, even the low-grade stimulants that are found in over-the-counter drugs. "A lot of the cold remedies that are available without a prescription contain ingredients that affect the heart," he says. "Most of them contain cardiac stimulants, and you'll see if you read the package that they shouldn't be taken by people with high blood pressure.

"Even people without heart disease can develop rhythm disturbances from these drugs," he adds, "and they definitely can scare people" who might experience sudden palpitation without knowing why.

Some heart drugs may backfire.

If an arrhythmia doesn't respond to changes in diet or lifestyle, a cardiologist may prescribe medication for them. These medications sometimes backfire and aggravate the very problem they were meant to solve, however. "Drugs are given to prevent a simple arrhythmia from developing into a more serious one," says Arthur Selzer, M.D., a San Francisco cardiologist. "But once in a while they can have the opposite effect." Other doctors have pointed out that "all the antiarrhythmic drugs that we have studied may aggravate arrhythmias."

Pacemakers are an option for those with a specific kind of arrhythmia called heart block, in which the heart's own electrical circuitry fails. Pacemakers are implanted in a heart patient's body, and they can run for several years. They're intended mainly for the heart patient who suffers frequent fainting spells. Some doctors feel that pacemakers are too often installed unnecessarily. Dr. Selzer points out that pacemakers are used twice as often in the United States as they are in Europe, and that anyone who hasn't fainted and feels generally healthy should get a second opinion before accepting a pacemaker.

Are you a candidate for a pacemaker?

Take Charge of Your Heart

Can the average person participate in relieving his or her own arrhythmia? Yes, says Dr. Gershen. The first step is to identify it. Sudden flushing is sometimes a sign of arrhythmia. So is fatigue, especially if it's accompanied by difficulty with sleeping on the left side, where the heart is pressed between chest and mattress. And there are other signs.

"If someone is constantly aware of his or her heart, and if the rhythm disturbances occur frequently—several times a week—or if they last a long time, for several hours or so, then the person should probably see a doctor," Dr. Gershen says.

How to deal with arrhythmias.

The next step might be to increase your intake of magnesium-rich foods, such as whole grains, dark green vegetables and beans. Giving up coffee and cigarettes, if you use them, is another tactic. Avoiding alcohol would probably be a good idea. And an attempt to resolve emotional stress may also help.

The most important strategy is the prevention of heart disease in the first place. Experts agree that cardiac arrhythmias are more common among heart disease sufferers, and that, when they do occur, arrhythmias are much more likely to damage a frail heart than a strong one. The way to keep the heart strong is to adopt a healthy, low-fat, high-fiber diet, a regimen of regular exercise, and a relaxed, positive attitude. That's also the best way to prevent cardiac arrhythmias.

Chapter 37

A Guide to Healthy Breasts

F inding a lump in your breast can be frightening. Even when it's happily resolved with the diagnosis of "benign," the experience can leave you feeling vulnerable about this part of your body, wondering what you can do to avoid being a victim of chronic breast pain, or worse, being the one in ten women who gets breast cancer.

Knowing about your breasts—how they function and their disorders—is a good way to minimize that feeling of vulnerability.

How hormones affect breast comfort.

Breasts consist mainly of fat, honeycombed with milk-producing glands and ducts that respond to changes in body chemistry. The milk-producing cells lining the glands are controlled cyclically by three major female hormones—estrogen, progesterone and prolactin. In a woman of childbearing age, each month these cells are stimulated to grow and to accumulate fluids. This makes many women's breasts feel heavy, and sometimes painful and lumpy, three or four days before their period. When menstruation begins, this hormonal stimulation stops. In a healthy breast, cell growth and fluids subside and pain disappears.

What Breast Pain Means

In some women, though, premenstrual pain is severe or becomes a month-long problem. Why this happens is something researchers are still figuring out. It's most likely related to imbalances in hormone levels—too much estrogen or too little progesterone, says Robinson Baker, M.D., director of the Breast Clinic at Johns Hopkins Hospital, Baltimore. And it may be influenced by other body chemicals produced by stress or stimulated by certain foods.

Lumpy, painful breasts are one of many ailments that doctors place in the catchall category "fibrocystic disease."

"Most doctors will agree that lumpy, painful breasts are perfectly normal," says Susan M. Love, M.D., director of the Breast Clinic at Beth Israel Hospital. "Sixty percent of women have breasts painful enough to go to the doctor sometime during their lives. Not because they want relief from the pain but because they're worried that they have cancer. If you can reassure them that this is okay and that they do not need treatment, most are perfectly happy."

The good news: Painful breasts are normal.

Other doctors *do* agree that painful, lumpy breasts are common. But, as we'll see later, they don't all agree that the condition is normal or necessarily healthy.

More severe forms of fibrocystic disease involve three separate types of breast conditions—fibrosis, the formation of cysts and changes in the cells lining the milk ducts, says Dr. Baker.

The facts about fibrocystic disease.

In fibrosis, the connective tissue that supports the milk ducts grows and thickens into scar tissue, perhaps as a result of too much estrogen, Dr. Baker says. In itself, fibrosis is not painful. But frequently it is accompanied by the formation of cysts. The milk ducts, blocked by tissue growth, are unable to drain properly and swell up into tender, fluid-filled sacs. Cysts can range in size from barely palpable to large enough to hold more than a quarter of a cup of water, and they can form in a week or two, Dr. Baker says.

Cysts Are Painful but Not Cancerous

Small cysts often shrink on their own; larger cysts are often punctured and drained with a needle. If they recur several times in the same spot, they may be removed surgically.

Does having fibrocystic disease increase your risks of developing breast cancer? For years, doctors had been saying it does increase your risk two to four times. Today, though, most say fibrocystic disease in itself does not lead to breast cancer—that is, cysts do not become cancerous.

More good news: Fibrocystic disease itself doesn't increase your risk of cancer.

Sometimes, though, some forms of this disease include overgrowth and abnormalities in the cells lining the milk ducts. This condition, known as proliferative, or hyperplastic, disease, can develop into a malignancy, although only a small number do, Dr. Baker says. The only way to diagnose this condition is by tissue biopsy.

Breast self-exams can detect problems in time.

All women, whether they are at risk for cancer or not, should examine their breasts each month. For a woman with fibrocystic disease, though, the question is how to distinguish all those lumps and bumps from one that might actually be cancerous. This is where regular breast self-exams are important. The idea is to become so familiar with your breasts, lumps and all, that when you find something different or unusual, you recognize it for what it is and have it checked out. "Any discrete [distinct] mass should be biopsied, regardless of a patient's age," Dr. Baker says. But there *are* ways to distinguish between benign and malignant lumps.

A cyst will be tender and move easily. It feels similar to an eyeball felt through an eyelid. A cancerous lump is often painless. It will seem to be anchored to the chest wall or to the breast tissue. Cysts can occur in both breasts simultaneously, but cancer usually occurs in one breast only, most often in the upper-right quarter nearest the shoulder.

Breast cancer: the family factor.

The greatest risks for developing breast cancer are, unfortunately, things you cannot control. If your mother, sister or grandmother developed breast cancer, your own chances of getting it are two to three times greater than those of the general population. If the cancer developed prior to menopause or was in both breasts, the risk is even higher. If you've already had cancer in one breast, your chances of getting it in the other breast are five times greater than if you'd never had cancer.

Breast cancer is unusual in women under age 30. Its incidence begins to rise in the early forties, but it's still relatively uncommon up to age 50. Most breast cancers are found in women ages 55 to 60.

A Diet to Discourage Breast Problems

There are ways, though, to decrease your odds, both for bothersome but benign breast ailments and breast cancer. More and more prevention-minded health professionals are observing, and researchers are confirming, that breast disease is influenced by one factor we can do something about—diet.

Fighting breast disease with diet.

"I believe in taking a broad approach," states Phyllis Havens, a registered dietitian with the Whole Health Group in South Portland, Maine, who counsels many women with breast tenderness and swelling and other premenstrual symptoms. "I recommend some major dietary changes and vitamin supplementation."

These include eliminating caffeine-containing foods and fat-rich dairy products, cutting back on red meats, sugars and fats, and adding safflower oil, fiber-rich vegetables and vitamins E and B complex.

The observations of Havens and others that this sort of diet relieves breast disease and problems with other estrogen-sensitive tissues like the uterus and ovaries are yet to be confirmed scientifically but are suggested in part by laboratory research.

Caffeine Is Out

John Minton, M.D., Ph.D., of the Department of Surgery, Ohio State University College of Medicine,

Columbus, has found that substances contained in certain foods can aggravate breast symptoms. These substances produce biochemical signals that activate enzymes that promote fibrous tissue and cyst fluid development in women with fibrocystic disease.

"I know that most women can reverse lumpy, painful breasts completely with changes in their diet," he says.

Dr. Minton discovered that eliminating foods containing substances called methylxanthines (which include caffeine and are found in coffee, tea, cola and chocolate) was associated with the disappearance of breast cysts in most women within a few months.

A change in diet meant fewer breast cysts.

But he also noted that some women who initially got much better on the diet later got worse. "We discovered that when they stopped drinking coffee, they were somehow attracted to other foods that were giving them the same biochemical kick," Dr. Minton says.

Can Vitamin E Help?

Christiane Northrup, M.D., a Yarmouth, Maine, gynecologist who refers some of her patients to the Whole Health Group for nutritional counseling, prescribes 400 to 800 international units daily of vitamin E for her patients with fibrocystic disease. "I find it sometimes helps a great deal to relieve pain and swelling, especially when the symptoms occur because of rapidly changing hormone levels that come with menopause," she says.

Can vitamin E counteract fibrocystic disease?

Preliminary research by Robert London, M.D., director of reproductive medicine at North Charles General Hospital in Baltimore, suggests that vitamin E may be of value in treating breast cysts.

In one study, 80 percent of the women responded to 600 international units of vitamin E daily for two months with decreased symptoms of pain.

His current work does not indicate that vitamin E lowers levels of estrogen or progesterone.

Vitamin A Offers Hope

What about vitamin A? Can this apparent cancer inhibitor protect against breast disease? The answers aren't in yet, but there's a tremendous amount of interest in its possible use, says Marc Lippman, M.D., director of the National Institutes of Health, Breast Cancer Division, Bethesda, Maryland.

"The data from animal studies is quite encouraging," Dr. Lippman says. "Forms of vitamin A can prevent the action of some tumor promoters, there's no doubt about it." In tissue cultures, vitamin A prevents the proliferation, or uncontrolled growth, of breast tissue cells.

Vitamin A: a force against abnormal growth of breast cells in the test tube.

One of the most promising forms of vitamin A for breast cancer, based on work done by Richard Moon, Ph.D., is a retinoid called 4-hydroxyphenylretinamide, which was surprisingly effective in the prevention of breast tumors in mice exposed to carcinogens, says Frank L. Meyskens, Jr., M.D., associate professor in the Department of Medicine at the University of Arizona in Tucson.

Researchers in Milan, Italy, may soon be conducting a trial using this and other vitamin A forms with women who have already had one breast cancer to see if it reduces the rate at which a second tumor appears.

In the United States, Maurice Black, M.D., of the Institute for Breast Disease of the New York Medical College, is using short-term high oral doses of both vitamins A and E in women who have had one breast cancer. This study arose as an offshoot of an ongoing investigation of the protective effect of specific cell-mediated immunity against the patient's own tumor. In the course of these studies, patients were identified who lacked this immunity. It was those nonreactive patients who participated in the high-dose vitamin studies.

These women don't naturally show the kind of immune response associated with good survival rates,

Promising results with vitamins A and E.

Dr. Black says. But with large doses of either A or E, 50 to 60 percent do show this immune response, and with both A and E 80 percent show the response, Dr. Black says. "We don't yet know if this induced response works as well as a spontaneous response. We haven't been following these women long enough to see if they have a reduced incidence of recurrent and/ or second primary breast cancer." (Large doses of vitamin A or E shouldn't be taken without medical guidance.)

Selenium Shows Promise

In mice, selenium seems to counteract breast cancer.

Selenium may have a protective effect. "The results of animal and human population studies continue to be encouraging that the risk of breast cancer does decline if selenium intakes are high," says Gerhard N. Schrauzer, Ph.D., professor of chemistry at the University of California at San Diego. In mice bred to carry a virus that puts them at high risk of developing breast cancer, those receiving extra selenium had an incidence of breast tumors that was 10 percent lower than those that received no additional selenium. "And there's increasing evidence that many human breast cancers have a similar viral influence," Dr. Schrauzer says. Mice that had been fed a high-fat diet and exposed to cancer-causing chemicals also had fewer, slower-forming tumors with selenium supplementation.

Can selenium fight breast disease in humans?

"Human studies with selenium and breast cancer have yet to be done on a large scale, but ongoing studies in Finland and Australia with women with benign fibrocystic disease are showing that selenium supplementation does seem to have beneficial effects," Dr. Schrauzer says. This is a hopeful sign that this unpleasant condition will, in the future, become preventable and treatable by nutritional means. Foods high in selenium include seafoods, liver, kidneys, meat and some whole grains. Supplements of more than 100 micrograms shouldn't be taken.

Cut Back on Fat

Your best bet against both benign breast disease and breast cancer may be the same thing that helps protect against heart disease—a low-fat diet. Population studies show a strong parallel between fat consumption and the incidence of breast cancer. Low-fat countries like Japan and Thailand have only about one-quarter the number of breast cancer deaths as the United States, Denmark and the Netherlands, where people consume up to twice as much fat.

And in animal studies, the evidence is "overwhelming" that a high-fat diet enhances the development of breast tumors, says Clifford Welsch, Ph.D., a tumor biologist with a special interest in breast disease and professor of anatomy at Michigan State University. Dr. Welsch and colleagues are trying to figure out just what it is that links fat with breast disease.

"One idea is that it promotes the secretion of hormones that stimulate the development of both hormone-responsive, normal and cancerous breast tissue," Dr. Welsch says. "It's my opinion that the evidence favors the theory that a high-fat diet increases the susceptibility of the breast tissue to hormone stimulus."

Theory: more fat, more hormones, more disease.

Forty percent of the calories in the average American diet come from fat, mostly in meat and dairy products like butter, cheese and milk. "I think we'd all do well to cut that by one-third to one-half," Dr. Welsch says.

Increase Fiber, Decrease Stress

And it might be a good idea to replace some of that fat with high-fiber foods, such as whole grains and vegetables. Chronic constipation, something few people eating high-fiber diets experience, has been associated with breast disease. Researchers at the University of California at San Francisco found that women with severe constipation (two or fewer bowel movements a week) were five times more likely to

A place for fiber in the healthy-breast diet.

show signs of possible abnormal cell proliferation in aspirated breast fluids than were women with normal bowel functions.

News Flash on Fat and Breast Cancer

Breast cancer is a major killer of American women, and among those age 40 to 44, it causes more deaths than anything else.

In 1942 a scientist demonstrated that there's a probable link between breast cancer and fat in the diet. And the evidence for that link has been getting stronger—and more complex—ever since. Now it seems clear that the more fat you have in your diet, the more likely you are to get breast cancer.

But there are some new wrinkles in the data. There's accumulating evidence that a low-fat diet may actually prolong the lives of women who already have breast cancer.

In one study of 953 women with breast cancer, researchers discovered that the women's risk of death increased 1.4 times for every 1,000 grams of fat eaten per month (equivalent to one extra pat of butter or margarine per day). This connection between life expectancy and fat intake was especially strong for women with cancers that were spreading.

Echoing the reports of other scientists, researcher Rashida A. Karmali, Ph.D., of Rutgers University, and her colleagues say that they were able to protect laboratory rats against breast cancer by feeding them fish oil. "Fish oil," says Dr. Karmali, "inhibited the growth of transplanted tumors, helped block development of chemically induced tumors and lowered levels of a biochemical indicator of cancer activity." Preventing cancer in rats is a long way from preventing it in people, she says. However, these preliminary findings hint at promising possibilities.

Do scientists now have enough information to devise a diet that prevents breast cancer, a diet including the right dietary fats in specific amounts?

Not yet. So far all they know is that cutting overall fat intake is likely to reduce the risk of breast cancer. The National Research Council advises that, to lower the risk of this disease and colon cancer, dietary fat should be reduced to 30 percent of total calories.

"Indeed," the council admits, "the data could be used to justify an even greater reduction."

"It may be that estrogen secreted by the liver is reabsorbed more readily by women with sluggish digestion," says Nicholas Petrakis, M.D., professor of preventive medicine at the University of California, San Francisco. "This could have a stimulating effect on the breasts."

One other thing the doctors who treat breast disease frequently mention is stress. "Most of the women I see feel their symptoms are aggravated when they're upset or overworked," Havens says. One of Dr. Love's patients, a politician, suffers from breast pain only when she is campaigning.

Can stress make breast symptoms worse?

"One's attitude, what we call the neuroendocrine aspect of tumorigenesis, can markedly control the development of breast disease," Dr. Welsch says. "It affects the entire central nervous system and can really throw it out of whack."

Preventing breast cancer with a new attitude.

What's a "good attitude" to have? It's not being so paranoid about getting cancer that you live in fear, but it's also not being negligent about checking your breasts for lumps each month—or taking other measures to reduce the risks, Dr. Welsch says.

Chapter 38

Bruises: What to Do When You're Black and Blue

D o you bruise easily, even when you can't recall hurting yourself? Do you wonder why you're black and blue? If so, you're not alone. Many people bruise easily. For most, it is not a serious problem, but tracking down the cause may be worthwhile. In some cases, bruising can be prevented. In others, bruises point to an underlying illness.

A blow to the body injures blood vessels and can make a bruise appear. Further bleeding is prevented through a process called hemostasis. First, the blood vessels narrow in response to the injury, and the clotting cells, or platelets, are attracted to the areas of blood-vessel damage. The platelets stick to these areas and cause a tight, but temporary, plug to form. Then proteins called clotting factors are activated, and the plug becomes permanent. This strong structural barrier is what prevents blood loss. If something goes wrong at any point in this chain of events, bleeding or bruising may result.

The appearance of bruises can sometimes suggest which part of the chain is functioning improperly. If your bruises look like clusters of small dots, you may have a platelet disorder. Bigger bruises generally indicate an abnormality in blood vessels or clotting factors.

Bruising Has Many Causes

If your bruises are larger than an inch across, if you've had no injury that you can recall and if you

The anatomy of a bruise.

When to worry about bruises.

haven't bruised easily in the past, your bruising may be caused by one of several factors known to interfere with hemostasis.

Drug-Induced Bruises

Certain common drugs can adversely affect the hemostatic process. A single aspirin can reduce platelet function for an entire week. Anti-inflammatory medications, antidepressants, asthma medications and substances found in many cough remedies also inhibit platelet action. The number of circulating platelets can be reduced by estrogen pills, diuretics and large amounts of alcohol. Steroids may weaken the supporting tissue of blood vessels in the skin, making them tear more easily. Spontaneous or easy bruising may result.

Cough remedies are one possible offender.

Nutrition-Related Bruises

Deficiencies in vitamin B_{12} and folate may cause a decrease in production of mature platelets and contribute to easy bruising. Drugs like Dilantin, a seizure-control medication, may inhibit folate absorption. Over a period of time, a poor diet could result in a vitamin B_{12} deficiency.

Vitamin C plays a major role in the synthesis of collagen, the main protein in the supporting fibers of the blood vessel walls. If you lack vitamin C, these fibers could weaken, making the blood vessels fragile. It's not certain whether increased doses of vitamin C will cure easy bruising. But it has been shown that vitamin C in doses eight times the Recommended Dietary Allowance (RDA) of 60 milligrams speeds wound healing, which also requires the production of collagen.

Vitamin C: a possible link to easy bruising.

Autoimmunity and Bruises

Easy bruising may result from viruses and autoimmune diseases. Viruses can occasionally cause a temporary drop in the platelet count. Lupus, an autoimmune disease in which the body attacks its own cell components, may cause a reduction in platelets and a production of substances that inhibit the clotting factors. Autoimmune diseases brought on by a reaction to certain hair dyes, insecticides, common drugs or quinine in tonic water destroy the circulating platelets.

Hereditary Bruising

Cautions for bruise-prone families.

If you have a family history of bruising or bleeding, you should consider having an evaluation for Von Willebrand's disease. This is an inherited disorder of one of the clotting factors. For unknown reasons, it affects women more often than men. Since the symptoms are often mild, this disorder may go unrecognized for a long time. You might notice prolonged bleeding after a wisdom tooth extraction, frequent nosebleeds, heavy periods or continued bleeding from a small cut. Individuals with Von Willebrand's disease should be especially careful to avoid aspirin and other drugs that inhibit hemostasis. Sometimes it may be necessary to treat this disorder by replacing the clotting factor.

Beating the Bruises

Three vitamins that may help.

It is comforting to know that bruising is usually not associated with serious disease and generally has no serious consequences. If you bruise easily, ask your doctor about discontinuing unnecessary medication, especially aspirin. Make sure you eat a well-balanced diet that includes plenty of folate and vitamins C and B_{12}. If your bruising persists, see your physician for evaluation for an underlying illness.

Ten Ways to Guard against Cancer

M any of us have lived with a feeling of help-lessness about cancer for so long that it's hard to change our thinking. But a massive body of research now refutes the long-held belief that we are at the mercy of cancer and instead shows that we can prevent it.

How much of an impact could we have if we all practiced prevention? "If it were possible that we could carry it out ideally, as much as 80 to 85 percent of all cancers today might not occur," says Charles A. LeMaistre, M.D., president of the American Cancer Society. "For too long we have regarded cancer as the dominant factor in its relationship with human-kind. Now, preventing this disease is becoming more and more realistic."

Eighty-five percent of all cancers could be prevented.

Hallmarks of an Anticancer Diet

By avoiding the things that are known to cause cancer and incorporating into our lives factors that protect against it, we can reduce our risk of develop-ing the disease.

"In some areas, the information is now so com-plete that it's unequivocal, such as the causal role of smoking in the development of cancer," says Dr. LeMaistre, who is also president of the University of Texas's M. D. Anderson Hospital and Tumor Institute in Houston. "In other areas, such as diet and nutrition, information is not yet complete, but it is sufficient to take action."

We now have enough in-formation to take action against cancer.

Seven Dietary Steps to Ward Off Cancer

The following steps, recommended by the American Cancer Society, summarize what we can do. Following these steps will also contribute to a healthier life in general.

1. Eat more high-fiber foods. There is a lot of evidence that colon cancer is less common in populations that eat a diet high in fiber, such as whole grains, fruit and vegetables. In a study comparing Finnish and Danish people, for example, colon cancer was much lower among the Finns. The diets of the two groups are similar, except that the Finns eat large amounts of high-fiber, whole-grain rye bread, while the Danes have a low-fiber diet.

How fiber works.

Fiber may work by hastening the travel time of fecal matter through the bowel, so that carcinogens (cancer-causing substances) are whisked away before they can do their damage. Another theory is that by increasing the bulk of the stool, fiber dilutes the concentration of carcinogens.

2. Eat more foods rich in vitamin A. Spinach, carrots, sweet potatoes and apricots and other sources of vitamin A may help protect you against cancers of the lung, esophagus and larynx. In a major study, Norwegian men whose intake of vitamin A was above average had less than half the rate of lung cancer of men whose intake of the vitamin was below average.

Vegetable "colors" that may stop cancer.

Right now it's unclear whether the effects are due to vitamin A itself or a precursor of vitamin A called beta-carotene, a pigment found in plants. The emphasis now is on the naturally occurring pigment because the precursors of vitamin A are the most probable agents that have this effect.

Beta-carotene is found in dark green and deep yellow vegetables and in deep yellow fruits.

3. Get plenty of vitamin C. Studies indicate that people whose diets are rich in vitamin C are less likely to get cancer, particularly of the stomach and esophagus.

We know that vitamin C can inhibit the formation of nitrosamines, cancer-causing chemicals, in the stomach. That may be how it protects against cancer.

Fruits and vegetables, particularly oranges, grapefruit, green peppers, broccoli, tomatoes and potatoes, are good sources of the vitamin.

4. Eat more cabbage-family vegetables. Broccoli, cauliflower, brussels sprouts, cabbage, kale and kohlrabi are known as cruciferous vegetables. Studies in large groups of people have suggested that consuming cruciferous vegetables may reduce the risk of cancer, particularly of the gastrointestinal and respiratory tracts. And tests in laboratory animals reveal that cruciferous vegetables may be highly effective in preventing chemically induced cancer.

A possible cancer fighter: the lowly cabbage family.

What is it about these foods that is protective? "We have to look upon these vegetables as a source of vitamins A and C and fiber, but there are other possibilities under investigation," Dr. LeMaistre says.

5. Trim fat from your diet. Studies in humans and laboratory studies point out that excessive fat intake increases the chance of developing cancers of the breast, colon and prostate. And it's not just one kind of fat that's a problem. Both saturated and unsaturated fats, whether of plant or animal origin, have been found to enhance cancer growth when eaten in excess.

The National Academy of Sciences recommends that we decrease the amount of fat in our diet to 30 percent of the total calories we eat. (Americans currently consume about 40 percent of total calories as fat.)

A healthy level of fat: 30 percent.

You can cut your fat intake by using less fats and oils in cooking, and by switching to lean meat, fish, and low-fat dairy products.

6. Control your weight. "The long-standing and repeated observation that obesity is correlated with cancer is sufficiently substantiated to take action," says Dr. LeMaistre. In one massive study con-

40 percent overweight and more likely to get cancer.

ducted by the American Cancer Society over 12 years, researchers found an increased incidence of cancers of the uterus, gallbladder, breast, colon, kidney and stomach in obese people. In that study, women and men who were 40 percent or more overweight had a 55 and 33 percent greater risk of cancer respectively than people of normal weight.

Regular exercise and lower calorie intake can help you avoid gaining weight. It's advisable to check with your doctor before embarking on a special diet or strenuous exercise routine, though.

7. Avoid salt-cured, smoked and nitrite-cured foods. Cancers of the esophagus and stomach are common in countries where large quantities of ham, bacon, hot dogs and salt-cured or smoked fish and similar foods are eaten.

Calcium against Colon Cancer

Colorectal cancer is the second deadliest cancer in the nation, killing about 60,000 people a year. (Lung cancer is number one, felling about 126,000 people a year.)

Among scientists there's a growing suspicion that manipulating certain factors in the diet may help prevent colorectal cancer. In addition to lowered dietary fat and increased fiber, researchers are now looking at a new possibility: calcium.

The idea that calcium might help deter colon cancer got a boost when researchers noticed that the disease seemed to strike more frequently in latitudes far from the equator—places with less sunshine. The hypothesis was that since sunlight helps the body make vitamin D, and vitamin D enables the body to absorb calcium, it was this nutritional pair that reduced colon cancer.

On top of this, scientists reported that in Scandinavia colon cancer occurs least where consumption of milk is greatest. And a 19-year study in Chicago revealed that men with the lowest intake of vitamin D and calcium had about three times the risk of colorectal cancer as those who had the highest intake.

Further evidence comes from researchers at Memorial Sloan-

Smoked foods absorb some of the tars from the smoke they're cured with. The tars contain cancer-causing chemicals similar to those in tobacco smoke. There is also good evidence that nitrates and nitrites can enhance the formation of nitrosamines in our food and digestive tracts.

Three More Important Precautions

In addition to diet, certain health habits can help stave off specific kinds of cancer.

1. Don't smoke cigarettes. "About 30 percent of all cancer is clearly and unequivocally due to cigarette smoking," says Dr. LeMaistre. "It's been 20 years

A deadly vice.

Kettering Cancer Center and Cornell University Medical College in New York City. They gave daily doses of 1,250 milligrams of calcium to people with family histories of colon cancer. The idea was to discover what effect the calcium might have on excessive proliferation (duplication) of cells in the lining of the colon. Excessive proliferation is often found in people prone to developing colon cancer. The researchers report that before the calcium supplements, cell proliferation was just what you'd expect in people susceptible to colon cancer, but that after two to three months of taking calcium, proliferation was lower—comparable to that of people with a lower risk of colon cancer. "Calcium modifies the environment in the colon," says chief researcher Martin Lipkin, M.D. "We think that calcium binds [captures] bile and fatty acids, reducing their irritation to the colon lining and thus decreasing the proliferation of cells. The result is a lower risk of colon cancer.

"We intend to conduct more research on calcium and colon cancer. We want to see what effect calcium might have on ulcerative colitis, familial polyposis and other conditions that may lead to cancer of the colon," Dr. Lipkin says.

since the Surgeon General's 'Report on Smoking and Health', without any significant findings having been refuted." Smoking poses a risk to the nonsmoker (passive smoking) as well, he points out.

It's never too late to quit smoking.

If you're a smoker and haven't quit because you think "the damage has already been done," take heart in the findings of a British study of over 18,000 people. Researchers found that people who had smoked for as long as 20 years—but who had been off cigarettes for 10 years or more—had no greater risk of lung cancer than people who had never smoked at all (*British Medical Journal*).

2. Go easy on alcohol. Heavy drinkers, especially those who also smoke, are at very high risk for cancers of the mouth and throat. Your risk of liver cancer also increases if you drink a lot.

3. Shield yourself from the sun. Too much sun causes skin cancer and other skin damage. "Like most other Americans, I'm learning that the tanning of hide is neither healthy nor beautiful," says Dr. LeMaistre. "I use maximum-strength sunblocks and also use hats and other ways of shading myself."

A sunscreen for maximum protection.

A sunscreen with a sun protection factor (SPF) of 15 or more gives maximum protection. Be especially wary during the midday hours—from 11:00 A.M. to 3:00 P.M.—when sunlight is strongest. And don't use indoor sunlamps or tanning booths—they're not safe, either.

Although they affect fewer people than the risk factors already mentioned, excessive x-rays, certain estrogen treatments and exposure at work to harmful chemicals and fibers like asbestos should also be avoided. "I think every effort should be made to protect a human being from excessive x-rays and from the other known causes of cancer, albeit they cause a very small percentage of cancer today," says Dr. LeMaistre. You can ask your doctor about the need for x-rays and estrogens and be familiar with proper safety procedures on the job.

Following all the preventive steps may reduce your risk of cancer dramatically. But there's another side to cancer prevention—early detection. Sigmoidoscopy, Pap tests and breast exams, for example, can catch cancers when there's still a very good chance of curing them. For details on these and other lifesaving early-detection methods, contact your local American Cancer Society chapter or ask your doctor.

Uncover cancers early—and live longer.

Chapter 40

One Doctor's Prescription for Cancer Prevention

By Charles B. Simone, M.D.

T here has been a great interest in nutrition and vitamins and minerals in the past several years. I got involved with nutrients as cancer-preventive agents in a very interesting way. While at the National Cancer Institute in Bethesda, Maryland, a young man with a rare cancer was referred to me for treatment. I was a medical oncologist (chemotherapist), radiation therapist and clinical immunologist.

Both he and his wife feared the word cancer, as most of us do. They knew that cancer is the number two killer in this country. He asked me why he got cancer: "Why me?" I told him I didn't know.

Why "cancer phobia" is widespread.

A Frighteningly Common Disease

One of every three people in America does get cancer. This young man was my age, and his wife was several weeks pregnant before his diagnosis was made. My wife was also pregnant for the same period of time. You can readily understand that an unusually close bond between us was inevitable.

In our initial conversation, he requested that I do all that was possible to cure him, but if that was impossible, he wanted to live long enough to see the birth of his child. As I said before, he had a rare

Charles B. Simone, M.D., is a radiation therapist and an associate professor of radiation therapy at Thomas Jefferson University Hospital's Bodine Center for Cancer Treatment in Philadelphia, Pennsylvania.

cancer that had spread to many parts of his body by the time I saw him. Both he and his wife were devoutly religious.

When he first came to me as a patient, I was very much involved with basic science. I had discovered the fundamental mechanism of how our white blood cells kill foreign cells like cancer. White blood cells are one army of our immune system. The immune system defends against infections and cancer. I was also heavily involved with administering chemotherapy. And in addition, I was on the road to discovering a new immunology technique to treat cancer victims. None of my interests or training "permitted" me to even think about nutrition as a therapy or as a preventive agent. Only a few short years ago, nutritional manipulation was considered quackery.

The nutritional approach to cancer prevention used to be considered quackery.

I began treating him with chemotherapy, and after a number of months, all of his cancer was gone. We were very encouraged. I continued on with the chemotherapy, as was standard practice. After about seven months he looked worse, but no cancer could be found. I had several different consultants see him, including a neurologist. No one could tell me why he looked so bad in spite of the fact that we could not detect any cancer. After several discussions, it was suggested that he looked as though he had pellagra (niacin-deficiency disease).

Since I had tried everything else, I decided, as a last resort, to put him on high doses of vitamins and minerals taken by mouth. He perked up within several days. I couldn't believe it. Because it was so hard for me to accept, I decided to stop the vitamins and minerals after three weeks to see what would happen. After I stopped them, he slumped down within days. Even then I was still a doubting Thomas, but I put him back on the same vitamins and minerals. Again, he perked up.

To my surprise, the vitamins and minerals seemed to work.

Ultimately, however, the cancer consumed him, but only after he had seen the birth of his son. Before he died, he asked me what his son and wife could do so that they would not get cancer.

Investigating Vitamins and Minerals

It was during that period of time that I began to investigate the effects of nutrition on cancer, but more important, the effects of nutrition and vitamins and minerals in the *prevention* of cancer. (I found that nutrition should not be used as the only treatment for cancer but rather as an adjunct to conventional cancer therapies.) Other important factors bolstered my interest also. I had heard estimates that nutritional factors account for 60 percent of all women's cancers and 40 percent of all men's cancers. That is a staggering amount of cancer related to what we eat or don't eat. Despite all of our various treatments for cancer, the results, in general, are quite limited.

The question asked by that patient has often been asked: "What can my family do so that they will not get cancer?" Since there was limited progress in treating cancer, I decided to turn some of my attention to preventing cancer.

After doing an extensive amount of research, I realized that the tremendous increase in cancer could be halted. Most cancers can be prevented, since the majority are related to preventable factors: nutrition and tobacco use. I wanted to share this information with people, so I wrote *Cancer and Nutrition*, which was published by McGraw-Hill. In it I outlined a "Ten-Point Plan to Reduce Your Chances of Getting Cancer." Point one discusses nutrition, and one important aspect of it concerns vitamins and minerals.

Vitamins and minerals have many important cancer-preventive functions. One of the major protective effects appears to be their ability to neutralize or scavenge free-radical chemicals. Free radicals are by-products of normal chemical reactions in your body that can make a cell develop into a cancer if not destroyed. They are also increased by harmful chemicals that are known to cause cancer. We all have natural protection against free radicals, thanks to cer-

I discovered that many, many cancers are related to what we eat or don't eat.

Most cancer can be prevented.

Vitamins and minerals against "free radicals."

tain vitamins and minerals called antioxidants, which are free-radical scavengers.

Other cancer-preventive properties or actions of some vitamins and minerals include killing cancer cells directly, reversing precancerous conditions, enhancing the immune system and neutralizing toxic chemicals. Here's a brief outline of each micronutrient's cancer-preventive properties.

Beta-carotene is heavy artillery. The body uses beta-carotene to make vitamin A. Over the years at least two dozen studies from around the world have found that people who consume higher-than-average amounts of beta-carotene and vitamin A have a lower incidence of cancer.

Beta-carotene may inhibit the development of cancer in the following ways:

1. It is a powerful antioxidant, or free-radical neutralizer.

2. It greatly enhances the immune system, which protects you from many diseases, including cancer.

3. It is the most powerful inhibitor of another very destructive molecule, called "singlet oxygen," which can cause cancer.

How beta-carotene may help your body deter cancer.

Vitamin A gets into the act. Vitamin A has many important functions. It decreases the growth of human breast cancer cells and exerts a protective effect for both smokers and nonsmokers against lung cancer.

Several clinical studies have used vitamin A to treat patients with skin cancer, lung cancer and cervix cancer. The results are very promising.

Vitamin A: a promising anticancer agent.

Robert Gallo, M.D., chief of the laboratory of tumor cell biology, and his associates at the National Cancer Institute have shown that high levels of a form of vitamin A (retinoic acid) suppress a certain oncogene. Oncogenes, very simply, are thought to cause cancer once they are triggered to act.

How vitamin E works. Vitamin E is a potent antioxidant. It inhibits the growth of certain cancer cells and neutralizes a potent chemical, called nitro-samine, that can cause cancer.

Teaming B vitamins and pantothenic acid. This group has been shown to be exceedingly important for the immune system.

Vitamin C protection. Vitamin C is a potent antioxidant that helps protect the body against bladder cancer. Researchers report a protective role of vitamin C in larynx cancer, cervical cancer and many animal cancers.

Vitamin C may have a protective role in viral illnesses. This may be important with a discovery that a certain human cancer of the lymph glands is caused by a virus. Also, AIDS seems to be related to a virus.

A deficiency in vitamin C causes a malfunction of the immune system.

Other vitamins play a basic role. Niacin, vitamins D and B_{12}, folate and biotin have no known direct anticancer or immune system effects. But they are important for maintaining a healthy body that can better fight off all diseases, including cancer.

Selenium and other defensive minerals. Selenium is a potent antioxidant. My own research shows that selenium protects the cell membrane from free-radical attack. Many animal studies show that high levels of selenium inhibit the growth of various cancers. The higher the selenium content of the soil, the lower the cancer rate.

Copper and zinc are other minerals that are free-radical scavengers. Zinc deficiency results in a malfunctioning immune system. Iodine deficiency has been related to thyroid cancer in several studies.

Marginal Intake
Means Marginal Protection

Vitamin or mineral deficiencies that are severe enough to cause diseases can be detected with our current capabilities. Marginal deficiencies, those

Vitamin C against bladder cancer.

Selenium: another force against destructive "free radicals."

which do not show any outward signs of disease, are very difficult to detect, however.

Many conditions (stress, smoking, advanced age) require higher amounts of vitamins and minerals. Also, it has been estimated that 25 percent of all households do not have nutritionally balanced diets. These circumstances may produce marginal deficiencies. These marginal deficiencies may result in less than full protection against free radicals and may inhibit the immune system from functioning properly, among other things.

Avoid marginal deficiencies and beef up your protection against disease.

Many people have advocated that taking certain vitamins and minerals may prevent cancer. R. Lee Clark, M.D., president emeritus of M. D. Anderson Hospital and Tumor Institute in Houston, has said, "Certain vitamins definitely help to prevent cancer." Raymond J. Shamberger, Ph.D., head of the enzymology section of the Cleveland Clinic, says, "There's no question that certain vitamins and minerals can help prevent cancer." And Dr. Heinrick Wrba, head of the cancer research institute at the University of Vienna, states, "Vitamin supplements along with proper diet can cut your risk of cancer."

Can taking supplements help you to prevent cancer?

I am advocating simple common sense. I believe that the following nutrients, if taken daily as part of a comprehensive plan, would be useful to all adults: beta-carotene (10 milligrams), vitamin E (500 international units), vitamin C (650 milligrams), selenium (200 micrograms), copper (3 milligrams), zinc (24 milligrams), vitamins B_1, B_2, B_6 and B_{12} (higher than average RDAs), plus vitamins A and D, niacin, folate, pantothenic acid, biotin and iodine in at least RDA amounts. (*Editor's note:* Many experts feel that people should get their vitamins and minerals from food rather than supplements, whenever possible.)

Keep in mind that while such a supplement program may modify an individual's risk of developing cancer, it has not been proved to prevent, mitigate or cure cancer. Furthermore, it is the total diet, not an individual dietary supplement, that establishes the

The total diet is what matters in fighting disease.

role of nutrition in determining health and reducing the risk of diet-related disease.

The nutrients listed previously could be taken daily unless otherwise specified by your physician. Pregnant and lactating women should take them only with the approval of their physician.

Heading Off Cancer Early

In closing, I would like to give an example of a precancerous condition and its relationship to possible vitamin/mineral marginal deficiencies. Precancerous conditions are not rare. If nothing is done about them, they can ultimately lead to a full-blown cancer. A certain kind of abnormal Pap smear, for instance, indicates a precancerous condition. A Pap smear is taken from the cervix in a woman's vagina as a check to see if that part of her body has cancer. There are five classes of readings for a Pap smear. Class V is outright cancer, for example, and Class III represents a precancerous condition.

Stopping precancer with supplements.

Several women who had Class III Pap smears representing precancerous conditions took the supplements mentioned earlier for four to six months. After that time, their Pap smears became completely normal. After a year, their Pap smears remained normal. This was obviously very encouraging.

If you read and follow the Ten-Point Plan, which is more fully described in my book, your chances of developing cancer and heart disease will be greatly reduced. Highlights of the plan include a low-fat, low-cholesterol, high-fiber diet, supplemented with vitamins and minerals, the elimination of all tobacco use, the reduction of alcohol intake, limited exposure to radiation (including sunlight), exercise and a physical exam every year beginning at age 35 or 40.

The Pap Test
and Nutrition:
Two Fronts against
Cervical Problems

I t has probably happened to someone you know, or perhaps it has even happened to you. Instead of a follow-up postcard or phone call from your gynecologist's secretary, you get an ominous call from the doctor himself. "Your Pap smear wasn't quite normal. I'd like to see you again in my office." Despite his reassurances, your mind spins with questions and dark imaginings. This is a time when you need all of the information you can lay your hands on.

The Pap smear is a scraping of cells from the cervix, the tip of the uterus that extends into the vagina. The sample includes cells from the cervix, vagina and uterine lining (called the endometrium). The cells are checked by a laboratory for any signs of abnormal change and classified according to the degree of abnormality found.

The Pap test: what it really means.

The Pap smear can usually detect inflammation or infection of the cervix and endometrium, which can occur with intrauterine devices (IUDs), pelvic inflammatory disease, or *Chlamydia* infections. It is not as useful for detecting cancer of the endometrium or ovaries.

But it is of great value in detecting possibly precancerous changes on the cervix long before any signs are visible to the doctor's eye. These changes are known as cervical dysplasia. (Dysplasia simply means "abnormal development of cells.")

The Pap test sees what the doctor can't.

Understanding the Pap Test

Currently, Pap smears are categorized in one of two ways—either they are divided into five classes and several subclasses, according to the severity of tissue change, or, increasingly, the abnormality found in the cells is more fully described.

How to "read" Pap smear results.

Class I is a normal smear with no abnormal cells. Class II is a kind of catchall category of minor cell changes that can include inflammation and infection or very early signs of dysplasia. Class III includes mild and moderate dysplasia. These are also known as cervical intraepithelial neoplasms (CIN) 1 and 2. (Neoplasm means "new and abnormal tissue growth," which may or may not be cancerous. Intraepithelial means "among the cells lining the cervix.")

Class IV Pap smears include severe dysplasia and cancer confined to the lining of the cervix, both called CIN 3. Class V is invasive cancer—cancer that has spread beyond the cervix to the uterus and possibly to other parts of the body.

While it's important to know into what class or category your Pap smear has been placed, it's even more crucial to know *why* it's been put there, says Ralph Richart, M.D., director of the Division of Obstetrics and Gynecologic Pathology and Cytology at Columbia Presbyterian Medical Center in New York City.

Get a full explanation of Pap test results from your doctor.

"The current classification system is simply not precise enough to keep up with new knowledge of the cause and process of cervical dysplasia," Dr. Richart says. "Every doctor should request from the laboratory a written description of the cell changes found in the Pap smear. And he should be able to explain in detail to his patient the reason for the abnormality, especially in the catchall Class II category."

The cervix may be reacting to a vaginal infection like *Trichomonas,* or to uterine inflammation from an IUD. More important, it may be showing signs of having been exposed to one of the viruses that cause venereal warts that have been associated with cancer. Since treatment varies in each of these cases, these distinctions are crucial. Unfortunately, they are not always made, Dr. Richart says.

The Link between Sex and Cervical Dysplasia

The whole school of thought concerning cervical dysplasia and cancer has been turned upside-down in the last year or two as the result of findings that many of these tissue changes are caused by a group of sexually transmitted viruses known as human papilloma virus (HPV) or, commonly, as the condyloma virus, Dr. Richart says. If they are allowed to flourish, all these viruses will cause abnormal tissue growth or breakdown. Some will form tiny flat warts that can grow undetected on the cervix or in the vagina, on the male urinary opening or on the penis. Others form large cauliflower-shaped warts.

"It is now generally agreed that the condyloma virus is the major agent responsible for abnormal Pap smears," Dr. Richart says. "The genetic material of this virus has been found in a large percentage of dysplastic tissue samples."

The primary cause of abnormal Pap tests.

The condyloma viruses are named by numbers according to their order of discovery. There are approximately 40 now known. "Several of them—particularly HPV 6 and 11—are thought to be essentially benign," Dr. Richart says. "Their association with neoplasia is not very strong."

On the other hand, HPV viruses 16, 18 and 33 are routinely associated with cancer and cancer precursors. The main sign of exposure to these viruses is the development of flat genital warts, which often go undetected until they're discovered during a gynecological examination in women or a penile exam in men.

Practically all abnormal Pap smears show signs of the condyloma virus. One percent of all women,

2.5 percent of women under 30 and about 4.5 percent of women in high-risk groups have the virus detected by the Pap smear.

"Recent studies have not confirmed the original suggestion that herpes is a factor in cervical dysplasia or cancer, and I believe most authorities now believe that herpes plays no role or only a minor role," Dr. Richart says.

Are You at High Risk?

What's a high-risk group? "The most important risk factor is multiple sex partners," Dr. Richart says. "It's just like any other sexually transmitted disease. Every time a woman climbs into bed with a new partner or a man climbs into bed with a new partner, they run the risk of that person being a carrier of this virus. Every other risk factor is secondary."

The statistics confirm that sexual activity plays a major role. Among nuns, cervical cancer is rare. Among prostitutes, it's almost an occupational hazard. And there's an unfortunate increased risk for the one-man woman whose mate tends to roam, as seen in Latin America. In those countries, tradition dictates that wives be strictly monogamous. But there's an equally strong tradition for men to frequent prostitutes. In those countries, cervical cancer rates are high.

Sexual activity: a big factor in cervical cancer.

And there's an especially disturbing risk factor for some other women. The wife of a man whose previous wife died of cervical cancer is herself three times more likely than normal to develop the disease.

Obviously, these findings point to the need for the woman who is diagnosed as having dysplasia to insist that her husband or boyfriend see a doctor, too. In fact, one study by researchers at Columbia University found that 53 percent of the male partners of women with cervical dysplasia had condyloma lesions on their penis or in their urinary opening. This could be especially important in cases where the virus returns again and again.

Cervical dysplasia: a man's concern, too.

"A woman who has recurrent infections probably should have her husband checked to see if he is a carrier, but that's ahead of where we are now," says Rosemary Zuna, M.D., director of cytopathology in the Department of Pathology at the State University of New York, Stony Brook. "It's probably the thing to do, but it's not being done routinely at this time."

The Pill Seems Safe, but Smoking Is Not

While researchers believe the condyloma virus triggers most dysplastic symptoms, they also think other risk factors may make some people more vulnerable to the virus, or may trigger forms of dysplasia that are not virus related. "We know that in some women, these lesions go away by themselves," says Dr. Zuna. "And we know that in some women, they develop into cancer. What we don't know is the real key that causes some lesions to actually invade the tissues and become malignant."

Tobacco is a known risk factor. Women who smoke more than 15 cigarettes a day are twice as likely as nonsmokers to have cervical dysplasia or cervical cancer. And they are 3.5 times more likely to develop invasive cancer (*British Journal of Cancer*). Samples of cervical mucus taken from women smokers contain chemicals that cause cancerous cell changes (*American Journal of Epidemiology*).

Women who smoke double their risk.

The daughters of women who took the drug diethylstilbestrol (DES) during pregnancy may be a high-risk group. But women using birth control pills or menopausal estrogen are apparently not at risk.

It's true that there have been one or two English studies linking the use of birth control pills with cervical dysplasia. But many top researchers contest their findings. "These studies are criticized because they did not adequately take into account the increased sexual activity that might be seen in women using birth control pills," Dr. Richart says. "When this factor is controlled for, these women seem to develop no more cervical dysplasia than normal."

Women who choose diaphragm and condom use may have lower-than-usual cervical cancer rates, possibly because the devices protect the cervix from contact. Male circumcision is no longer considered a factor. Neither is the number of children you have had nor a family history of cervical cancer.

Condoms may protect against cancer.

Vitamins That Lower Risk

Until recently, eating habits were not considered an important factor in cervical dysplasia. Now, though, researchers are finding that nutritional status apparently plays a role in the development of cervical dysplasia and cervical cancer, just as it may with other cancers or precancerous conditions. Poor nutrition may make cervical cells less able to withstand the mutagenic effects of some viruses or the carcinogens found in the cervical mucus of women who smoke. It can also weaken the body's immune system, making it less able to fight infection.

Poor nutrition may weaken defenses.

Lower-than-normal intake of selenium, vitamins C and A and the B-complex vitamin folate have been found in women with cervical dysplasia or newly diagnosed cancer.

Researchers at the Albert Einstein College of Medicine in New York City found that women whose intake of vitamin C was less than 30 milligrams daily (only half the Recommended Dietary Allowance, and equal to about half a medium orange or two ounces of juice from concentrate) had a risk of developing cervical dysplasia ten times greater than that of women whose daily intake was higher (*American Journal of Epidemiology*).

A lower intake of vitamin C meant a greater risk of developing cervical dysplasia.

They also found that women were three times more likely to have severe cervical dysplasia or cervical cancer if their vitamin A intake was below the group median of 3,450 international units daily (equivalent to about a third of a cup of shredded carrots or four dried apricots).

Cervical problems: a possible link to vitamin A intake.

"Whether nutritional factors and their interaction in cervical epithelial cells have antitumor properties that may influence the host's immune system or even influence the maturation or development of normal cervical epithelium is a challenging scientific problem," says Seymour Romney, M.D., director of gynecologic cancer research at the Albert Einstein College of Medicine.

Dr. Romney is involved in two research projects. In one, women with mild or moderate dysplasia are being given supplemental vitamin C to see if their condition improves. In another, they are being treated with topical applications to the cervix of a synthetic form of vitamin A, retinyl acetate gel. "We have no results yet on these studies," Dr. Romney says. But researchers at the University of Arizona may have an inkling of what to expect. They did a study very similar to Dr. Romney's vitamin A study, using a different form of vitamin A, transretinoic acid. The treatment showed encouraging activity in preventing worsening of the condition in women with mild to severe cervical dysplasia.

Folate also seems to play a role in dysplasia, especially in women using birth control pills who may have lower body levels of this vitamin, according to researchers at the University of Alabama at Birmingham. Their research involved 47 young women with cervical dysplasia. Half were given ten milligrams of folate (25 times the Recommended Dietary Allowance) each day, while the other half received a placebo (dummy pill). After three months, the cervical dysplasia had regressed to normal in four of the women in the folate group. There was no improvement in the placebo group. In fact, the dysplasia had worsened in four of the women. (*Note:* Large doses of vitamins require a doctor's supervision.)

If you're on the Pill, make sure you get enough folate.

"Just what kind of nutritional recommendations will come out of further research is yet to be seen," Dr. Romney says. But the indications are now that preventing cervical dysplasia is yet another good reason to make sure you're getting plenty of fresh fruits

A diet for preventing dysplasia.

and vegetables rich in vitamins C and A and folate-rich dark leafy greens.

Why Yearly Checkups Are Vital

It may be frightening to find yourself in the high-risk group. But there are two important—and reassuring—things to remember about Pap smears. First, quite a few women at some time in their lives will have smears showing mild, moderate and even severe dysplasia, but they won't go on to develop cancer. Their condition will be successfully treated.

Second, if you're getting Pap smears every year, it's very unlikely that you'll suddenly discover you have cervical cancer. Most cell changes in the cervix follow a long, slow continuum. Most cervical cancers take about ten years to develop and appear years earlier as treatable dysplasia. The women who end up with invasive cancer either do not get yearly Pap smears or are among the unlucky few who develop a rapidly growing cancer.

Regular Pap tests can detect problems early.

How your doctor treats your cervical dysplasia depends on several factors—the classification of your smear, whether you intend to have children, other risk factors, your doctor's own opinions and experience, even how reliable you are at coming in for follow-ups. Nevertheless, there are some generally accepted procedures for diagnosis and treatment, Dr. Zuna says.

If your smear is Class II, your doctor should determine the reason for the classification and treat it. Inflammation or infection can be treated with antibiotics or other drugs.

If you have the condyloma virus, don't take chances.

If your smear shows signs of the condyloma virus, however, treatment is needed, whether the dysplasia is mild, moderate or severe. "Some doctors will wait a few months and do another smear, but I'd rather get a firm diagnosis and treat," Dr. Richart says. "It's a sexually transmitted disease, whether you currently have symptoms or not. Why risk infecting someone else?"

Biopsies Tell the Story

Treatment is basically the same for all classifications of dysplasia. First, your doctor will view the cervix with a colposcope. This instrument provides a magnified view of the cervix, allowing the doctor to see growths, from which he will take a small bit of tissue for biopsy. "A biopsy is important, because it's the only way to rule out invasive cancer," Dr. Richart says.

A biopsy can rule out cancer.

If no growth is seen, but another Pap smear still shows abnormal cells, your doctor will probably want to do a conization, Dr. Richart says. "Conization is usually done when you cannot absolutely rule out the possibility of invasive cancer." In this procedure, a cone-shaped piece of tissue is cut from the center of the cervix for analysis. This may reveal a lesion in the cervical canal. The procedure usually does not affect your ability to bear children.

If either of these procedures confirms dysplasia or exposure to the condyloma virus, the treatment is the same—the lesions are removed. They are treated just as some forms of skin cancer are. They can be coated with chemicals that make them slough off, frozen in a procedure called cryosurgery, vaporized with a laser beam or, less frequently, burned off with cauterization.

The recommended treatment for dysplasia or the condyloma virus.

Several months later, you have a follow-up Pap smear. If it is not normal, the treatment may be repeated. If it is normal, you and your doctor will determine a schedule of smears to monitor for possible recurrences. Even though your condition is cured, you are now in the high-risk group and should have Pap smears at least once a year.

How Often
Are Pap Tests Necessary?

The American College of Obstetrics and Gynecology recommends a Pap smear every year. The

A smart choice.

American Cancer Society recommends an annual Pap smear and pelvic exam for all women who are 18 years or older or who are sexually active, with less frequent exams after three satisfactory tests, at the discretion of the woman's physician.

There are two good reasons for an annual Pap smear. One is the remote possibility that you may develop a fast-growing cancer. The other is that the Pap smear does have a 15 to 30 percent rate of error of false negatives—that is, it indicates your cervix is normal when it isn't. More frequent tests minimize your chances of walking around with an undetected dysplasia.

Dysplasia occurs most often in women ages 25 to 35; cancer *in situ* (confined to the uterus) in women 30 to 40; and invasive cancer, in women ages 40 to 60. Women who have had a hysterectomy should still be getting regular Pap smears, Dr. Zuna says. The cells in the upper vagina can develop cancer, and sometimes a partial hysterectomy is done, leaving the cervix. A Pap smear doesn't always detect cancer of the endometrium or ovaries. Always inform your doctor of any abnormal bleeding or pain, even if your Pap smear is normal, Dr. Zuna says.

No More Cramps
and Kinks

New York City Ballet dancer Patrick Hinson was in the middle of a pirouette-packed performance when, suddenly, his calf kinked out.

His show-must-go-on attitude kept Hinson on his toes. "I just kept telling myself, 'If you can get through this to a point where you can put your foot down flat, the cramp will go away.' " That's just what happened, and not a moment too soon.

Most of us can sympathize with the agonized dancer. We've all had muscle cramps in the calf of a leg, the arch of a foot or just under the ribs. It's a few moments of intense, grabbing pain that then begins to ease off. Reach down to rub that recalcitrant calf and you can actually feel a knot or thickening in the lame leg. Severe cramps, like those that sometimes occur during convulsive seizures, can be so strong they snap bones. Even ordinary cramps frequently tear muscle tissue. That's why they so often leave a lingering ache.

Muscle cramps may seem to strike out of the blue, but that's only because their warning signals go unnoticed. If you're a frequent victim, you may be putting yourself into a position or situation where a cramp is unavoidable.

A common ailment: muscle cramps when you least expect them.

How Muscles Cramp

Many cramps, especially those that strike your legs at night, occur because your body has assumed a compromising position, says Israel Weiner, M.D., assistant professor of neurological surgery at the University of Maryland School of Medicine, Baltimore. Perhaps you've let your foot point downward, which automatically contracts the calf muscle somewhat. Then, consciously or unconsciously, you've tensed your calf muscle, contracting it still more. This position is the ideal setup for a cramp.

Looser blankets can prevent cramps.

"When you contract the muscle, if there is nothing counteracting that movement, like another muscle or a tendon being stretched in opposition, the contracted muscle can shorten beyond its normal limit and go into an uncontrollable shortened state—in other words, a cramp," Dr. Weiner says. In bed, heavy or tucked-in blankets may push your feet down. Then, if you tense your leg muscles, as you inevitably do when you stretch or turn over, it's . . . *gotcha!*

Older people seem particularly prone to nighttime cramps, and they are sometimes overtreated for this problem, Dr. Weiner says. "It's important for them to know that this problem is usually not serious and that it can almost always be resolved without drugs." How? By loosening bed covers or using a board to keep the weight of the covers off your feet. If you sleep on your stomach, hang your feet over the edge of the bed. And keep your feet flexed upward toward your head when you're stretching your legs. That makes the muscles on the front of your legs contract, providing opposition to the calf muscles.

How high heels instigate cramps.

High heels also throw the legs and feet into a cramp-prone position, as some fashion-conscious women have discovered. The plump and shapely calf is actually a contracted muscle. In fact, women who wear high heels constantly may so shorten their calf muscles that when they take the shoes off, they're unable to touch their heels to the ground. Their leg muscles act like they are constantly walking around on tiptoe, which is exactly what they are doing.

Relieve Cramps in Seconds

Doctors, coaches and sufferers agree that the fastest, surest cure for a cramp is to stretch the affected muscles. If your calf cramps, for example, you can simply stand firmly on your flat foot and press down as hard as you can, or you can do more elaborate stretches.

Cramps actually start when the nerves that control the muscles are prompted to misfire, for any number of reasons. Stretching, apparently, changes neural impulses, making the nerves change their signal from "contract" to "relax." Usually stretching relieves a cramp within seconds. And staying fit and limber can help prevent cramps.

Stretch a muscle, kill a cramp.

Cramps that occur when you are active can be due to bad positioning, but they frequently have other causes, like an insufficient blood supply to the tissue, muscle fatigue or mineral depletion. When the cramp occurs can be the tip-off to what's causing the problem, says Mona Shangold, M.D., director of Georgetown University's Sports Gynecology Center and co-author (with husband Gabe Mirkin, M.D.) of *The Complete Sports Medicine Book for Women.*

What about Minerals?

"Cramps that occur when you first start to exercise are usually due to a mineral imbalance, such as a calcium, sodium or potassium deficiency or excess," Dr. Shangold says. "Abnormal blood levels of these minerals usually allow the muscle to contract but prevent it from relaxing."

How minerals affect cramps.

The minerals work in fairly complex ways that are not entirely understood, says James Knochel, M.D., chief of medical services with the Veterans Administration Hospital in Dallas, who has spent many years studying mineral-related muscular disorders.

"Mineral deficiencies can affect blood flow to muscles," Dr. Knochel says. "When you contract a muscle, for instance, it releases potassium into the surrounding tissue, where it acts as a dilator of arteries in the muscle bed. This doesn't occur in someone who is potassium deficient. It's equivalent to putting a tourniquet around your arm and then attempting to use the arm, which produces a cramp." Perhaps that's one reason ballet dancer Patrick Hinson swears by potassium-packed bananas and baked potatoes.

Potassium deficiency: an invitation to muscle cramps.

A potassium deficiency also impairs the ability of the muscles to use glycogen, a sugar that is their main source of energy, Dr. Knochel says. This makes them weak and cramp-prone. Potassium and other mineral deficiencies may also affect the "excitability" of nerves—their tendency to fire off a series of muscle-cramping messages. And they may affect the muscles' "fatigue threshold"—their ability to do more work without becoming tired and spasm-prone.

Body mineral levels may be affected by hormonal changes or unusual physical demands. Pregnancy, too, can make women particularly prone to leg cramps.

Magnesium helped reduce cramps in pregnant women.

In one study, researchers at Brigham Young University in Provo, Utah, found that 266 milligrams a day of supplemental magnesium reduced cramping in all their groups of pregnant women. The women were followed during the final two months of their pregnancy. The group with the most cramps—women over age 27 who already had at least one child—was helped the most by the magnesium. Their cramps were reduced by 57 percent.

Some clinical studies seem to indicate that additional calcium may reduce muscle cramps in pregnant women and growing children who may be deficient in these minerals because of increased nutritional needs. Calcium and magnesium work closely together in the muscles, Dr. Knochel says.

An uncommon cause of cramps: too little sodium.

While sodium deficiencies are another well-known cause of muscle cramps, most doctors no longer recommend salt tablets, since most people's diets already contain more than adequate salt. But, Dr. Knochel says, if you are on a low-sodium diet and find you have muscle cramps, especially when you sweat heavily while working or exercising, too little salt may be your problem.

In any case, it's good to check with a doctor if you suspect a mineral deficiency is causing your muscle cramps. Mineral imbalances aren't particularly common, Dr. Shangold says. At risk are those taking diuretics or steroids, heavy drinkers, pregnant women and older people who may not be eating well.

Who's at risk for mineral imbalances?

Other Causes—and Cures— for Cramps

Cramps that occur after you have exercised for a little while are most frequently caused by an inadequate blood supply to the muscle, Dr. Shangold says. "At rest, your arteries may be large enough to transport the small amount of blood that your muscles require to function properly. When you exercise, however, your muscles require large amounts of oxygen-rich blood. If your arteries are not large enough to transport enough blood, your muscles suffer from lack of oxygen and go into spasm."

What some older people mistake for a leg cramp is a condition known as intermittent claudication. It's a cramplike pain that comes on after a bit of exercise. It makes the leg feel heavy and weak.

The exercise cramp.

Intermittent claudication is caused by clogged arteries in the leg, and its symptoms are similar to angina in the heart muscle, says Robert Layzer, M.D., professor of neurology at the University of California at San Francisco. It's important to see a doctor if you have such symptoms, or any cramping pain in the legs accompanied by numbness or coldness in the affected leg or foot.

Most doctors recommend exercise, stopping smoking, a low-fat diet, and drugs for this condition when it occurs in the lower leg. In some studies, vitamin E has also relieved symptoms, perhaps by reducing the tendency for red blood cells to clump together and form clots. In one study, supplementa-

A possible remedy for intermittent claudication: vitamin E.

tion with 600 international units of vitamin E daily for at least three months provided improvement for a number of patients. Those who got the vitamin E required far fewer leg amputations than those treated with placebos (dummy pills) or other drugs. They were better able to walk. Blood circulation improved in their legs, although it sometimes took up to 25 months of supplementation before this result was apparent (*Vasa*).

Exercise-Related Cramps

Cramps that occur after you have been exercising for a long time are most often due to dehydration, Dr. Shangold says. "When you exercise for a long time, particularly in hot weather, you lose a lot of fluid. During a vigorous tennis match, for instance, a player can lose as much as two quarts of water per hour. Your blood volume is reduced, and there may not be enough blood to supply oxygen to all your exercising muscles. As a result, the most actively exercised muscles may not get enough blood, and they can go into spasm and hurt."

Drinking water can prevent cramps.

You can protect yourself from developing these kinds of cramps by drinking a glass of water before you exercise and at least every 15 minutes while you exercise, Dr. Shangold says.

Side Stitches and Swimmer's Cramps

A stitch, or a side sticker, is a cramp in the diaphragm, the large muscle that separates your chest from your gut and controls breathing. The cramp occurs when this muscle doesn't get enough blood during exercise, Dr. Shangold says. "When you run, you lift your knees and contract your belly muscles, so that the pressure inside your belly increases and pushes on the diaphragm from below. At the same time, if you're breathing heavily, you are expanding your lungs, which presses down on the diaphragm from above. This dual pressure squeezes the diaphragm and shuts off blood flow to it. The muscle can't get enough oxygen and goes into spasm."

How to get rid of a "stitch in the side."

If you develop a stitch, stop exercising, Dr. Shangold says. Push your fingers deep into your belly just below your ribs on the right side to stretch the diaphragm muscle with your hand. At the same time, purse your lips tightly and blow out as hard as you can. This should release the pressure on your diaphragm and stop the stitch.

It's true that if a swimmer gets an abdominal cramp, he may have trouble reaching shore safely. But contrary to popular belief, swimmer's cramps don't seem to depend on how recently you have eaten. They're more likely to be caused by fatigue or extreme exertion. "It's true that digesting food requires that some blood be shunted away from the heart and muscles," Dr. Shangold says. "But no healthy person should have trouble digesting food and swimming at the same time." In fact, the Red Cross no longer recommends that you wait for an hour after eating before you hit the surf.

It's okay to swim shortly after eating.

Unknotting an Unexpected Cramp

Preventive measures should keep most cramps at bay. But if an occasional one still sneaks up on you, try stretching it away with the simple exercises mentioned earlier. Then, doctors say, if the area still hurts, treat it as you would an injured muscle, which is exactly what it is.

Rest the limb to avoid pain from further cramps or spasms and to keep from injuring the muscle even more. Apply ice to reduce swelling and pain.

Avoid getting a cramp in the first place by checking your body posture. Don't point your toes or let your feet get pushed over by bed covers. Don't set yourself up for a muscle injury, which may make you more susceptible to cramps. Train carefully. Avoid intense, jerky movements. Stretch to warm up and cool down. Don't bounce. Don't exercise beyond the point of fatigue. But do exercise. Sedentary people are prone to cramps, too. And see a doctor if you think a mineral deficiency may be your problem.

Good posture prevents cramps.

Chapter 43

How to Stop Diabetic Complications with Good Nutrition

Most of the 11 million Americans who suffer from diabetes know that the worst part of their illness isn't their blood-sugar imbalance itself but the complications that arise from it. Hardening of the arteries, stroke, blindness and kidney damage—older diabetics are much more likely to come down with those and other afflictions than are their nondiabetic friends and neighbors.

But surprisingly little has been done to remedy this state of affairs. Synthetic insulin and the so-called oral agents give diabetics day-to-day protection from their disease. But neither drugs nor do-it-yourself urine tests offer the kind of long-range protection that diabetics really need.

Three reasons nutrition works.

That's why more and more diabetics and their doctors are turning to nutrition. It makes perfect sense, for three reasons: Diet control is already the primary form of therapy for the 10.5 million non–insulin-dependent diabetics; nutrition may help prevent heart disease (the real killer in diabetes); and supplements may let diabetics stock up on nutrients without violating their special diets.

Diabetes and Heart Disease: Breaking the Deadly Link

For every diabetic, avoiding complications means avoiding atherosclerosis, or hardening of the arteries. This is the primary complication, the one that sets the stage for the rest. Diabetics develop this form of heart disease much faster and earlier than the average person, and their risk of heart attack or stroke is roughly double the average. If someone could break the link between atherosclerosis and diabetes, the plight of diabetics would be halfway solved.

Actually, that is exactly what a pair of researchers at the University of Mississippi's Atherosclerosis Research Laboratories think they have finally done after more than a decade of hard work. Anthony Verlangieri, Ph.D., and John C. Kapeghian, Ph.D., believe that vitamin C (ascorbic acid) can prevent hardening of the arteries in diabetics—and perhaps in everyone else.

The role of vitamin C.

"Up until now, there's never been a good explanation why diabetics develop atherosclerosis so much faster than the rest of the population," Dr. Verlangieri says. "But we think we now have evidence that shows why. Ultimately, we think vitamin C might prevent some of the renal [kidney] and retinal [eye] progression of the disease."

Sugar molecules and vitamin C molecules, he explains, seem to "compete" with each other as they circulate in the blood. Like two pedestrians flagging down the same taxi, they vie for the same molecular "transport system" that will carry them out of the blood and into the endothelial cells that line every blood vessel.

When sugar levels are high in diabetics, less vitamin C reaches the endothelial cells. If too little of the vitamin gets through, Dr. Verlangieri says, the "cement" that holds the cells in place on the arterial walls may deteriorate. If that happens, single cells may break off and fly loose. Each missing cell, apparently, can leave behind it a hollow space that quickly provides a toehold for cholesterol. One chunk of cholesterol leads to another, until eventually the arteries are almost choked. The stage is then set for high blood pressure, stroke or heart attack. In theory, vita-

A cellular cement that may stop cholesterol buildup.

min C supplements can interrupt this process before atherosclerosis sets in.

While Dr. Verlangieri's conclusions about the powers of vitamin C are still controversial, he is not alone in recommending this nutrient to people with high blood sugar. In fact, Stanley Mirsky, M.D., former president of the New York affiliate of the American Diabetes Association and author of the book *Diabetes: Controlling It the Easy Way*, agrees with him.

Possible Rx for diabetics: 500 milligrams of vitamin C daily.

"We tell our diabetes patients to add 500 milligrams of vitamin C to their daily regimen," Dr. Mirsky says. "It's part of our belief that controlling the diet is the primary goal in preventing diabetic complications. Diet is more important than insulin or other oral agents."

Those diabetics who plan to take ascorbic acid supplements must keep one thing in mind, however. Vitamin C can skew the results of certain at-home urine tests. In one of the many test kits marketed to diabetics, vitamin C can trigger a false-positive reading, while in another test kit it can produce a false-negative reading. "If you seem to be getting unreliable test results, stop the vitamin C for a few days and see if your results are different," Dr. Mirsky says.

Before taking vitamin C for diabetes, check with your doctor.

Nutrition for Nerves

Dr. Mirsky has also found that good nutrition can soothe neuropathy, another common complication of diabetes. Pain, burning, itching and numbness are typical of this mysterious nervous system disorder, whose symptoms appear and disappear without apparent reason at spots all over the body. It can attack any part of the nervous system without warning. It can even disrupt the nerves of the digestive tract or the bladder, causing constipation, diarrhea or urinary tract infections.

The feet, however, seem to be the most common target for neuropathy. Indeed, diabetics have to take exquisite care of their feet, washing them daily, softening them with special creams, checking for any sign of a cut or blister, and seeing a podiatrist often. Poor circulation in the feet means that something as minor as a stubbed toe can lead to an uncontrollable infection. No wonder diabetes accounts for 20,000 foot and leg amputations in the United States every year.

Thiamine for Foot Pain

Dr. Mirsky prescribes thiamine, or vitamin B_1, for those of his patients who are kept awake at night by pain or sensitivity in their feet.

"Even though lots of people say that it won't work, I've found that about 80 percent of my patients improve by taking B_1," he claims. "I prescribe between 50 and 100 milligrams a day. A week or two after they start taking it, they find that their feet don't bother them, and they can enjoy their sleep.

Vitamin B for foot pain in diabetics.

"We don't know exactly why this vitamin works," he adds. "Thiamine has always been used to treat nervous disorders, and I think it just improves the tone of the nerves. A lot of doctors give their patients Dilantin [a seizure-control medication that's sometimes used to help diabetics] even though it has potentially harmful side effects and often doesn't work at all. With B_1, the worst thing that can happen is that it won't work. But it usually does." Vitamin E supplements can also help the diabetic, Dr. Mirsky claims. "I often recommend vitamin E in capsules of 400 international units, three times a day. I don't know exactly how it works, but I think it acts as an antioxidant, which helps prevent harmful peroxide molecules from damaging healthy cells. I prescribe it when I need everything I can get to control the disease." (By comparison, the U.S. Recommended Daily Allowance for vitamin E is 30 international units.)

Can vitamin E help diabetics?

E for Better Circulation

Harvey Walker, Jr., M.D., Ph.D., of Clayton, Missouri, agrees. "We also use vitamin E in our therapy for diabetic patients who have circulation problems," he says. "Let me explain. There are two pulse sites in each foot. A diabetic patient may lose one or both pulses, which is an indication of reduced circulation in the foot.

"Now, loss of a pulse has always been thought to be irreversible, which, of course, has serious consequences for the diabetic. But using a year of vitamin E and lecithin supplementation, we have actually restored the pulse at one or both sites in one-third of the 150 patients we've treated this way."

A suggested remedy for "loss of pulse" in diabetics' feet: vitamin E and lecithin.

Magnesium for the Eyes

Perhaps the most frightening of all the complications of diabetes is retinopathy. Nine out of ten diabetics who've had the disease for 20 years or more begin to show pinpoint hemorrhages on the retina, the area at the back of the eye that receives incoming light and relays it to the brain for interpretation. The hemorrhages sometimes lead to a loss of vision. Diabetic retinopathy, in fact, is the leading cause of blindness in Americans over age 20.

There is some evidence that a deficiency of magnesium might cause or at least aggravate the development of diabetic retinopathy. A study conducted a few years ago in England showed that retinopathy patients had low blood levels of magnesium. Those results suggested that "low concentrations of magnesium may be an additional risk factor" for the eye disease. Since then, there have been a few reports of doctors prescribing magnesium for their diabetic patients. Dr. Mirsky, for example, tells his patients to consume plenty of magnesium-rich foods, like whole grains, nuts and meat.

Retinopathy patients had low magnesium levels.

Most recently, researchers in Japan also concluded that "a derangement of magnesium metabolism may have some relationship to the onset and/or development of diabetic retinopathy." Of 109 diabetics studied, those who failed to keep their blood sugar levels under control tended to have low blood levels of magnesium and tended to excrete more of the mineral in their urine. Those with the lowest magnesium levels of all were the patients who suffered from "proliferative" diabetic retinopathy, the most serious stage of the disease (*Magnesium Bulletin*).

A strong link between low magnesium levels and diabetic retinopathy.

Fiber Flattens Sugar Curve

While it's important to stress the prevention of diabetic complications, it would be wrong for a diabetic to forget that controlling the rise and fall of his or her blood sugar level after a meal is the first concern. "The major complications—kidney failure, heart disease, blindness, neuropathy—can all be prevented by keeping blood sugar levels as close to normal as possible all the time," Dr. Mirsky says.

Making sure that there's plenty of fiber in your diet is one excellent way to do that.

While fiber comes in many forms, one type of fiber that has excited researchers lately is guar gum. Extracted from the bean of a plant that grows in India, guar gum has in the past been used as a thickener in products such as ice cream. In the future, however, it may be added to granola bars or pasta as an extra boost of fiber.

A possibly important dietary fiber for diabetics: guar gum.

Like some other kinds of fiber, guar gum delays the rise in blood sugar that ordinarily follows a carbohydrate-rich meal of, for instance, spaghetti. To demonstrate this effect, researchers in Italy recently fed five diabetics a meal of *spaghetti alla carbonara* (a pasta dish made with eggs, Parmesan cheese, butter and ham) and later an identical meal in which the regular pasta was replaced with pasta that was 20 percent guar gum.

Comparing blood samples after each meal, the researchers discovered that sugar levels rose more slowly after the meal made with guar gum spaghetti. In fact, glucose levels at 60 minutes after the guar gum meal were roughly equal to the glucose levels at 30

After a meal with guar gum, blood sugar levels were "flatter."

minutes after the meal with ordinary spaghetti. The researchers aren't sure why it happened this way, but they feel confident guar gum may someday be a valuable tool for the diabetic, whether insulin-dependent or not, who wants to control his or her blood sugar while still enjoying high-carbohydrate foods (*Annals of Nutrition and Metabolism*).

Think Positive

Fiber and nutrients aren't the only tools available to the diabetic who wants to avoid heart disease and other complications. The many diabetics who are obese or who smoke would be wise to lose weight and crush their nicotine habits as soon as possible. Starting an aerobics or jogging program is an excellent idea. One therapist even suggests stair climbing for exercise. But whatever you do to counteract diabetes, you need to discuss it with your doctor, especially if it concerns nutrition.

Other steps to help control diabetes.

A positive mental attitude can make a big difference, too. Many people are at first depressed and bewildered when they learn they are diabetic—depressed by the fear that it may shorten their lives and bewildered by the complexly cautious lifestyle they must adopt. However, with proper care, including good nutrition, a diabetic can lead a full, happy, productive life.

Chapter 44

Lower Your Blood Pressure with Diet

You begin your day with a juicy half-moon of cantaloupe, a glass of freshly squeezed orange juice and a bowl of bran cereal with half a cup of skim milk.

Lunch is broiled mackerel, parsley potatoes and a side salad of watercress, carrot medallions and almonds, tossed with your own dressing made of fresh garlic in corn oil and apple-cider vinegar.

The perfect diet for lowering blood pressure?

Midafternoon, you calm your rumbling stomach with a cup of low-fat yogurt into which you've sliced half a banana.

For dinner, you whip up a luscious casserole of brown rice, onions, broccoli, cashews and melted part-skim mozzarella, lightly seasoned with garlic.

If you have high blood pressure, theoretically you've just done everything right. Your one day's menu contains every nutrient known to help *lower* blood pressure. Today, medical research has uncovered a way to fight hypertension that's more positive than just avoiding salt and saturated fat. There are actually foods you can eat more of that help you win this often-deadly numbers game.

Your blood-pressure "medication" may be in many of the foods you eat.

And if you didn't know already, high blood pressure can be deadly. According to Michael Rees, M.D., author of *The Complete Family Guide to Living with High Blood Pressure*, hypertension is the single most important cause of strokes, a major cause of diseases of the brain, kidneys and eyes and, in fact, is the cause of an estimated one-third of all heart disease. Some 60 million Americans have blood pressure that is too high—blood pressure that might just respond to some dietary fine-tuning. They might want to start with this menu.

Potassium-Rich Foods

Cantaloupe, winter squash, potatoes, broccoli, orange juice, some fresh fruits, and milk contain hefty

---

What Type of High Blood Pressure Do You Have?

Did you know there's more than one type of high blood pressure? And that the kind you have should determine the type of treatment you receive? Rather than treat all high blood pressure the same (with weight loss, salt restriction and drugs), doctors need to be able to determine what category you fit into—a tricky affair to say the least.

Two Cornell University doctors have found that a simple, two-minute blood test may make that task a bit easier, at least if low calcium levels are part of your problem. "The test measures levels of free calcium in the bloodstream," explains Lawrence M. Resnick, M.D., assistant professor of medicine at Cornell. Other routine tests for calcium measure total calcium, which includes the free (available to tissues) as well as that bound to protein (which is not available to tissues).

"People who are low in free calcium are the ones whose blood pressure is most likely to respond favorably to calcium supplements," Dr. Resnick says. And he estimates that about one-third of all hypertensives are "calcium sensitive." "Also, people with low free-calcium levels are more sensitive to sodium—eating salt raises their blood pressure. We can also predict which drugs will work better. Calcium-sensitive patients, for example, respond better to diuretics, alpha-blockers and calcium channel blockers, whereas beta-blockers work better in people who have higher free-calcium levels to begin with.

"Our goal," says Dr. Resnick, "is to be able to find out what type of high blood pressure a patient has, so that treatment can be individualized according to his or her needs. This blood test is a good start in that direction."

amounts of potassium. The fact is, how much potassium you have in your diet may be just as important as how little sodium you eat. Studies of vegetarians, who tend to have lower blood pressures than meat eaters, found that their sodium intake was no different from that of hypertensives, but their potassium intake was significantly higher.

Which one is more important to your blood pressure—sodium or potassium?

A group of scientists in Israel looked at the eating habits of 98 vegetarians whose average age was 60 and compared them to a similar group of meat eaters. What they found was a very low prevalence of hypertension—only 2 percent—among the vegetarians, although they lived in an adult population where the expected prevalence was 20 to 25 percent. The vegetarians ate as much salt as their neighbors and had the same genetic predisposition to developing hypertension. But they didn't. The researchers concluded that it was their potassium-rich diets of vegetables, fruits and nuts that kept them from developing hypertension (*American Journal of Clinical Nutrition*).

Just how does potassium protect the body from hypertension, even when sodium intake isn't restricted? No one really knows, although there are a number of theories. For one, potassium is an effective diuretic—and has been used as one for nearly four centuries. But in addition to helping the body rid itself of water, potassium also helps slough off sodium, an effect called natriuresis. Potassium also appears to act on several important physiological systems that regulate blood pressure and control the workings of the vascular system.

Potassium helps the body get rid of excess water and sodium.

In both animal and human studies, potassium seems to have little effect on people whose blood pressure is normal. But it can produce a significant drop in both systolic and diastolic pressures of hypertensives.

And there may be one group of people for whom potassium is literally a shield against the ravages of excess sodium. According to George R. Meneely, M.D., emeritus professor of medicine at Louisiana

The danger zone: more than four grams of salt a day.

State University Medical Center in Shreveport, there may be "a substantial fraction of the population worldwide, including primitive societies, who develop elevation of the blood pressure if they eat more than four grams of sodium as sodium chloride [everyday table salt] a day.

"There is extensive animal evidence," says Dr. Meneely, "that the hypertensogenic [hypertension-causing] effect of excess sodium is counteracted by extra dietary potassium. There is pretty good literature on its effect in humans, too."

For anyone who wants to increase his or her dietary potassium, here's a cooking tip from a group of Swedish scientists: To avoid potassium loss in cooking, steam rather than boil vegetables. When doctors at a Swedish hospital tested the two cooking methods with potatoes, a rich source of potassium, they discovered that boiled potatoes lose 10 to 50 percent of their potassium, while steamed potatoes lose only 3 to 6 percent. They had similar results with carrots, beans and peas (*Lancet*).

How to preserve potassium when you cook.

A Calcium Bounty in Your Refrigerator

Dairy products, leafy green vegetables like kale and watercress, and nuts contain calcium. If you've been scrupulous about cutting sodium out of your diet, you may be cutting out calcium, too. There's a convincing amount of evidence from all corners of the world indicating calcium can lower your blood pressure. Unfortunately, the best sources of calcium—dairy products—also have a fair amount of sodium. A two-ounce serving of Swiss cheese contains 544 milligrams of calcium (the Recommended Dietary Allowance is 800 milligrams), but there's a hefty 148 milligrams of sodium in there, too. But the evidence is too overwhelming in favor of calcium as an antidote to hypertension for anyone to give up milk and cheese entirely.

Calcium may help lower blood pressure, too.

Consider, for example, a study of 82 percent of the adult residents of Rancho Bernardo, an upper-middle-class community in Southern California. What separated male hypertensives from normotensives, according to researchers at the University of California, San Diego, was milk. Milk consumption was lower in borderline, untreated and treated hypertensives (*American Journal of Clinical Nutrition*).

In an even larger study, involving 20,749 people across the country, calcium was the only one of 17 nutrients evaluated that differed in the hypertensives. Those people with high blood pressure consumed 18 percent less calcium (*Annals of Internal Medicine*).

People with high blood pressure were getting less calcium than others were.

That figure alarms researcher David McCarron, M.D., professor of medical nephrology in the Division of Nephrology and Hypertension at the Oregon Health Sciences University in Portland. He conducted that particular study—and several others linking calcium and blood pressure—and he's convinced that a good hypertensive diet has to contain dairy products, regardless of the fact that they contain sodium and cholesterol.

"If you have to, switch to low-sodium or low-cholesterol cheeses, which are an excellent source of calcium and low in saturated fatty acids," he says. "If you don't have a cholesterol problem and you're near your ideal body weight, you don't necessarily have to worry about the cholesterol."

As for sodium, Dr. McCarron's work indicates that calcium may actually negate the harmful effects of salt on the system. An increased calcium load tends to facilitate the body's excretion of sodium, he notes.

Calcium works on blood pressure in another way—by relaxing the blood vessels. "You'll rarely hear a doctor say that because the most doctors are ever taught in medical school is that calcium makes blood vessels contract," he says. "When blood vessels contract, blood pressure goes up. But calcium actually regulates contraction *and* relaxation of the blood vessels."

Dr. McCarron: Calcium helps lower blood pressure by relaxing blood vessels.

Balancing minerals to lower blood pressure.

But one of the most interesting things to come out of Dr. McCarron's research is not how calcium works alone to lower blood pressure but how it works with potassium, sodium and magnesium to regulate pressure. "It's the proportions of these minerals in the body that seem to be the most important thing," says Dr. McCarron. "The possibility exists that the more you want to eat of one, the more you'd better eat of the others. We, of course, consider calcium the most important. But if you're not taking in enough sodium, potassium and magnesium, the probability is that you're not getting enough calcium either."

And, not coincidentally, the foods that are abundant in one tend to be abundant in the others.

Vitamin C: A Role in Preventing High Blood Pressure?

Since high blood pressure is a risk factor for heart disease, it's important to get it down to normal levels. Preventing its occurrence in the first place is better yet. Now a group of Japanese researchers has suggested that high vitamin C intake may, in fact, help prevent high blood pressure from developing.

The researchers tested a group of healthy men (aged 30 to 39) to determine both their blood pressure and their blood levels of vitamin C. They found that the higher the vitamin C levels, the lower the incidence of high blood pressure. These results, say the researchers, could help explain why some populations with high dietary intake of vitamin C have a low mortality rate from heart disease and atherosclerosis, or hardening of the arteries (*International Journal for Vitamin and Nutrition Research*).

Magnesium as a Partner in Health

Nuts, brown rice, molasses, milk, wheat germ, bananas, potatoes and soy products provide magnesium. Inadequate dietary magnesium has been shown to increase blood pressure in animals and humans both. Though the exact mechanism isn't known, there is some indication that magnesium exerts its pressure-lowering effect by regulating the entry and exit of calcium in the smooth muscle cells of the vascular system. Together, the two minerals produce the regular contraction and relaxation of blood vessels.

Magnesium: a blood-pressure lowering agent?

In a test involving untreated, newly diagnosed hypertensives, Dr. McCarron found that they consumed less calcium and magnesium than a similar group whose blood pressures were normal. Their sodium intake didn't seem to matter (*Annals of Internal Medicine*).

"The interaction of magnesium and calcium gives the calcium the ability to get where it has to in a cell," says Dr. McCarron. "Magnesium facilitates calcium getting to the right place where it can have this relaxing effect."

Some Fats Are Good for Your Blood Pressure

In a pilot study of healthy people in Italy, Finland and the United States, researchers discovered that the level of dietary linoleic acid—polyunsaturated fats—was associated with incidences of high blood pressure. There were more hypertensives among the Finnish population than among the Italians and Americans. The Finns consumed more saturated and less polyunsaturated fats than the others.

When a group of Finns aged 40 to 50 was placed on a low-fat diet high in polyunsaturated fats and low in saturated fats, even when salt consumption wasn't

The power of polyunsaturates.

reduced, blood pressures dropped significantly. When they returned to their old eating habits, their old blood pressures returned, too (*American Journal of Clinical Nutrition*).

What's the magic? James M. Iacono, Ph.D., director of agricultural research services at the U.S. Department of Agriculture's Western Human Nutrition Research Center in San Francisco, and other researchers have one theory. They believe polyunsaturated fats lower blood pressure because when they're metabolized by the body, they yield a substance that is essential for making prostaglandins. These are fatty acids that seem to control blood pressure by aiding in the sloughing off of water and salt from the kidneys (*Hypertension*).

Fish Are Helpful, Too

A new antihypertension possibility: fish.

Mackerel and other marine fish are high in eicosapentanoic acid, one of the omega-3 fatty acids. Tests in Germany involving 15 volunteers on a mackerel diet provided some heartening results. After only two weeks, serum triglycerides and total cholesterol dropped significantly, mirrored by "markedly lower" systolic and diastolic blood pressures.

The Germans didn't simply pull mackerel out of their hats. They were attempting to approximate the diet of Greenland Eskimos and Japanese fishermen, who enjoy a very low incidence of cardiovascular disease. The key appears to be the omega-3 fatty acids found in many fish (*Atherosclerosis*).

Cod-liver oil may have lowered blood pressures.

Another study tested the effects of cod-liver oil on the Western diet. Cod-liver oil also contains omega-3 fatty acids. A group of volunteers added three tablespoons of cod-liver oil a day to their normal diets and wound up with lower blood pressures (*Circulation*).

Fiber Up, Blood Pressure Down

Bran, fresh fruit and vegetables, beans and whole grain breads supply fiber. There are some early indications that plant fiber can significantly lower blood pressure, though precisely why is still a mystery.

Researcher James W. Anderson, M.D., chief of endocrinology at the Veterans Administration Medical Center in Lexington, Kentucky, placed 12 diabetic men on a 14-day diet containing more than three times the dietary fiber (and fat) of a control diet. Average blood pressures dropped 10 percent. In patients whose blood pressures had been normal, systolic pressures were 8 percent lower, and diastolic figures had dropped 10 percent.

A 10 percent drop in blood pressure.

The news was even better for the men who had high blood pressure to begin with. Their systolic pressures dropped by 11 percent and diastolic pressures by 10 percent (*Annals of Internal Medicine*).

Dr. Anderson was pleased with his results, but he's not sure why he got them. "My strongest hunch is that it's related to certain changes in insulin. The patients' insulin needs were low on the high-fiber diet. There's a lot of evidence that insulin contributes to high blood pressure. It's basically a salt-retentive hormone. We also reported a small increase in sodium loss in feces. I didn't think at the time it was meaningful, but thinking about it later, having two different mechanisms working together like that—the insulin and the sodium excretion—you can get a synergistic effect."

What makes the results even more significant is that salt use was not restricted during the diet. "In fact," says Dr. Anderson, "there was a 50 percent increase in sodium intake. But potassium also went up, so the sodium:potassium ratio stayed the same."

Fiber may help to lower blood pressure.

Onions and Garlic Benefit Your Blood Pressure

The old wives were right. Their tale of onions lowering blood pressure was on target. They do. What the old wives didn't know was why. According to Moses Attrep, Jr., Ph.D., formerly a chemist at East

Why onions are a friend of the heart.

Texas State University, it may be a hormonelike substance called prostaglandin A_1, which he isolated in yellow onions and which also occurs in the human kidney. When injected into humans and animals, prostaglandin A_1 lowers blood pressure, at least for brief periods.

Low-Fat Diets and High Blood Pressure

There's mounting evidence that dietary fat can have an effect on blood pressure.

A recent study—one of a long line of similar investigations—suggests that it may actually be possible for people to lower their blood pressure by cutting back on (or changing the type of) fat in their diet. In the three-month trial, middle-aged men with normal blood pressure followed either a low-fat diet (25 percent of calories from fat, equal amounts of polyunsaturated and saturated fats) or a more typically American diet (about 40 percent of calories from fat, mostly saturated). They all consumed the same kinds of foods, but the low-fat group ate leaner fare—like meat trimmed of fat, low-fat milk and margarine.

And in line with the results of other studies, there was a 9 percent drop in blood pressure in the group that was on the low-fat diet.

Researcher James M. Iacono, Ph.D., director of the U.S. Department of Agriculture's Western Human Nutrition Research Center, says that the data he gathered suggest a cause for the decrease in blood pressure. "The bodies of the men in the low-fat group excreted 4 percent more sodium and 11 percent more potassium than those in the normal-fat group," he says. "The excretion of these two minerals, one of which is known to sometimes raise blood pressure with higher daily intake, may be what triggers the reductions in blood pressure."

If such low-fat diets can pull down blood pressure as well as research suggests, they may soon become as crucial as low-salt eating in the nondrug treatment of hypertension.

"Until scientists can define the most effective low-fat diet for reducing blood pressure," says Dr. Iacono, "the wisest approach is to follow the current recommendations to reduce your overall fat to about 30 percent of total calories and to maintain equal amounts of polyunsaturated and saturated fats."

The old wives were right about garlic, too. The Japanese and Chinese have used garlic to lower blood pressure for centuries. Its effect is possibly similar to that of onions, since it might also contain prostaglandins.

Note: If you are being treated for high blood pressure, consult your doctor before making any dietary changes. He or she may need to adjust your medication.

Chapter 45

Fighting Mental Disorders with B Vitamins

Three typical cases of B vitamin deficiency.

Aunt Mary wasn't all that old when her husband died—only 65—but in the past 3 years it seems as though she's aged 20 years, at least as far as her mind goes. She's forgetful, irritable and tired. And some days she's so confused, it's heartbreaking. You hate to think she's becoming senile, but what else could it be?

Teenagers are supposed to be rebellious, it's true, but you're beginning to wonder if your 14-year-old daughter's moodiness and hyperactivity aren't above and beyond normal adolescent turmoil. You're also wondering how anyone can live on french fries and soft drinks, which are about the only foods she'll eat these days. Could that be part of the problem?

The divorce was hard on Tim, but he was determined to pick up and go on with his life. Instead, though, he began feeling so emotionally and physically exhausted he found it hard to do his job, much less look after himself. Instead of getting better, Tim is slowly getting worse and worse. Could the stress be catching up with him?

Nutrition-oriented doctors see these kinds of cases again and again, in different combinations of the same factors—aging, long-term stress, poor eating habits, even special metabolic needs. They also see the unfortunate consequences. Aunt Mary could end up in a nursing home before her time, that wall-climbing teenager might become a high-school dropout, and perhaps Tim will find himself severely depressed, even suicidal.

But all three share a common problem—a B-complex vitamin deficiency. And they all could have gotten relief from their mental woes—perhaps prevented them altogether—if they'd been getting enough of these nutrients to meet their personal needs.

When Stress Runs High, B Vitamins Run Low

"Take someone who's just a little depressed or a little stressed because of things going on in his life. That person might find himself eating poorly. And that could lead to nutritional deficiencies that push him over the brink, into true depression or mental problems," says Charles Tkacz, M.D., medical director of the North Nassau Mental Health Center in Manhasset, New York. The center's specialty is finding and correcting nutritional deficiencies in psychiatric patients, an aspect of treatment that's all too often overlooked in traditional medical care.

Could you fall into the dangerous cycle of nutrient depletion?

Robert Picker, M.D., a Walnut Creek, California, psychiatrist, agrees. "I've run into this kind of situation too many times to count," he says. "The body's nutritional needs are increased during times of stress. What may normally be adequate suddenly becomes a deficiency. And that deficiency could begin a vicious circle of mental symptoms that the person just doesn't seem to be able to shake. In fact, as a psychiatrist, I am painfully aware that many of these people are in psychotherapy for long periods of time without ever realizing that the correction of a nutritional deficiency could have significantly helped or possibly cured their problem, or perhaps have prevented it in the first place."

What is normally adequate is suddenly a deficiency.

Overall nutrition is essential, but doctors should take a special look at the B-complex vitamins, especially B_6, B_{12}, thiamine, niacin and folate.

Why are the B vitamins important for our mental health? The brain, it seems, is more sensitive to fluctuations in dietary nutrients than neurologists once thought. It has a special need for B vitamins to perform at its best.

B vitamins help supply the brain with its energy source.

The role of B vitamins is extensive and complex. They are co-enzymes, or catalysts, in many of the body's most basic functions, including the process of oxidation, or the body's burning of food to provide fuel. What this means is that they're needed to supply the brain with its energy source, glucose. Without enough glucose, the brain begins to perform poorly. Fatigue, depression, even hallucinations can be symptoms of a low glucose level in the brain. B_6 and niacin are the B vitamins most involved in this process.

Depressed People May Have a B_6 Deficiency

Seriously depressed patients may have another problem to contend with, according to Jonathan W. Stewart, M.D., of the New York State Psychiatric Institute and Columbia University College of Physicians and Surgeons. "About 20 percent of the depressed patients we looked at showed neurological symptoms as well—numbness and tingling in the hands, like 'pins and needles' or 'electric shock' sensations. And those with the symptoms had significantly lower vitamin B_6 levels than did those without symptoms.

"I feel quite certain that low vitamin B_6 levels are responsible for those neurological symptoms," Dr. Stewart says. "What we don't know yet is whether the low vitamin B_6 levels are in fact causing the depression. It's conceivable that B_6 has a role because the enzyme processes that convert foodstuffs into neurotransmitters [chemicals in the body that carry electrical signals from nerve to nerve] require vitamin B_6 at several critical stages. In B_6 deficiency, patients might not produce enough neurotransmitters, which in turn could lead to the symptoms of depression."

If a patient is admitted with both depression and neurological symptoms, the possibility of B_6 deficiency should be considered, says Dr. Stewart. "B_6 may relieve the neurological symptoms, and we suspect it may even have a positive effect on depression."

Low Levels of B Vitamins Can Lead to Confusion

But the B vitamins play a second crucial role in our mental health. Several are known to be involved in the production of neurotransmitters, biochemicals that allow the brain cells to pass messages along their nerve pathways.

"B_6 is needed for the production of serotonin, a major neurotransmitter in many body functions," says Eric Braverman, M.D., of the Princeton Brain Bio Center in Skillman, New Jersey. "Folate helps produce catecholamines, which control many body functions. B_{12} is needed to produce acetylcholine, another neurotransmitter. In other words, all the chemicals produced by the brain cells depend on nutrients taken into the body, and in many cases, they seem to depend on certain B vitamins."

What happens when they're not there?

"We know that people who aren't getting enough of these nutrients get a whole host of psychiatric and neurological symptoms, like depression, confusion, fatigue and psychosis," Dr. Tkacz says.

It was seeing that volunteers deprived of B_6 soon sunk into a funk, that prisoners of war fed thiamine-poor polished rice lost muscle coordination and reasoning power, and that diets short on B_{12} or folate could cause symptoms of senility or psychosis that led doctors to begin thinking backward. If nutrient deficiencies caused such problems, perhaps people with these symptoms could be helped with doses of the nutrients they seemed to be missing.

That's exactly what doctors like Dr. Tkacz, Dr. Braverman and Dr. Picker are doing. "We take blood samples for special nutritional testing, then initially put most patients on therapeutic doses of many nutrients, including 40 to 50 milligrams a day of all the B vitamins," Dr. Tkacz says. When the nutritional tests have been evaluated, the patient may be given more

B vitamins help the brain cells transmit information.

Doctors want to know: Can doses of B vitamins clear up psychological symptoms?

of a specific vitamin, mineral or amino acid that's been found to be lacking in his body.

"We've found, and studies confirm, that many depressed patients are low in B₆," Dr. Tkacz says. "A certain number are helped to recover from their depression by taking B₆ under medical supervision."

Can taking B₆ help cure depression?

Bad Nerves? Check for Thiamine

Derrick Lonsdale, M.D., a Cleveland physician with a special interest in biochemistry and nutrition, found that one of the first signs of a thiamine deficiency was changes in behavior—neurotic symptoms like depression, insomnia, chest pain and chronic fatigue. All 20 of the patients he studied improved with additional thiamine.

Not incidentally, these nervous patients also had poor diets. They were eating lots of "empty calories," usually refined carbohydrates or sugar-laden drinks, foods that used up their thiamine reserves without putting any back, Dr. Lonsdale reports.

Folate Deficiency and Depression

And several doctors are looking into folate deficiency as a cause of depression, insomnia, irritability, forgetfulness and some supposedly psychosomatic disorders.

A lack of folate may cause various emotional and psychological problems.

In reviewing medical literature, A. Missagh Ghadirian, M.D., of the Royal Victoria Hospital, Montreal, found folate-deficiency depression in people taking medications for rheumatoid arthritis, antibiotics, birth control pills and anticonvulsants. "Sometimes the deficiencies are quite severe, but sometimes they are more marginal and might even escape notice," he says. "If the depression is due to deficiency, making sure the patient gets enough additional folate works well to relieve the condition."

Mental Woes Linked to Low B$_{12}$

Doctors are realizing now, too, that sometimes the first sign of a B$_{12}$ deficiency can be bizarre mental misfirings that resemble psychosis or senility. One 47-year-old woman who had been "seeing" flying saucers was found to have low B$_{12}$ levels. Four days after starting B$_{12}$ supplementation, her hallucinations were gone (*American Journal of Psychiatry*).

Hallucinations: a possible sign of a B$_{12}$ deficiency.

Low on B Vitamins?

How many of these risk factors for a B vitamin deficiency fit you?

- You eat a diet that's high in sugar.
- You seldom eat liver, brewer's yeast or whole grains.
- You've been under a lot of stress lately.
- You have digestion problems or have had stomach or small intestine surgery.
- You take any one of these: birth control pills, diuretics, cholesterol-lowering drugs, antibiotics, psychoactive or anticonvulsant drugs.
- You drink alcohol regularly.
- You drink a lot of coffee.
- You smoke cigarettes.

Do you have any of these symptoms?

- You feel more tired, irritable, depressed, emotional, irrational, or anxious than you'd like or than you think is normal.
- You are older and have suddenly developed emotional or mental problems, especially depression, even though you have no prior history of any mental problems.
- Counseling and psychotherapy haven't helped you.
- You have skin rashes that won't go away.
- You have sores inside your mouth or cracks around the corners of your mouth.
- You have numbness, tingling, twitching in your legs, or your feet burn.
- You suffer from premenstrual tension or from postpartum depression.

Note: These problems may well have causes other than, or besides, B vitamin deficiency. Work out the solution with a good physician.

One of Dr. Tkacz's patients was a confused, forgetful woman in her early sixties. She'd been diagnosed as senile, but her family had decided to check for a nutritional deficiency. It turned out the woman had a very low level of B_{12}, and with just a few injections she recovered completely, Dr. Tkacz says. She'll have to have B_{12} injections for the rest of her life, but that's certainly better than being prematurely consigned to a nursing home.

Is it Alzheimer's disease—or a nutrient deficiency?

"A lot of families would have simply written off her symptoms as part of aging, but that's not usually the case," Dr. Tkacz says. "That's why it's so important to be careful when you're dealing with a possible diagnosis of dementia or Alzheimer's disease. You want to make sure you're not dealing with a B_{12} or a folate deficiency. I'd say 5 to 10 percent, easily, of elderly people with mental problems really have nutritional deficiencies, and many involve the B-complex vitamins."

Beware the "Tea and Toast" Syndrome

It's the borderline B vitamin deficiencies that are most likely to slip through the cracks of traditional medicine—those that might present themselves only as depression, fatigue, irritability, which are symptoms for which most doctors would find no cause.

"I think the borderline deficiencies are extremely common," Dr. Tkacz says. "It's what's called the 'tea and toast' syndrome. Older people living on Social Security or a pension find themselves short of money and don't eat as well as they should." Add to that teenagers subsisting on fast foods and people of any age who let life's stresses overtake their daily intake of B vitamins, and you've got quite a crowd.

The best sources of B-complex nutrients.

So what's the best protection against a deficiency? Eating foods rich in the B-complex vitamins is important. (See the table, Best Food Sources of Vitamin C, on page 130, for a list of good sources of B-complex vitamins.) Whole grains, peanuts, seeds and beans also contain good amounts. An alternative is B_{12}-fortified brewer's yeast or a good B-complex supplement.

"I have my patients take from one teaspoon to one tablespoon of brewer's yeast a day," Dr. Picker says. He also has them follow a diet that's high in fiber and complex carbohydrates and low in fats and sweets. "I advise them to minimize or eliminate alcohol or caffeine intake, and I always give them a big lecture about smoking. All three of those are big users of the B vitamins."

"Just one simple step of providing B complex or brewer's yeast in the diet can eliminate a whole host of potential neurological and psychological problems," adds Dr. Tkacz.

Caution: Alcohol, coffee and cigarettes burn up vitamins.

Chapter 46

Psychiatric Symptoms: The B$_{12}$ Connection

The patient's behavior changed quite suddenly and became increasingly bizarre. He was irritable and agitated. He was hardly sleeping at all and was hyperactive. And he had delusions that he was of great importance. In fact, he was convinced that his hometown was planning a day of celebration in his honor and that several Hollywood celebrities would attend. When he was finally admitted to a hospital, it took six men to restrain him. And the patient was 81 years old!

His doctor performed all of the proper physical and neurological tests, but the results were normal. And all of his blood tests were normal, too, except for one. The test for vitamin B$_{12}$ showed that he had an abnormally low level of the vitamin in his blood.

The doctor prescribed daily B$_{12}$ intravenously, and by the end of one week, the patient's mental status had returned to normal. He continued to receive weekly B$_{12}$ by injection and six months later was still completely normal.

B$_{12}$ deficiency is a possible cause of mania.

"That particular syndrome, called mania, has never before been traced to B$_{12}$ deficiency, so most general physicians may not be aware of that possibility," says Frederick Goggans, M.D., the doctor who treated that patient. "But what makes the case even more unusual is that the patient's mental problems appeared before any other signs of B$_{12}$ deficiency."

The Secret Signs of a B$_{12}$ Deficiency

Usually, a B$_{12}$ deficiency is easy to spot, because even though it's needed only in tiny amounts (the Recommended Dietary Allowance, or RDA, is three *micrograms*), B$_{12}$ works for us in a big way. It's needed for the production of healthy red blood cells and for the proper functioning of the nervous system.

When there's not enough B$_{12}$ to go around, the nerves and spinal cord are affected, leading to numbness and tingling in the hands and feet and an unsteady gait. The red blood cells become enlarged and misshapen and are unable to carry oxygen properly, which is their main job. The condition is called pernicious anemia, and other symptoms are pallor, weakness, fatigue and diarrhea. Mental problems can eventually occur, but not until much later. Or that's what doctors used to think. New reports are proving that's not always true.

The physical signs of low B$_{12}$.

At the University of North Carolina, doctors recently described the cases of two patients with psychoses (severe mental disorders) caused by vitamin B$_{12}$ deficiencies. Both of the patients had no other symptoms of B$_{12}$ deficiency, and both returned to normal after receiving B$_{12}$ injections.

The doctors warn that "psychiatric manifestations may be the first symptoms of a vitamin B$_{12}$ deficiency," and they recommend that all patients with psychoses caused by brain-tissue dysfunction be checked for a B$_{12}$ deficiency (*American Journal of Psychiatry*).

"Even though most doctors are aware that B$_{12}$ deficiency can lead to psychiatric symptoms, they may not be aware that it can happen before any signs of anemia," says Lorrin Koran, M.D., an associate professor of psychiatry at the Stanford University Medical Center.

In B$_{12}$ deficiency, psychiatric symptoms can show up before anemia.

"So upon finding normal red blood cells, a doctor may be likely to dismiss the possibility of B_{12} deficiency prematurely," adds Dr. Goggans.

Not Necessarily Senile

How does a doctor know when to check further? "Severe mental disorders usually begin when people are in their twenties," explains Dr. Goggans, who is medical director of Charter Hospital of Fort Worth, Texas. "So when an older person comes into the hospital with mental problems and has no prior history of a mental disorder, I'm sure to screen for B_{12} deficiency."

Other, more common, psychiatric problems can be caused by B_{12} deficiency, too. "Depression and dementia in the elderly are the two syndromes most classically associated with B_{12} deficiency," says Dr. Goggans. "Dementia closely resembles senility, with its loss of intellectual function. But when it's caused by B_{12} deficiency, it's reversible." Unfortunately, many elderly people may be written off as senile when their condition is actually treatable.

Is "senility" sometimes caused by lack of B_{12}?

"Biochemical depression is also very common in the elderly," adds Dr. Goggans. "It causes sleep and appetite disturbances, lack of energy and intellectual decline. But it's also easily treatable by standard antidepressants and is exceptionally responsive to B_{12} replacement therapy."

Older people take note: You're at risk for B_{12} deficiency.

"We're careful to check for B_{12} deficiency in older people," says Todd Estroff, M.D., former assistant director of neuropsychiatric evaluation at Fair Oaks Hospital in Summit, New Jersey. "They're especially susceptible because they don't eat well. The older person with poor teeth who tries to survive on tea and toast is more likely to develop a deficiency."

One study of 49 patients in the geriatric psychiatry unit of a Massachusetts hospital found B_{12} deficiency more than any other undiagnosed medical problem. "None of these patients had frank pernicious anemia . . . nor was there evidence of peripheral neuropathy [nerve damage]," say the researchers (*Journal of the American Geriatrics Society*).

In another study, published by three doctors from Denmark, low values of B$_{12}$ were found in one out of every three patients admitted to a geriatric center (*Acta Medica Scandinavica*).

But the elderly aren't the only ones at risk. "I've seen teenagers with B$_{12}$ levels so low you wonder how they can be walking," says Charles Tkacz, M.D., medical director of the North Nassau Mental Health Center in Manhasset, New York. "It's amazing they didn't need to be carried in on a stretcher. They're getting into trouble because of a junk-food/fast-food diet."

Also at risk for B$_{12}$ depletion: teenagers.

Reliable Dietary Sources of B$_{12}$

Beef liver packs in a big wallop of B$_{12}$, but it's also found in other meats, fish, dairy products and eggs. Because B$_{12}$ is found almost exclusively in foods of animal origin, anyone who avoids those foods runs the risk of developing a deficiency. That's why vegans, strict vegetarians who eat no eggs or dairy products, can become deficient if they're not careful.

A special caution for vegetarians.

But even those of us who aren't vegetarians should be extra sure to get enough B$_{12}$. One government study showed that the amount of B$_{12}$ we're eating has decreased dramatically over the last two decades. According to the researchers, our intake of B$_{12}$ dropped by 8 percent during that period, more than any other vitamin. The reason? A lower consumption of liver and dairy products, say the researchers.

The trouble is, even if you *do* eat plenty of B$_{12}$-rich foods, you may still end up with a deficiency. Some people can't absorb B$_{12}$ from their digestive system because they lack what is known as intrinsic factor, a molecule that latches onto B$_{12}$ and escorts it to the site on the intestinal wall where it is absorbed. Because intrinsic factor is produced in the stomach, people who have had stomach surgery are also likely candidates for B_{12} deficiency. They remain healthy only as long as they receive B_{12} injections, which bypass the digestive problems.

Are your medications interfering with B_{12} absorption?

Other factors can upset the precarious balance of this vitally important substance, too. Cholesterol-lowering medications, potassium-replacement agents and anticonvulsants can all interfere with B_{12} absorption. And studies have shown that antiulcer drugs can have the same effect because they reduce stomach acidity, which is important for B_{12} absorption. "Certain parasites, such as some tapeworms, can also steal B_{12}," Dr. Koran says.

"Luckily, vitamin B_{12} deficiency is usually among the easiest deficiencies to correct," says Dr. Tkacz. "And since depression is so common, we check everyone who is admitted to our hospital."

"My chief job is to screen patients for underlying medical illness, so everyone in my hospital gets

---

Zinc and B_{12} May Halt Brain Disorders

Doctors have known for years that a vitamin B_{12} deficiency can lead to all kinds of psychiatric problems. A Dutch study has taken that one step further. Doctors there evaluated patients who had Alzheimer's-type senility and alcohol-related brain damage, and they found low levels of B_{12} and zinc in both groups. On top of that, the low zinc levels threw off the zinc-to-copper ratio, creating a relative copper toxicity.

The researchers believe that early recognition and adequate treatment with B_{12} and zinc can possibly prevent irreversible damage in patients with these disorders (*Journal of Orthomolecular Psychiatry*).

checked for B$_{12}$ deficiency," says Dr. Estroff. "They must get by me before they can be called psychiatric patients."

A Deficiency That's Often Overlooked

Unfortunately, if you go to your family doctor because of a mental problem, he probably won't check for B$_{12}$. "When most doctors see behavioral symptoms, they refer the patient to a psychiatrist," Dr. Estroff says.

"They tend not to look for physical disorders. And most psychiatrists don't look for B$_{12}$ deficiency because they rely on the general practitioners to clear the patients medically. The way it ends up, nobody covers it.

"The result is that the patient may not receive the proper treatment. They may be given shock treatments, antidepressants or other medication because their problems are mistakenly labeled as psychiatric."

Dr. Tkacz has found the same thing. "Some doctors don't check for vitamin deficiencies in psychiatric patients. I've seen patients who've been to four or five other doctors or hospitals before coming to our center, and it's not unusual for us to find that they have B$_{12}$ deficiencies."

Lack of B$_{12}$: an easily overlooked diagnosis.

"And if you don't look for it," says Dr. Estroff, "you don't find it."

The problem is that even if the doctor does check for B$_{12}$ deficiency, the test results may not be accurate. Several studies have shown that the usual test for B$_{12}$, called the radiodilution assay, is unreliable.

"The standard test measures B$_{12}$ as well as some similar but inactive forms," Dr. Estroff explains. "So the test may show a normal result when the patient is actually deficient. That fact is not widely known by physicians and psychiatrists. There is another, more

Checking for B$_{12}$ depletion.

reliable test, but it's more difficult to do, takes longer and is more expensive, so most labs don't use it."

No one is sure how many people may be suffering needlessly because of undiagnosed B_{12} deficiency.

"Psychiatric symptoms *can* be caused by medical illness," Dr. Estroff maintains. "B_{12} deficiency is one cause, but it's just the tip of the iceberg. It's a small aspect of a highly neglected area of medicine and psychiatry."

Chapter 47

Calcium versus Osteoporosis

There are knowledgeable people in the world who are, for lack of a better phrase, slightly bone dumb—people who think milk is for children and that fibula and tibia are Shakespearean characters; people who believe that brittle bones and the "dowager's hump" are inevitable aspects of growing old. Young women shrug off that clinical-sounding word "osteoporosis" as something that afflicts only grandmothers, and young men tune out talk of the bone-degenerating condition because it's a woman's problem.

It is these people, those whose knowledge of bones comes from cutting apart a frozen chicken, who should consider the words of experts like Jon Block, M.D. "Worrying about osteoporosis after it shows up is like closing the barn door after the horse has already gone. We need to take precautions earlier because you can do very little to reverse the condition once it occurs," says Dr. Block, a member of the osteoporosis research program in the University of California at San Francisco's Radiology Department.

Stopping osteoporosis before it starts.

Previously, medical efforts have concentrated on treating osteoporosis, but today there's more attention paid to prevention. The target audience is young women, preferably in the teen years, and the goal is to make them aware of changes they can make that could help them avoid the crippling bone condition.

A new approach to the bone-thinning disease.

A "Modern" Disease

Osteoporosis was once scarcely recognized because most people didn't live long enough for their bones to deteriorate. As average life expectancy increased, however, doctors noticed that older women broke their wrists more often than older men, which one German surgeon in 1882 blamed on tripping on long skirts. Wiser men have since put fashion aside and learned that menopause's hormonal changes trigger the loss of bone strength. That's because following menopause, there is a dramatic decrease in the production of estrogen, a sex hormone that maintains bone strength.

Menopause—when women are at highest risk for osteoporosis.

Today, the average woman will live to see at least 78 candles on her birthday cake, which means she will also spend more than one-third of her life in the postmenopausal stage, when osteoporosis is a high risk. "More women are getting older and living longer, as are men, so the situation for both sexes stands to get much worse unless something is done," says James A. Nicotero, M.D., director of the Osteoporosis Diagnostic Center at St. Francis Medical Center in Pittsburgh.

Almost 20 million people have some form of osteoporosis, and at least 1 million people annually break bones that are weakened by osteoporosis. About 50,000 people die each year from complications due to osteoporosis, and many victims are incapacitated for life.

What Your Mother Didn't Know

How osteoporosis occurs is clearer now than in your mother's day. Calcium, a silver-white metal that's a dominant element in bone, is stored in the skeleton. When more is needed to maintain bones, teeth and bodily functions than is taken in, a calcium deficiency is created. A federal survey shows that up to 50 per-

Many men and women don't get enough calcium.

cent of males between 18 and 34 have diets deficient in calcium, while two-thirds of women between 18 and 74 fail to take in enough calcium each day.

When the reserves are taxed day after day without being adequately restocked, bones become porous and brittle (hence the name "brittle bone disease") and break easily. Vertebrae can collapse, and the resulting dowager's hump can cause severe back pain. Once bone weakens, it is difficult to rebuild it to its original strength; there's no cure per se, and the objective is to keep the deterioration from worsening.

Latest Theory:
Salt Contributes to Calcium Loss

As if there weren't already enough reasons to take the saltshaker off the table, there's now evidence that sodium may play a role in calcium loss.

Ailsa Goulding, Ph.D., senior research officer, Department of Medicine at the University of Otago in New Zealand, believes that consumption of common table salt increases the amount of calcium lost through the kidneys. In one study, animals given salt supplements lost more calcium and phosphate—another element in bone—in their urine and had less of the minerals in their skeletons than those animals not receiving salt. Another study found that adding a teaspoon of salt to the daily diet of young women increased the amount of calcium lost. Dr. Goulding also found that a single teaspoon a day can cause enough of a calcium loss to decrease bone mass 1.5 percent a year.

The relationship between salt and calcium excretion may be one reason why women in primitive societies that add no sodium to food suffer less bone loss than U.S. women, even though their calcium intakes are low by our standards. It may also help explain the relationship between low-calcium intake and high blood pressure in countries with high salt consumption, such as the United States.

Why women have more trouble holding onto calcium.

Women have more trouble with calcium than men and lose bone mass faster, which is why osteoporosis is eight times more common in women. There are plenty of factors: Because of smaller body size, women generally have less bone mass to start with; bone loss begins at an earlier age; pregnancy and breastfeeding appear to take a heavy toll, since one skeleton supplies calcium for two lives; women are more likely to go on weight-reducing diets that typically are low in calcium; and women live longer than men.

The calcium thieves.

There are also social factors: Women smoke and drink alcohol more than their grandmothers did, and both have been implicated in calcium loss; soft drinks and fast foods low in calcium are dietary staples; the think-thin mentality keeps many women away from calcium-rich foods; and although activity appears to stimulate bone development, many women live sedentary lifestyles. For a more detailed discussion of the risk factors, see chapter 48.

Bone Loss Starts Earlier than Expected

"Some bone loss is going to occur in men and women, which is a normal part of the aging process," says Robert Recker, M.D., who has conducted bone research at the Creighton University School of Medicine in Omaha. "But if lifestyle changes are made early and not just when the prospect of osteoporosis looms ahead, then there's a good chance fractures can be avoided."

Getting your bones ready for the future.

Bone mass stops developing at age 35, and bones slowly start losing calcium thereafter, until menopause occurs at about age 50 and triggers a more drastic calcium drain. "The strength of a woman's bones at age 35 will determine how she handles the high-risk years," says Stanton Cohn, Ph.D., former professor of medicine, School of Medicine, State University of New York at Stony Brook, and head of the Medical Physics Division of the Brookhaven National Laboratory, New York. "The years before age 35 are crucial. A woman can increase calcium intake and exercise between ages 35 and 50 and have some impact, but by that time, all she's trying to do is maintain what's already there."

The amount of calcium needed daily depends on several factors. The government's Recommended Dietary Allowance (RDA) is 800 milligrams. Experts generally agree, however, that the calcium allowance should be higher, possibly 1,200 milligrams for teenagers, 1,000 milligrams for women age 20 through menopause, 1,200 milligrams for pregnant and lactating women, and anywhere from 1,000 to 1,500 milligrams after menopause, depending on whether estrogen is also being taken.

How much calcium do you really need?

How to get the necessary calcium depends on personal preference. A glass of low-fat milk contains about 300 milligrams of calcium, so several would meet the RDA. But there are plenty of other sources: low-fat cheeses, yogurt and ice cream; red kidney beans, lima beans and soybeans; blackstrap molasses; fruits such as watermelon, oranges, raisins and strawberries; fish, especially sardines and salmon when they have soft bones that can be eaten; Brazil nuts, almonds and sunflower seeds; and green, leafy vegetables, which is where the cow gets the calcium for milk in the first place.

Enough calcium can be obtained from food alone. A report in the *New England Journal of Medicine* concluded that the calcium intake of hunter-gatherer tribes still roaming the earth and living lifestyles similar to people who lived in preagricultural days is more that 1,500 milligrams a day, which exceeds the current highest suggested daily requirement. They ingest no dairy products and assure sturdy bones just by eating what they pluck, pull or catch.

Diet is the best source of calcium.

Some people have trouble sticking to a balanced diet, and others just don't like dairy products, in which case calcium supplements may be in order. The most widely recommended are calcium-carbonate tablets, which contain almost three times more calcium than other types of supplements (and that means fewer tablets to swallow).

Some people prefer to take their supplements with meals, while others take them at bedtime; both approaches seem to work, although the experts question whether taking large doses at once is wise. "It's probably best to take it slowly throughout the day instead of in a sudden shot all at once. If you overload, there's a chance that a good bit will be lost through body wastes," says Dr. Cohn.

Don't take more calcium than you need.

Moderation is the watchword. Megadoses of calcium that exceed 2,000 milligrams a day can in rare cases lead to kidney stones and constipation.

Develop an Appetite for Exercise

Swallowing isn't the only activity that's fundamental in osteoporosis prevention. Exercise is stressed, since the evidence suggests that activity strengthens bone mass. In the younger years, almost any form of exercise is beneficial, experts say. For the elderly, brisk walking is recommended. Enjoyment is the key, since the activity must become a routine part of everyday life.

Keep moving to strengthen your bones.

Ironically, it appears that too much exercise can lead to an early onset of osteoporosis. "Young women who exercise to extremes and reduce their body fat levels down to 17 to 20 percent seem to trigger normal changes that alter their regular menstrual cycle and cause calcium loss," says Henry A. Solomon, M.D., professor of medicine and cardiology at Cornell University Medical Center. "This applies to any actively menstruating woman. Most of the cases that have been seen are women in their twenties and thirties."

The Debate over Drug Treatments

Taking preventive steps early in life could spare a woman from becoming entangled in the debate over medical treatments of osteoporosis in later years. At the center of the controversy is estrogen. Some physicians routinely prescribe the drug to postmenopausal women, along with progestogen, which is supposed to protect the uterine lining from cancer that could be caused by the estrogen. Others in the medical community say the treatment hasn't been proved safe.

The pros and cons of hormone therapy.

Meanwhile, sodium fluoride has joined the fracas. This experimental drug has some practitioners anxiously waiting because there is initial evidence that whereas calcium and estrogen only prevent further bone loss in postmenopausal women, sodium fluoride may make bones stronger.

A new diagnostic device may help prevent women from reaching the stage where any of the synthetic bone drugs are needed. In a 15-minute office procedure, the bone densitometer measures the mineral content of the wristbone at two precise locations, which correspond respectively to both the hipbone and spinal column. The densitometer uses only one one-hundredth the radiation of a standard forearm x-ray and concentrates the radiation in an area of only two inches; an x-ray scatters radiation to other organs, says Dr. Nicotero, whose diagnostic center includes a densitometer.

A better way to detect osteoporosis.

"Conventional x-rays can't detect osteoporosis until 30 to 40 percent of the bone mass is lost, in which case bone loss is so extensive that fractures may occur. At that stage, estrogen is often prescribed. The beauty of the densitometer is that we can detect as little as a 2 percent change in bone mass, which means we can initiate therapies before too much damage is done," he says. "So this device could decrease the use of estrogen because a woman wouldn't be given estrogen if she were found to have excellent bone density at the time of her menopause."

Osteoporosis: Not a Simple Calcium Deficiency

With all the information that's surfacing, it would seem that avoiding osteoporosis is simply a matter of drinking milk while exercising in the sun. In this case, however, simplicity is confusing.

Calcium is only part of the solution.

"One of the big problems is that the issue of calcium and osteoporosis has been blown out of focus," says David Fardon, M.D., a Knoxville, Tennessee, orthopedic surgeon and author of *Osteoporosis: Your Head Start on the Prevention and Treatment of Brittle Bones.* "We've paid a lot of attention to the fact that there's not enough calcium in the diet, but the situation has been oversimplified. It's not just a calcium-deficiency disease, because there are other factors involved. Some people assume that getting extra calcium will automatically shield them from osteoporosis, but it's not that simple."

To fight osteoporosis, consider all the factors.

Robert P. Heaney, M.D., who has conducted joint research with Dr. Recker at Creighton University School of Medicine, agrees: "If you go out and buy a bottle of calcium supplements without considering the importance of the other factors, you'll realize some benefit. But if you're striving for the maximum results, you must make sure the other pieces of the puzzle are there also."

Researchers at the University of Iowa College of Medicine, for example, found that calcium intake alone wasn't related to bone density, but bone density was greater when calcium and vitamin D were adequate (*American Journal of Clinical Nutrition*). But be aware that vitamin D supplements, if taken in excess (the Recommended Dietary Allowance is 400 international units), can build up to toxic levels.

Other mysteries of osteoporosis are just beginning to unravel. In a case involving young and middle-aged men, two groups thought to be safe from osteoporosis, researchers at a Veterans Administration hospital in Illinois found extensive bone loss in those who were chronic alcoholics. The finding enhances previous theories about alcohol interfering with the integrity of the bone.

Does alcohol confound calcium metabolism?

Of all the questions that remain, one may be the hardest to answer: How do you get a teenager to drink enough milk?

Is It Possible to Reverse Bone Loss?

Scientists have reported that calcium supplements are likely to help slow down bone loss and thus put the brakes on osteoporosis. That's why so many doctors prescribe calcium (up to 1,000 milligrams a day) to their patients with the disease, along with vitamin D (400 international units a day), plus estrogen, exercise and fluoride.

But there's been precious little evidence that calcium supplements could actually help *reverse* bone loss. Until now.

In a study conducted by Paul D. Miller, M.D., of the University of Colorado School of Medicine in Denver, 21 patients with osteoporosis actually *gained* bone mass after a year of taking daily doses of 1,500 to 2,000 milligrams of calcium plus vitamin D.

In fact, by the end of the year, their bones had returned to normal mass. And instead of showing a continuing decline in mass, the bones of another 29 patients showed no change.

Dr. Miller reports that the calcium and vitamin D therapy seemed to work for some women regardless of whether they took estrogen.

And taking fluoride along with the nutrients didn't seem to have any effect on bone loss at all.

"The increase in bone mass was very unusual," says Dr. Miller. "We are quite excited about the apparent reversibility of osteoporosis."

Up to this point, osteoporosis has been regarded as merely treatable, not curable. But if Dr. Miller's findings are corroborated by other research, calcium (with vitamin D) may emerge as the core ingredient in a long-awaited cure.

Until then, we can heed current advice from a growing medical consensus: Make sure you're getting enough calcium.

"Brittle bones just don't make a profound impression on the public," says Dr. Fardon. "Also, people want results. They want the satisfaction of seeing their efforts work, and it's not as rewarding to change your lifestyle in the hope of preventing a broken hip decades down the road."

The answer? "Instill good habits while they're children, then they won't have to make any drastic changes later in life when they are set in their ways," Dr. Fardon says. "The best place to start is in the womb, so the child has strong bones when born."

A prime deterrent against osteoporosis: early detection.

Adds Dr. Block, "Women are flocking to get mammograms because they realize there is the likelihood they could get cancer. But this wasn't always the case, and it took time to get the message out. Today, you don't find women asking doctors to measure their bone mass, even though there's a good chance they'll develop osteoporosis. Women don't realize that some of these diagnostic techniques exist. Family physicians will have to do a lot of the motivating, and groups like the Osteoporosis Foundation should help get the message out. The awareness will come, but it will take time."

Who Gets Osteoporosis?

Y̲ou lock your doors, buy a smoke detector and perhaps install a security system to protect the valuables in your home. Do you give the same protection to the valuable strength in your bones?

You may be in greater need than others of prevention against osteoporosis, a disease that gradually steals strength-building calcium from bones.

Take Stock of Your Skeleton

To get an idea whether you'll be standing tall in years to come or whether you'll be one of the millions for whom even a simple task could be backbreaking, see if any of the following risk factors of osteoporosis fit you.

Advancing age means bone strength retreats. It usually isn't until after age 50 or so that neglected bones start demanding attention—usually by fracturing or shortening your stature. Menopause occurs around this time, taking the biggest toll of all on the skeletal system. The diet of an older person is often too poor to maintain bone integrity. And with increasing age, the intestines become less efficient at absorbing what calcium there is in the diet. The number of people over age 65 in the United States is expected to reach 22 percent of the population by the year 2050, making osteoporosis one of the medical profession's top research priorities.

If you're over age 50, your bones are at risk for calcium loss.

If you're a woman, you should be concerned about your bones. While both sexes unavoidably lose some bone mass simply due to aging, most of the 15 to 20 million cases of advanced osteoporosis are in women. The fact that women have smaller frames than men may be one explanation for the inequity—when the body needs calcium elsewhere and calls on bones to give up part of their supply, men's bones simply have more on reserve.

Menopause, either natural or surgical, means increased risk. Estrogen, the multitalented hormone produced by a woman's ovaries, helps maintain bone mass and strength in addition to its sex-related duties. When menopause shuts down the supply, bones are more susceptible to fractures. Scientists confirmed this estrogen/bone-strength link when they began seeing premature osteoporosis in premenopausal women who had had their ovaries removed. Hormones may also help account for the female bias in osteoporosis. Testosterone, a male hormone helpful for bone mass, has a more gradual decline in production than estrogen's somewhat here-today, gone-tomorrow departure. Women who have spent years taking estrogen-containing birth control pills are thought to enjoy greater protection from osteoporosis, also.

Caucasian and oriental women are at greater risk than black women. Large-scale studies have repeatedly shown much higher rates of osteoporosis in fairer-skinned races. Two theories may account for this, says Diane Meier, M.D., co-director of the Osteoporosis and Metabolic Bone-Disease Program at Mount Sinai Medical Center, New York City. She's conducting a study of 150 white women and 150 black women, ages 26 to 65, to see if the former have a genetic predisposition to excessive bone loss, or if nutritional habits and body composition are the key. "Blacks, at least in the North American population, tend to have higher obesity rates. And obesity is protective against bone loss," Dr. Meier explains.

The hormone/bone-strength connection.

Two theories why black women have a lower risk.

(Very thin people, then, are also at greater risk.) Black people may have larger and denser bone structures, too, which may give them an advantage against osteoporosis.

A diet short on calcium will mean bone loss in the long run. Scientists found women who had a calcium-rich diet in childhood and early adulthood built a bone mass more able to withstand osteoporosis in later years. Lactose, a carbohydrate in calcium-laden milk, may help the body absorb calcium. Major health organizations are urging people to start getting the Recommended Dietary Allowance (RDA) of calcium (800 milligrams for children 1 through 10 and for adults, and 1,200 milligrams for children 11 through 18 and for pregnant and lactating women) early in life, but most Americans obtain barely half these amounts.

Optimum calcium intake should start early.

Constant dieters lose more than pounds. They risk losing bone mass, too, after years of passing up high-fat (but also high-calcium) dairy products. Low-fat dairy products like skim milk and cottage cheese can help dieters meet their calcium needs.

Strict vegetarians may restrict their bones' strength. "Pure vegetarians who don't eat any dairy products have a hard time getting adequate calcium," says Dr. Meier. "The green vegetables they eat, like broccoli and spinach, do have calcium, but they also contain oxalates, which block the absorption of calcium in the gut."

A meat-eater's diet may eat away at bone strength. A culinary love affair with red meat puts overindulgers at greater risk. Studies indicate high protein levels speed up the excretion of calcium in urine and keep the mineral from making its way to bones.

Too much protein could be a problem.

A vitamin D deficiency could mean low-grade bone strength. Vitamin D is normally obtained in adequate amounts through a healthy diet and through the skin with 10 to 20 minutes of sun exposure daily. It's crucial for intestinal absorption of calcium and bone remodeling. But older people may run into a vitamin D shortage due to poor nutrition and long housebound periods due to illness or injury. The sunshine/vitamin D connection is also why people who live in rainier, cloudier climates are thought to be at higher risk than those on whom the sun always shines.

A family history of osteoporosis is related to your risk of getting the disease. A woman's grandmother, mother and aunt may be a clue to what may be in store for her. One theory behind this: If female relatives reached menopause at a rather early age, they may pass along that tendency. So more years are spent without estrogen's bone protection.

A lazybones lifestyle leads to thinner bones later. One of the many beneficial effects of exercise on the body is the way it helps build bones. Any weight-bearing exercise stimulates the skeleton to put down new bone. Tennis players, weight lifters, ballet dancers and other athletes show wider bones and more cortical, or outside-layer, bone in limbs involved in their particular sport. And astronauts are prime examples of gravity's usefulness—when they're weightless in space, they lose a significant amount of bone mass. Patients confined to bed face a similar situation and can lose as much as 1 percent of their trabecular, or inner, bone per week. Resuming normal weight-bearing activity gradually restores the bone.

Stimulate your skeleton.

Certain substances make calcium seep away. Prolonged use of aluminum-containing antacids, prednisone- or cortisone-containing drugs and diuretics can increase the risk of bone loss. Excessive sodium in the diet is also being explored as a possible cause of calcium excretion, but this research is still very preliminary.

Three types of drugs that can erode bones.

Medical disorders may be additional risk factors for bone loss. Diabetes, hyperthyroidism, hyperparathyroidism, Cushing's disease, rheumatoid arthritis and gastrectomy have been reported to cause osteoporosis, but scientists note the need for more research in this area.

Cigarette smoking may weaken bones. Smoking is suspected of exerting a possibly toxic effect on bone mass. Women who smoke have lower estrogen levels, tend to be thinner than nonsmokers and undergo menopause at an earlier age. Overall, women smokers appear to have lower cortical bone mass.

Alcohol may abuse bones. Heavy alcohol use is one of the few things that puts a man at risk for osteoporosis. Alcoholic men have lower bone mass and lose bone more rapidly than nonalcoholics. In women, the incidence of hip fractures increases as alcohol intake rises. These associations could stem from a direct toxic effect of alcohol, poor nutrition, lower body weight, liver disease or other alcohol-related factors.

One risk factor for men.

Chapter 49

Vitamin D:
Another Force
against Bone Disease

Sunshine: your best source of vitamin D.

One of the best friends your bones ever had just traveled 93 million miles to get here. It's sunlight, and if you aren't outside welcoming it, well, maybe you don't know what you're missing. But your bones do.

The sun, that untiring nuclear furnace, brightens our days, warms our cold bodies and melts the snow. But the sun is more than just a pretty face. The sun's rays also trigger an ingenious biochemical process in our skin that stimulates the production of vitamin D, and that's good for our bones, too.

Get enough sunlight—just 10 to 20 minutes a day, experts say—and your skin will manufacture all the vitamin D your body needs.

An Urgent Need for Vitamin D

Fortunately, most Americans get plenty of vitamin D. But a number of the nation's elderly—though no one knows exactly how many—live in the shadows, locked away from the light of Earth's shining star. As a result, their bodies don't make enough vitamin D. Neither do they get enough vitamin D in their diet, a secondary but important source of the vital nutrient.

Why is vitamin D so important?

Think of vitamin D as a bus. Every day, calcium—an essential mineral—takes a ride on that bus. Its destination: your bones. Calcium makes your bones strong and hard. Without calcium, your bones can become dangerously soft or brittle. But calcium has to have a way of getting from your gastrointestinal tract to your bones. That's where vitamin D comes in.

Vitamin D's job is to transport calcium into your bones.

Vitamin D formed in the skin is converted in the liver to a prohormone, 25-hydroxyvitamin D. It's then converted once again in the kidney to an active hormone, 1,25 vitamin D, or calciferol. This hormone is what moves calcium along on its way to your waiting skeleton.

"The main thing vitamin D does is help the gastrointestinal tract absorb calcium," says Patrick Ober, M.D., of the Bowman Gray School of Medicine in Winston-Salem, North Carolina. "Calcium won't be absorbed, and it won't ever be utilized unless it can be transported into the bloodstream. And that's the function of vitamin D."

D Deficiency Can Be Crippling

Exactly how much vitamin D does the average person need? The U.S. Recommended Daily Allowance (USRDA) of vitamin D is 400 international units daily.

Thanks to the sun, most of us get enough vitamin D without even trying. But for those who spend little time outdoors or who cover up every available patch of sun-receptive skin, vitamin D deficiency can be both painful and potentially crippling.

In adults, prolonged vitamin D deficiency may lead to osteomalacia (soft bones) or osteoporosis (brittle bones).

There's more to osteomalacia and osteoporosis than just a reduction in the amount of calcium going to your bones. Your body needs calcium for other purposes—to keep your heart beating rhythmically, to regulate muscle contractions, to promote blood coagulation and, in general, to keep your body's cells glued together. When your body doesn't get enough vitamin D, the bones don't get calcium, but neither

A shortage of vitamin D and calcium means trouble.

does the rest of your body. So it responds to immediate calcium needs by siphoning calcium from the bones.

Know the warning signs of osteomalacia.

The early warning signs of osteomalacia are bone tenderness or pain, back pain, irritability and weakness. These symptoms often are dismissed as the inevitable consequences of old age. But it's not necessarily so. Left undiagnosed, osteomalacia sufferers ultimately may have trouble making it up a flight of stairs and, in the worst cases, might not be able to walk.

Other Conditions Can Threaten D Status

The link between vitamin D deficiency and osteoporosis is not as clear. Osteoporosis patients are believed to suffer a calcium deficiency. Some patients do absorb calcium more efficiently with the administration of vitamin D in its hormonal form. Research suggests, however, that not all cases of osteoporosis respond as well to increased vitamin D. An estimated 20 million Americans, most of them postmenopausal women, suffer from osteoporosis, believed to be a result of reduced production of estrogen in the body. This condition interferes with the conversion of vitamin D to a hormone, so the bones are deprived of calcium.

Certain illnesses make it hard for some people's bodies to process vitamin D. These include liver, kidney or parathyroid disease, and vitamin D-dependency rickets, a hereditary disorder. Vitamin D along with calcium has been found useful in treating these problems, but in doses well beyond the USRDA of 400 international units.

Some drugs and vitamin D don't get along.

Certain anticonvulsant drugs—phenobarbital and phenytoin, for instance—also can abnormally speed up the breakdown of vitamin D. Supplementation is required to reverse osteomalacia caused by these drugs but, again, in doses that must be medically prescribed.

Nursing mothers and pregnant women also may require additional vitamin D and calcium. In these cases, however, supplements should *not* be taken without a doctor's recommendation.

Children can also suffer vitamin D deficiency, and their bones, too, can turn soft. This condition in young people, characterized by bowlegs and pigeon chest, is called rickets.

Sunshine-Shy Oldsters Face Trouble

In the early days of the Industrial Revolution, as soot, smoke and dust rose high into the sky, blocking sunlight, rickets emerged as a serious problem among children. Today, thanks in large part to vitamin D-fortified dairy products, vitamin D deficiency is uncommon among American children.

Among American kids, vitamin D deficiency is rare.

Of growing concern, however, are reports of vitamin D deficiency among senior citizens, even in the midst of America's Sun Belt.

"What we see happening in our society is that people, particularly as they get older, have a tendency to avoid sunlight purposely," says John L. Omdahl, Ph.D., a biochemist in the University of New Mexico School of Medicine.

All things being equal, says Dr. Omdahl, a 70-year-old man shouldn't need more vitamin D than a man 50 years younger. As a practical matter, though, many older Americans *do* need more vitamin D because their bodies don't make enough to begin with.

Why not?

There are a variety of reasons, Dr. Omdahl explains. Many older people worry that exposure to sunlight may lead to skin cancer. Or perhaps they just have trouble getting around, so they remain indoors. And in the winter, in particular, they are reluctant to venture outside into the cold.

Why many older people don't get enough sunshine.

Contributing to the deficiency is insufficient vitamin D in the diet. Many older people have trouble digesting milk products, says Dr. Omdahl, so they don't consume enough dairy foods to meet nutritional requirements.

It also is believed that as we get older, our bodies become less able to absorb calcium. Likewise, blood levels of vitamin D hormone also diminish.

Are you getting enough vitamin D?

Particularly telling is a 1982 study of elderly residents in Albuquerque, New Mexico. According to the study, which Dr. Omdahl coauthored, elderly Americans appear to be getting less vitamin D than the USRDA of 400 international units. Sixty percent of the elderly New Mexicans took in less than 100 units a day. Most were not taking vitamin D supplements, and they avoided sunlight, which was abundantly available.

Vitamin D deficiency is uncommon in the United States, says Dr. Omdahl. But among the elderly, particularly city dwellers, vitamin D deficiency *does* occur. "What percentage of the elderly that is, we're still trying to determine," says Dr. Omdahl. "But it is something that should be of concern to the general population."

Less Sunlight, Lower Vitamin D Intake

How climate can influence your vitamin D levels.

In the winter, getting enough vitamin D can be a problem for anyone living in the northern latitudes. One reason is that the sun is lower in the sky. The sun's ultraviolet rays have trouble punching through the atmosphere, which is thicker at that low angle. There are also fewer hours of daylight and more clouds. Also, when it's cold outside, few of us are inspired to sunbathe. Sitting next to a nice, sunny window doesn't help, either. Glass filters out Sol's ultraviolet rays.

Suppose you live in West Thumb, Wyoming, and it's been snowing there continually since October. Can you still get enough sunshine to meet your needs?

Maybe not. "In the winter, in the northern part of the United States, I'd say the chances are you *aren't* going to get enough vitamin D by skin," says Hector DeLuca, Ph.D., chairman of biochemistry at the University of Wisconsin.

For the vulnerable elderly, some of whom may get very little sunlight even in the summer, the need for vitamin D can be particularly acute.

Fortunately, the sun is not the only source of vitamin D. There are some simple ways for the elderly—and the rest of us—to get enough vitamin D while we're huddled up next to the radiator waiting for spring.

We can consume more dairy foods. If you're tallying up international units of vitamin D, a quart of fortified milk holds 400. Vitamin D also is abundant in certain oily fish, such as salmon, mackerel and sardines. You'll find 500 international units of vitamin D in a 3½-ounce helping of salmon and 575 units in the same size serving of mackerel.

Good food sources of vitamin D.

Fish-liver oils are very rich in vitamin D. There are, for example, 1,000 international units of vitamin D in a tablespoon of cod-liver oil. Other foods contain vitamin D, including liver, butter, cheese, eggs and beef. Some cereal products also are fortified. Vitamin D, however, is not plentiful in vegetables.

How Not to Overdose on Vitamin D

Be aware that because the body can store excess vitamin D in fat, large doses of vitamin D, taken over time, can cause serious health problems. That's a very unusual problem but something to keep in mind. When vitamin D dosage hits the level of thousands of international units, that's when trouble can begin.

If too much vitamin D in the diet can cause illness, what about sunshine? Can you overdose on vitamin D after a relaxing afternoon on the golf

Multivitamins may supply all of the vitamin D you need.

course? Not to worry. At a certain point, your body knows when to turn off the vitamin D tap. It's self-regulating, like a thermostat.

"Sunshine is the way you were meant to get your vitamin D," says Dr. DeLuca. "The amount of vitamin D that can be made in the skin is limited." We can safely get all the vitamin D most of us require in a multivitamin tablet, which Dr. Ober and Dr. DeLuca recommend as "insurance."

"Most of these vitamins have 400 units of vitamin D, which is a safe amount. But I really wouldn't want most people going beyond that," says Dr. Ober.

Put Senility
in Reverse
with a Better Diet

W hen asked a few years ago to name three wishes, scientist and novelist Isaac Asimov answered: to live so happily and effectively that no one would mourn his passing, to leave this world knowing that civilization would survive into the 21st century and beyond and, finally, not to outlive his intelligence—that is, to remain productive and quick-witted to the end, without senility.

Like Dr. Asimov, most of us worry about the possibility of mental decline in later life. We can tolerate the predictable aspects of the aging process—mild forgetfulness, blurred near vision, difficulty hearing—but none of us wants to be among the estimated 15 percent of those over 65 who suffer from some degree of senility.

And for the most part, there's nothing that says we must. Doctors once accepted senility as one of the irreversible penalties of old age, but some now say the opposite: that in many cases the symptoms of senility can be prevented or reversed.

Antisenility Nutrients
in the Spotlight

If there were a contest for the antisenility "nutrients of the year," the prize might be awarded to vitamin B_6 and copper. Two University of Texas nutritionists reported the remarkable news that a deficiency of

A link between senility and low copper or B_6.

B$_6$ or copper in young rats causes some of the same kind of brain cell abnormalities as those seen in senile humans.

The researchers found, among other things, that in rats and humans, the dendrites—delicate, branching roots that carry electrical impulses from one brain cell to another—tend to shrivel up and die when deprived of B$_6$ or copper. Without the all-important dendrites, brain circuitry breaks down (*American Journal of Clinical Nutrition*).

Though the rats were fed a diet skimpier in the two nutrients than any comparable human diet would be, the researchers said that a mild deficiency of

---

It Takes Zinc to Think

According to British physician Roy Hullin, M.D., the difference between a sharp mind and a fuzzy one could depend on the amount of zinc in your diet. When Dr. Hullin studied 1,200 patients over 65, he found that the 220 senile people in the group had significantly lower zinc levels than those who were not senile. And, he says, he got similar results in a younger group (under 65) who were just starting to show signs of senility.

"It is not generally appreciated," says Dr. Hullin, "that as much zinc as iron is required in the diet." The fact is, over 80 enzymes require zinc to work, many of them involved in the function of the central nervous system.

But the elderly may not be getting an adequate supply, since many can't afford the foods (such as meats and seafoods) that are high in this nutrient. Dr. Hullin says there's a "strong case" for more work in this area and possibly for "zinc supplementation to the population at risk."

those nutrients over the years could have the same devastating effect. The Texas researchers, Elizabeth Root, Ph.D., and John Longenecker, Ph.D., recommended getting adequate amounts of B_6, copper and other nutrients into the diet as soon as possible for the sake of prevention. (Liver is a fine source of both.)

Liver, for example, is high in "antisenility" nutrients.

"If you catch these changes early, then you might prevent some of the neurological damage from occurring," Dr. Root says. "But it's not just B_6 and copper. People who have a poor diet in general are the most likely to get in trouble. We're starting some more experiments on the possible effects of deficiencies in magnesium and folate, two nutrients that also come up low in most diet surveys."

Experiments with rats are one thing, but what about studies of people like you and me? What about people who feel fairly fit mentally but who want to be even sharper in the years ahead? What about people who want to learn how to use a home computer or write a book when they retire—or just keep their bridge game sharp? Can nutrition give them the extra edge they want?

Can nutrition give your brain an edge?

Keeping a Keen Mind

Actually, there's recent evidence that physically healthy people over age 60 can be measurably keener of mind than their peers if they maintain sufficient dietary levels of vitamins B_{12} and C, folate and riboflavin (B_2). Even mild, virtually unnoticeable deficiencies of those nutrients can mean less-than-optimum brain function.

For maximum brain power, avoid deficiencies of vitamins B_{12} and C, folate and riboflavin.

At the University of New Mexico, senility experts Jean M. Goodwin, M.D., and her husband, James S. Goodwin, M.D., and others placed advertisements in newspapers and on TV and radio in the Albuquerque area asking for volunteers for an experiment. Each volunteer had to be at least 60 years old, free of all serious diseases and not on medication. After a screening process, the Goodwins chose 260 men and women between the ages of 60 and 94 from various social and income levels.

All the volunteers gave a sample of their blood and filled out a three-day food diary, stating exactly what they had eaten during that period. Taken together, the blood test and diet survey showed the researchers almost exactly what each person's levels of most vitamins and minerals were.

After this process, the volunteers underwent two mental performance tests. In the first one, a researcher read a one-paragraph story to each person and asked him to repeat it as quickly and accurately as possible. A half hour later, the volunteers had to recite the paragraph from memory, with no cues. The second test measured each person's ability to solve nonverbal problems and to think abstractly.

The people with the lowest nutrient levels had the lowest mental test scores.

The researchers fed all the test scores and nutritional profiles into a computer and waited to see if good nutrition would correlate with quicker thinking. It turned out that the volunteers with the lowest B_{12} and C levels scored worst on the memory test. Those with the lowest levels of B_{12}, C, folate and riboflavin did worst on the problem-solving test (*Journal of the American Medical Association*).

"We showed that in a population of healthy older people, those people who had a deficient intake and low blood levels of certain vitamins scored significantly worse on the tests," says Dr. Jean Goodwin, who is now at Milwaukee City County Medical Complex in Milwaukee, Wisconsin. "Our recommendation is that everyone maintain an adequate intake of those nutrients."

Vitamins Separate the Sharp and the Not-So-Sharp

"Giving older people extra vitamins sounds to us like a sensible course," Dr. James Goodwin adds. "Studies in nursing homes have shown that when you put half the residents on a multivitamin and the other half on a placebo [dummy pill], the staff will eventually be able to tell, with great accuracy, which half was supplemented and which wasn't. The group on the vitamins is always 'doing better.' "

Scientists say that, in nursing homes, multivitamins may make the difference.

One of the nursing home studies referred to above took place at a long-term-care hospital in Leeds, England. It showed that a supplement of vitamin C could, in many cases, help even people who are weak and listless to actually improve mentally and physically.

The trial involved 115 men and women, ages 59 to 97, half of whom received a plain soft drink every day and the other half a soft drink with 1,000 milligrams of vitamin C added to it. The experiment lasted 28 days, and the medical staff, not knowing which group was which, observed the patients to see whose appetite, interest in the life around them and general demeanor changed for better or worse.

It turned out that in less than a month, there was greater improvement in the supplemented group. On the average, they gained more weight and became more active than usual. Some of the patients who had seemed beyond help surprised the staff with their improvements (*Lancet*).

Vitamin C seemed to improve the well-being of nursing-home residents.

Confusion Cleared Up

Thiamine (B$_1$) may also keep the brain thinking straighter and younger. An orthopedic surgeon in England thinks that thiamine deficiency can cause confusion, and that confusion can lead to stumbles and broken bones.

The surgeon, M. W. J. Older, M.D., had noticed that people who came to him for hip and thighbone surgery all experienced a dip in their thiamine levels as a result of the stress of the operation. He also noticed that until the thiamine shortage passed, the patients suffered a bout of confusion.

A surgeon's opinion: Thiamine deficiency can cause mental confusion.

Digging a little deeper, Dr. Older found that patients who came in for *elective* hip surgery—planned in advance, that is—weren't thiamine deficient before the operation, and their postsurgical thiamine deficiency didn't last as long. But the patients with *emergency* fractures, he discovered, were deficient before, during and after their operations. That raised the possibility that preoperative thiamine-related confusion may even have helped cause the emergencies.

"Mental confusion in the elderly awaits further study," Dr. Older notes, "but our data support the concept that thiamine deficiency may be a contributory factor to postoperative confusion. We suggest that the causation of the fracture itself may be attributable to thiamine deficiency, with confusion precipitating the fall" (*Age and Aging*).

A link between thiamine deficiency and bone fractures.

Can Vitamin C Boost the Immunity of the Elderly?

Your body generally puts up a good fight against incoming germs—when it can. But sometimes, keeping up your immunity isn't so easy, especially when you're old.

Now help may be on the way in the form of vitamin C, according to researchers in Belgium. The doctors there found that a 500-milligram daily injection of the vitamin significantly bolstered the immune system in a group of people over 70. The group receiving the placebo shot, they report, had no improvement.

In a similar experiment, the researchers tested a 500-milligram *oral* dose of vitamin C and found that it worked nearly as well as the injected form. The researchers conclude that vitamin C should be considered as a possibly "successful, nontoxic and inexpensive" means of improving the immunity of the elderly (*Gerontology*).

Heading Off Alzheimer's Disease

Good nutrition may even help people suffering from Alzheimer's disease. This most-feared form of senility strikes in middle age and gradually destroys its victims mentally and physically. Alzheimer's is regarded as unexplainable and untreatable, but there is hope.

"Let's say that someone has a mild case of Alzheimer's," geriatric specialist Charles H. Weingarten, M.D., of McLean Hospital in Massachusetts, says. "They may fall into poor dietary habits that make the situation worse. You may not be able to reverse the disease. But good nutrition might enable that person to function better. It might make a significant difference in the amount of care a person requires—perhaps even allowing someone to stay at home rather than being institutionalized," says Dr. Weingarten.

Can better nutrition help people with Alzheimer's disease?

Be Alert to Signs of Pseudosenility

Nutrition aside, people who want to avoid mental decline in themselves or their relatives would be wise to learn that certain conditions can masquerade as senility but aren't senility at all. In the past, many people have been diagnosed as demented and wrongfully sent to institutions because their families and physicians didn't know the real cause of their strange behavior.

The side effects of certain prescription drugs, for example, can imitate senility. In one case, a 66-year-old man became disoriented and obsessed with events that had happened 20 years before, and he lost most of his short-term memory. He recovered after being taken off propranolol, a drug that stops angina pain in heart patients (*Journal of the American Medical Association*).

Warning: Certain conditions (including medication side effects) can pass as senility—but aren't senility at all.

"The high frequency of adverse drug reactions causing central nervous system symptoms in the elderly is well documented," Dr. Weingarten says. He stresses the importance of "scrutinizing all medications to search for reversible factors in psychiatric illness requiring hospital care." He also feels that undetected physical illnesses can look like mental illness in older people (*Journal of the American Geriatrics Society*).

Is it dementia or just depression?

Depression, which is treatable, may also disguise itself as senile dementia. Both illnesses, says one authority on psychiatry and aging, are marked by poor concentration, loss of interest, disorientation, self-neglect, weight loss and slow, shuffling gait. "Dementia is sometimes more apparent than real," he says (*Medical Journal of Australia*).

One lesson is clear: If any elderly relative or friend of yours is diagnosed as having irreversible senile dementia, don't accept the doctor's verdict automatically. Ask the doctor to make sure there are no hidden illnesses, no vitamin deficiencies, no side effects of drugs and no milder, more treatable mental illnesses to blame. Get a second opinion, if necessary. And remember that senility in late life is the *exception*, not the rule.

A Nutritional Formula for Healthy Teeth and Gums

Three out of four people over age 35 have periodontal (gum) disease to some extent, the American Dental Association says, and almost 40 percent of all 60-year-olds have lost several teeth because of it. Tooth decay is what ruins children's teeth, but for adults the enemy is gum disease.

The disease starts when a coating of plaque forms on the teeth. Plaque is a sticky film of food and bacteria that accumulates between teeth, along the gum line and behind poorly fitted dentures. If you don't carefully remove all of the plaque every day, the overlooked bacteria will attack your gums. The gums may start to bleed and pull away from your teeth, and when they do, you're in trouble: The infection can strike at the tooth sockets (called the alveolar bone), and the teeth may eventually loosen and fall out.

How gum disease begins.

The scary part of periodontal disease is that, like glaucoma, it can sneak up on you. One doctor says, "You don't know you have it until your teeth get loose." Actually, there are warning signs. Bad breath is one, and so are bleeding gums. But the bleeding may stop, and there may not be any pain, even when the disease is silently progressing. Antibiotics are sometimes used to halt infection, and surgery might be needed to repair the damage.

Gum disease is sneaky, with few warning signs.

Unfortunately, the treatment is painful, expensive and time-consuming. The process of stripping away the infected gums can take six to eight months and cost hundreds—even thousands—of dollars. But that's less than half of it. Only skin grafts can replace the lost gums, and if any teeth come out, the price of fancy gold and porcelain bridgework can be astronomical.

Indeed, nature has been unfair to the gums. Not only are they continuously bathed in an infectious mixture of bacteria and food particles but they also may be the last to get their share of indispensable vitamins and minerals. Even when the rest of the body has enough vitamin C and folate, the gums may still be deficient, and, when the blood needs more calcium, it robs the tooth sockets first. As a result, the gums need extra amounts of those three nutrients.

Holding the Line with Vitamin C

There is some evidence that vitamin C protects gums from infection, but no one knows how exactly. Some researchers think that vitamin C makes white blood cells tougher and faster and better at killing bacteria. Others say that vitamin C promotes the formation of healthy new gum tissue. And still others think that it latches onto iron molecules, thus depriving bacteria of one of its essential foods.

A possible protector of the gums: vitamin C.

One dentist who uses vitamin C in his practice is Robert C. Miner, D.M.D., of Hancock, New Hampshire.

One dentist's Rx for periodontal disease: vitamin C and calcium.

"If I see someone with periodontal disease, I recommend vitamin C, along with calcium," Dr. Miner says. "As far as results go, it's hard to document the effects. But I know that if people with trench mouth [a gum disease caused by poor nutrition and stress] start taking a gram of vitamin C a day and take a short course of antibiotics, I know that the condition will improve."

Dr. Miner inherited a good deal of his expertise from his father, who was also a dentist. "He was dean of the Harvard School of Dentistry between 1919 and 1944," Dr. Miner says, "and he was a pioneer in the use of nutrition in dentistry. At the time, he was a maverick, but today the things he suggested have become common practice. I grew up with those ideas, and I've tried to carry them further.

"My feeling is that if the body has adequate nutrition, it is more likely to resist disease. In people who are well-nourished, you don't see the kind of breakdown that you see in people who are undernourished. And I should add that 80 to 85 percent of the people who wear dentures are undernourished, because they avoid most of the foods they have trouble chewing."

Saving Your Gums

Experimental data suggest the importance of vitamin C in gum disease. Researcher Millicent Goldschmidt, Ph.D., for instance, of the University of Texas Health Science Center at Houston, has mixed vitamin C in liquid and given it to monkeys. The vitamin reduced to very low levels the population of one of the disease-promoting types of bacteria in the monkeys' mouths. The bacteria need iron to survive, and the vitamin C may somehow keep it away from them.

In monkeys, vitamin C seemed to help kill off disease-promoting bacteria in the mouth.

Similar research has been going on in Seattle and in Europe. In Seattle, Olav Alvares, D.D.S., Ph.D., and a team of researchers put a group of monkeys on a vitamin C-deficient diet for 25 weeks and discovered that it made their gums easy prey to inflammation. The "pockets"—that is, undesirable pouches between teeth and gum where bacteria like to hide and flourish—were larger than normal in the vitamin C-deficient animals. A diet low in vitamin C apparently elevates the risk of gum disease, they conclude (*Journal of Periodontal Research*).

In Yugoslavia, experiments have shown that vitamin C might be able to reverse the kind of gum breakdown seen in periodontal disease. Researchers there looked at samples of cells taken from the gums of 21 volunteers whose diets contained very little vitamin C. Under an electron microscope, the researchers saw the biological equivalent of a tumbled-down brick

Can vitamin C actually rebuild deteriorated gums?

wall. Collagen and other structural components, which are the bricks and mortar of healthy tissue, were literally broken and disheveled.

But after the volunteers were given 70 milligrams of vitamin C daily for six weeks, the cells pulled them-

---

Eight Tips for Tougher Teeth

Getting enough of the right nutrients is one way to help head off dental problems. Here are eight others, culled from the best advice of leading experts in the field.

1. Brush your teeth, but don't obliterate them. Doctors discovered why one man's teeth were almost hanging by threads when they asked him to demonstrate how he brushed: He was scrubbing hard enough to bend his toothbrush's handle. "I call it the dental-chainsaw massacre," says Michael Lerner, D.M.D., who sees signs of "dental abrasion" in about one-third of his new patients. The problem arises with a too-firm brush being used in a too-firm horizontal, back-and-forth fashion. It can wear off not just a tooth's protective enamel but also skin along the gumline, exposing the unprotected root of a tooth. So brush regularly (at least daily), but brush gently, preferably in a circular motion.

2. Don't forget flossing. It may be a bit awkward at first, but flossing is the best way to remove plaque and stubborn food parti-cles from between teeth and away from sensitive gum lines. Flossing is also a good way of "massaging and stimulating the gums," says Vincent Cali, D.D.S. Dr. Cali recommends flossing *before* brushing (so that brushing can sweep away the plaque and food particles that flossing has loosened), and he says not to be alarmed by the sight of a little blood. It's normal for the first week or two after starting to floss, and it's a sign that you're doing a good job.

3. Treat your teeth and gums to the "exercise" of heavy-duty chewing. Just as flossing can stimulate and strengthen the gums, so can chomping on fresh vegetables, fruits and whole grain breads. These foods also encourage healthy saliva flow. And there's even evidence that vigorous chewing, especially in children, can help teeth come in straight by increasing growth of the jawbone.

4. Eat sweets (if you must) with meals rather than between them. Sweets subject your teeth to a decay-causing process

selves together and began to look organized and vigorous. The changes "correspond to a very early phase in tissue regeneration," say the researchers. They note that vitamin C is necessary for the formation of collagen, which is a protein, and that collagen is a critical

Too little vitamin C can make periodontal disease worse.

that lasts about 20 minutes; at that point, enough saliva has been mustered to shut the process down. But if you restrict sweets to mealtimes, you minimize the damage because saliva flow during a meal is at its peak. (You also keep the number of decay-causing episodes to a minimum of three a day.) The worst time to eat sweets, say experts, is before bed, when saliva production is almost at a standstill.

5. Don't smoke. In a study of women over the age of 50, scientists found that a far greater number of smokers than nonsmokers wore dentures. "The study confirms the association between [tooth loss] and cigarette smoking," says a summary of the findings. Smoking's ability to interfere with the body's uptake of calcium may be the reason, researchers say.

6. Use mouthwash. Bacteria cause tooth decay, and those bacteria can thrive on the tissues of the mouth as well as on the teeth. "I recommend using a mixture of hydrogen peroxide and water—a 3 percent solution of hydrogen peroxide with an equal amount of water," says Dr. Cali. "Swish it around in your mouth for 30 seconds or so. Two or three mouthfuls should do the trick." Do *not* swallow, however.

7. Brush your tongue. "Dentists often refer to the upper palate as the roof of the mouth," Dr. Cali says, "but we seldom think of the tongue as the floor." That's what it is, though, and it can attract a lot of dirt in the form of bacteria. For that reason, Dr. Cali recommends giving the tongue a light brushing.

Brushing your tongue can go a long way toward tidying the breath, too.

8. Make regular visits to your dentist and hygienist. Every six months is what's recommended; it gives the hygienist a chance to clean the plaque you may have missed. But are you afraid the dentist will find a target for the drill? Well, if you've been heeding the above advice, you should have nothing to worry about, right?

building block for the gums and a lot of other tissues. Vitamin C deficiency alone won't cause periodontal disease, the researchers say, but it can make it worse (*International Journal of Vitamin and Nutritional Research*).

Calcium and Folate, Hard at Work

Calcium is the other key ingredient in the prevention or arrest of periodontal disease. A growing number of researchers say that calcium deficiency can weaken the alveolar bone, making it more vulnerable to infection and ruining its ability to grip and anchor the teeth.

Another nutrient that is crucial to dental health: calcium.

"Calcium has nothing to do with the teeth, actually," says Anthony Albanese, Ph.D., past director of research at the Burke Rehabilitation Center in White Plains, New York. "It has to do with the alveolar bone, which surrounds the tooth. This is the most active bone in the body; it turns over its calcium frequently, picking up calcium from the blood and giving it back."

Women should be especially conscious of their calcium intake. Like the rest of the bones in a woman's body, the alveolar bone tends to become more fragile and calcium deficient after menopause. "We find that women's teeth become loose after they've had two or three pregnancies," Dr. Albanese says. "That's because the unborn child needs 400 milligrams of calcium a day, and its needs take precedence over its mother's. Beyond that, women frequently go on diets, which limit their calcium intake, and when they reach menopause, they lose even more." He recommends extra calcium along with a vitamin D supplement to improve calcium utilization.

Why women may need extra calcium for better teeth.

"We start our women patients on calcium as early as we can," agrees John M. Cusano, D.D.S., a nutrition-oriented dentist in West Hempstead, New York. "We tell them that even the American Medical

Association recommends a gram of calcium a day for postmenopausal women."

Dr. Cusano is something of a model among nutrition-minded dentists. "We started using nutrition in our practice about seven years ago, and we've had excellent results," he says. "We explain to our new patients what it means to eat a balanced diet. When they first come in, more than half of them are eating an inadequate amount of vegetables. We try to get them to eat more vegetables, and we try to get the big coffee drinkers and smokers to cut down.

"Then we put them on a supplement program. At first, we 'shotgun it' by giving them a small multivitamin supplement. After the body acclimates itself to the vitamins, we start them on 1,500 milligrams of vitamin C per day, or 500 milligrams with each meal. Then, if they have periodontal disease, we start them on calcium supplements. After four to five weeks, we have them on the full program, which includes all the B vitamins, vitamin C, vitamin E and calcium.

"Some of the patients ask me why they need more than the minimum daily requirement of the vitamins. I tell them that the minimum daily requirement is fine if they're looking for minimum daily health. But we're looking for maximum daily health. A lot of it depends on whether we can motivate the patients. We have a microscope here, and we let them look at the bacteria that are damaging their teeth. When they see them, they believe it," Dr. Cusano says.

The B vitamin folate also seems to play an important role in stopping the advance of periodontal disease. According to one theory, the gums themselves can be deficient in folate even when blood tests show that the rest of the body has enough. And a lack of folate apparently weakens the gums' ability to fend off bacteria.

Folate: an important nutrient for healthy gums.

Under experimental conditions, folate deficiency has been corrected with a mouthwash that contains folate. At the New Jersey Dental School in Newark, researchers asked a group of 15 volunteers with in-

A mouthwash containing folate may aid inflamed gums.

flamed gums to gargle twice a day—after breakfast and right before bed—with some folate-rich water. After 60 days of gargling, the researchers examined the group's gums.

The gums soaked up folate like a sponge, and the volunteers' gums were much less inflamed. They were also less inflamed than the gums of a 15-member control group that had been asked to gargle with plain water for 60 days (*Journal of Oral Medicine*).

The Telltale Signs of Gum Disease

Healthy teeth depend on healthy gums. And yet it's been estimated that more than half of all adults over the age of 18 do not have healthy gums. They have periodontal (gum) disease to some degree. Even children as young as five can have beginning stages.

What causes gum disease?

The same demon that causes tooth decay: dental plaque, that sticky film of food particles and bacteria that is the bugaboo of mouths everywhere. The bacteria in plaque produce by-products that can irritate the gums and, in time, seriously damage the structures that hold teeth in place. Gum disease is the number one reason teeth fall out. (As a result, one out of five adults wears dentures.)

Fortunately, many of the same procedures for protecting your teeth can help protect your gums (regular brushing and flossing, eating a balanced diet and avoiding smoking and chewing tobacco), but to play it safe, be alert for the signs of gum disease listed below. Dentists warn that symptoms can progress to serious levels before any pain is experienced, so keep on the watch for all or any of the following, and see a dentist immediately if you think you're developing a problem.

Look for the following:

• Gums that bleed when you brush.

• Gums that are red, swollen or tender.

• Gums that have pulled away from the teeth.

• Pus between the teeth and gums when gums are pressed.

• Permanent teeth that are loose or separating.

• Any change in the way your teeth fit together when you bite.

• Any change in the fit of partial dentures.

• Inescapably bad breath.

Chapter 52

Nutrients: Experimental Treatment for Impaired Vision

Research supports the theory that cataracts can be caused by an excess of free radicals in the lens of the eye. Free radicals are highly reactive chemicals that are generated by a normal chemical process in the body called oxidation. Left unchecked, free radicals can initiate reactions that result in unwanted tissue changes. Because light also promotes oxidation, the transparent tissues of the eye are particularly susceptible to free-radical damage.

Shambhu D. Varma, Ph.D., professor and director of research in the Department of Ophthalmology at the University of Maryland Medical School, is investigating the role of free radicals in cataract formation and cataract prevention by antioxidant nutrients. In test-tube experiments, Dr. Varma maintained rat lenses in a fluid that generates free radicals when exposed to light. He found that the lenses lost their transparency. "Oxidation is one of the factors contributing to the pathogenesis of cataracts," says Dr. Varma, "although there might be other causes, too."

Because vitamin C is an antioxidant, Dr. Varma and his colleagues wanted to see if it would have a beneficial effect. Again, rat lenses were maintained in a special mixture that caused free-radical damage. But lenses maintained in the same mixture fortified with vitamin C were significantly protected from damage by free radicals. According to the researchers, that may explain why there is such a high level of vitamin C in the eye (*Proceedings of the National Academy of Sciences*). In a similar study, Dr. Varma and his co-

Another possible cause of cataracts: oxidation.

Vitamins C and E protected animal lenses against oxidation.

workers found that vitamin E also offered protection against cataracts (*Photochemistry and Photobiology*).

Good nutrition is essential to healthy, clear lenses.

"I did one study with a strain of mice that have a tendency to develop cataracts. I found they don't develop them as much as expected if they're given vitamin E," Dr. Varma says. "A good diet is established to be necessary for the maintenance of a healthy, transparent, pliable lens. If your diet is deficient in antioxidant vitamins E and C, chances of developing cataracts might be accelerated," he says.

Preventing Retina Damage

The retina, the membrane at the back of the eye that receives the image formed by the lens, may also be susceptible to free-radical damage. After seven years of ongoing study, Ely J. Crary, M.D., of Austell, Georgia, says he has found a way to retard the progression of diabetic retinopathy, a disease of the retina that frequently leads to blindness. He uses a combination of the antioxidants selenium and vitamins E, C and A.

Vitamin C and other antioxidants prevented further loss of vision.

He theorizes that in diabetics, decreased metabolism in the cells of the eye's blood vessels is caused by a buildup of free radicals, or oxidants. This weakens the capillary cell walls, leading to blood leakage. It's this vascular leakage that's responsible for the early loss of sight. Antioxidants remove the oxidants, he says, preventing further damage.

Dr. Crary: Nutrients may curb diabetic retinopathy and senile macular degeneration.

"I've worked with close to 1,000 patients with diabetic retinopathy and senile macular degeneration," Dr. Crary says, "and have seen the diseases retarded in about 70 percent of the cases. This program of nutritional supplementation has shown no adverse effects, either. If someone has early diabetic retinopathy or senile macular degeneration, they should at least consider this program in addition to regular therapy—under a doctor's care, of course. The earlier the treatment is started, the better the response. I'm still amazed at the results we get from this method."

Take E and See?

Many research studies have tied vitamin E to the health of the retina. In a study at Cornell University, dogs fed diets deficient in vitamin E were found to develop damaged retinas. Damage could be detected after only three months of the E-deficient diet. "Night blindness and eventual severe day visual impairment" followed, say the researchers (*American Journal of Veterinary Research*).

Vitamin E deficiency is linked to damaged retinas.

Retrolental fibroplasia (RLF) is a disease of the retina that occurs in premature infants and causes blindness. In the 1950s, it was discovered that oxygen therapy in incubators was the cause, and careful monitoring of oxygen levels caused a decline in the incidence of severe RLF. There was resurgence of the disease, however, as more very small premature infants were able to survive.

More recently, researchers from the Department of Newborn Medicine at the Royal Alexandra Hospital in Edmonton, Alberta, found that vitamin E can prevent RLF in infants given oxygen. In the study, 17 percent of the tiny infants who received no vitamin E developed RLF, while none of the infants given oral vitamin E within 12 hours of birth developed RLF. Say the researchers, "It is recommended that vitamin E be given within 12 hours of birth to all [low-birth-weight] infants . . . who require supplemental oxygen" (*Ophthalmology*).

Researchers use vitamin E to treat a rare visual disorder in premature infants.

Chapter 53

A Pioneering Approach to Better Vision

Can you solve eye troubles with changes in lifestyle?

Most patients would probably think it strange for an eye doctor to ask them how often they exercise, the last time they had a chocolate bar or whether they enjoy their job. After all, what could any of these things possibly have to do with cataracts, glaucoma or even a simple case of dry, itchy eyes?

But for Joseph M. Ortiz, M.D., a suburban Philadelphia ophthalmologist, getting answers to questions about diet, exercise, stress and allergies is an important part of the detective work involved in tracking down the cause of an eye problem, or, better yet, stopping one before it starts.

That is because Dr. Ortiz believes that the most important requirement for healthy eyes is a healthy body. "You can never forget that your eyes are connected to the rest of your body," he says. "The two are inseparable."

He's seen the connection again and again—an uncontrollable twitch, traced to the stress of a new job and aggravated by too much coffee; a bad case of dry eyes, caused by an extremely low-fat diet; computer-induced eyestrain, relieved by a new prescription for reading glasses and a no-glare screen. And it goes beyond that.

Your eyes can be hurt by whole-body diseases like high blood pressure, heart disease and diabetes. In fact, looking into the eyes is a good way to see signs of those illnesses. They are the only place in the body where blood vessels can be viewed directly. Clogged, bleeding or scarred vessels in the back part of the eye, called the retina, mean the same problems are occurring elsewhere in the body, Dr. Ortiz says. "They say the eye is the mirror of the soul. Well, it's also a window to look in on the rest of your body." That's why it's no surprise to him that some of his patients who start out treating an eye problem end up with lower blood pressure or extra energy—and a new faith in whole-body healing.

A Whole Body Approach to Better Vision

Dr. Ortiz is one of a still-rare breed of preventive ophthalmologists. His training is traditional, with a medical degree from New York Medical College and a residency and research work at Yale and the University of Pennsylvania. He helps supervise a resident-staffed eye clinic at the Hospital of the University of Pennsylvania and admits many of his surgical patients to Wills Eye Hospital of Scheie Eye Institute in Philadelphia.

The making of a preventive ophthalmologist.

But his conversion to preventive medicine is wholehearted. After a bout with hepatitis during his freshman year in medical school left him wondering if he would survive to grow old, he gradually changed his diet to emphasize whole grains, vegetables, fruits and some dairy products. Along the way, he monitored the effects of dietary changes with blood tests. "Those tests really helped me see how cutting out red meat, sugar, coffee, white flour and alcohol improved my blood cholesterol and overall health," he says. And no one can accuse him of not preaching what he practices. He suggests the same menu for his patients.

Every one of his patients, whether they have an eye problem or not, is encouraged to change his or her diet toward whole grains and fresh produce, to

**The doctor's orders:
whole grains, fresh pro-
duce, exercise, rest, nu-
trients and no smoking.**

stop smoking and to get plenty of exercise and rest. He recommends vitamin supplements to patients with special problems and to older patients.

"If I see previous eye damage—scar tissue or injured blood vessels in the retina—I'll recommend vitamin E and zinc to help maintain the health of the blood vessels and the cells of the retina," he says. "If someone is old, has dentures, or doesn't eat much meat, I'll suggest B vitamins, since they may not be getting enough. I think most people get enough vitamin A in their diet, so I reserve that for people with absorption or storage problems—colitis, cirrhosis or a history of alcoholism."

**Extra vitamins and min-
erals prepare patients
for eye surgery.**

His surgical patients are "prepped" with 2,000 milligrams of vitamin C, 50 milligrams of zinc and 200 international units of vitamin E daily for a week before their operation, and they stay on those supplements until they heal. "This reduces inflammation after surgery and cuts up to two weeks off their period of recuperation," Dr. Ortiz claims.

For night blindness, the inability of our eyes to adapt to the dark, Dr. Ortiz prescribes vitamin A and zinc. Vitamin A is essential for the health of the cells lining the retina, which are called rods and cones. And in low-light situations, the chemical impulses of those cells, which send visual images to our brains, require vitamin A to form a light-sensitive pigment known as rhodopsin, or visual purple. Without the pigment, we become virtually blind after dark.

**Why vitamins A and E
and zinc are important
to healthy eyes.**

Zinc, Dr. Ortiz says, enhances the eye's ability to use vitamin A. It is important in the conversion of vitamin A to its active form, retinaldehyde. Vitamin E also has an important effect on how much vitamin A is available for use in the eye and has been found to be of help as a cataract fighter, Dr. Ortiz claims.

Slowing or Reversing Cataracts

Cataracts, the clouding of the eyes' lenses, are an inevitable feature of aging, Dr. Ortiz admits. "Anyone who lives long enough is going to get them." But his own work with some of his patients and laboratory studies with animals have shown that cataract formation in its early stages may be significantly slowed and, in some cases, even reversed.

Most researchers believe that a type of cataract found in the aging eye (radiation cataracts) is caused by years of exposure to the sun. "Sunlight absorbed by the lens reacts with an amino acid called tryptophan, breaking it up into particles called free radicals," Dr. Ortiz explains. These destructive, unpaired electrons bind with proteins in the lens, forming the dense pigment that blocks sunlight from the eye and gives it a yellow-brown color.

But laboratory studies have shown that vitamins E and C and the trace mineral selenium block free radicals' destructiveness. Instead of attacking the proteins, free radicals combine with these nutrients and are neutralized.

Vitamins that neutralize the hazards of sunlight.

In patients at an age where cataracts are likely to occur (starting at around 55), Dr. Ortiz suggests vitamin C and vitamin E. If they have high blood pressure, he recommends that instead of vitamin E they get more selenium—preferably in the form of two or three bulbs of garlic each week. (Selenium supplements should not be taken in amounts of more than 100 micrograms daily without the guidance of your physician.)

The doctor's prescription for people likely to get cataracts includes vitamins E and C and selenium.

In patients already showing signs of cataracts, Dr. Ortiz may prescribe vitamin C, vitamin E, selenium if needed and riboflavin (vitamin B_2). Vitamin E may enhance glutathione, a substance that apparently protects the proteins in the eyes' lenses from free-radical damage.

A Sight-Saving Regimen

One of Dr. Ortiz's cataract patients is spry, 80-year-old Dr. Ibraham Marker. This man lost the use of one eye several years earlier when blood vessels in his retina burst. When he realized cataracts were destroying his remaining vision, he was determined to find a doctor who would help him without requiring surgery. After three months of Dr. Ortiz's eye regimen, Dr. Marker's eyesight had improved dramatically. With glasses, visual acuity in his "good" eye had improved from 20/100 to 20/60. Even his retina-damaged eye showed an improvement—from 20/400 to 20/200.

A remarkable improvement in vision.

"This man is a remarkable example of how nutritional supplements can work to improve the health of the retina," Dr. Ortiz says. "You have to use total body care to help your eyes. This man is in good health. He eats carefully, is very active and does a lot of walking. I think the reason supplements helped him so much is that he takes such good care of himself. Eventually he may need cataract surgery, but at this time both he and I are satisfied with his improved vision."

Special Advice for Diabetics

Dr. Ortiz's diabetic patients, because they are especially prone to cataracts and retinal damage, receive additional advice and supplements.

A recommendation for diabetic patients: better diet and chromium.

"I tell them to bring their blood glucose level down to 140, not by increasing their medication but by changing their diet. I also recommend daily chromium. Chromium makes insulin work more efficiently in the body and so helps lower blood sugar levels." A too-high blood sugar level can damage blood vessels in the retina, creating a condition called diabetic retinopathy, which eventually leads to blindness.

To further protect the eyes' blood source, Dr. Ortiz recommends a supplement of eicosapentanoic acid (EPA, a substance in fish oil that helps lower blood cholesterol and triglyceride levels and prevents clumping of blood platelets). This helps to lessen the fatty buildup, clotting and hemorrhaging that can destroy the retina, Dr. Ortiz claims.

In some cases, he also recommends bioflavonoids, nutrients that are found in the white peel of citrus fruits. Bioflavonoids keep capillary walls strong, helping to prevent leakage from blood vessels. Some bioflavonoids may also work to inhibit an enzyme, aldose reductase, that promotes some kinds of cataracts.

Sidney Cohen, 69, of Philadelphia, a diabetic for 30 years, came to Dr. Ortiz in 1983. "My vision was failing fast," he says. "I'd been to a number of eye clinics, and they all said the same thing. They could control my insulin and perform laser surgery to cauterize the leaking blood vessels in my eyes. They never said I could get better."

"My vision was failing fast."

With Dr. Ortiz's help, Cohen started on nutritional therapy for the first time in his life. From his regular diabetic diet, he eliminated dried fruits, grapes, concentrated fruit juices, white flour and red meat. He added whole grains, fish, vegetables and low-fat dairy foods. In addition to chromium, EPA and two grams of bioflavonoids, he took vitamin C, vitamin E, selenium, zinc and vitamin A.

"And you know what? My vision has improved by at least 40 percent. I can see better in the day and at night. My blood cholesterol is lower, I have much more energy, and I sleep better at night."

Forty percent better eyesight, day or night.

Vitamin C and Glaucoma

Glaucoma, a dangerous buildup of fluid in the eye, which can permanently damage the retina, is another condition that can respond to nutritional therapy, though it usually first requires traditional medical treatment.

"I never start off using vitamins to treat glaucoma," Dr. Ortiz says. "The main thing is to get the pressure down as quickly as possible, using eyedrops sometimes supplemented by laser surgery to 'drill' pinpoint holes in the eye through which the fluid can drain."

The first step in treating glaucoma is to reduce the pressure.

Then, if the pressure has to be brought down a little further, Dr. Ortiz will suggest vitamin C. This treatment is effective only in large doses. "The vitamin C acts as an osmotic agent," he explains. "It draws fluid away from the eye."

Using vitamin C is Mrs. Catherine Laws, an 82-year-old widow from Media, Pennsylvania, who proudly says she can see well enough to drive, even though she only putters around town.

"I still use my eyedrops, but I'm also taking vitamin C every day now," she says. "I take it in divided doses, four or five times a day, as crystals mixed with water."

Vitamin C helps, too.

The eyedrops lowered the pressure in her eyes by about 10 millimeters of mercury. Dr. Ortiz says that vitamin C lowered them an additional two to four points, putting her eye pressure within normal limits.

"I feel the vitamin C helped me a great deal," Mrs. Laws says. "I've had this condition about 20 years, and now it's getting a little better. Something has to be responsible for that, and I think it's the vitamin C."

Retraining the Brain to See Better

Echoing thoughts similar to those of Mrs. Laws is another of Dr. Ortiz's patients, Myrna Miller, who saw her eyesight improve for the first time in her life when she began going without her glasses several hours each day.

"In the beginning, I could hardly see at all, but after three or four months, I noticed my vision had become much clearer and that my glasses were too strong," she says. "By the end of four months, I wasn't wearing my glasses around the house at all." An examination showed her sight had improved from 20/400 to 20/200, without glasses. And that improvement has remained even though she wears her new, weaker glasses most of the time.

In myopia, or nearsightedness, glasses can cause the tiny muscles that focus the eyes' lenses to become very strong, thereby stretching the outer layer of the eyes, Dr. Ortiz explains. Removing the glasses makes the muscles work less, and the eye stretching is decreased. This may stabilize the myopia. It also trains your brain to interpret visual messages even though they're not clearly in focus.

Sometimes, not wearing eyeglasses helps.

"My glasses had gotten thicker and thicker, and I always thought the end result of it would be that I would go blind or something," Mrs. Miller says. "It's really heartening when you can put that in reverse and keep it there."

With patience, vision can improve.

Mrs. Miller had the time and patience to go without her glasses. Not everyone can do that or have the results Mrs. Miller had, but they still can be active participants in their eye care, Dr. Ortiz says.

"The saddest people I see are those I can't do anything for, those who are blind," he says. "You can't turn back time, but you can make the most of the time you have. The main thing people must realize is that they are the masters of their own health."

Chapter 54

Nutritional Therapy: More Positive Evidence

Today, the role of vitamins and minerals in the treatment of disease is being investigated in countless ways. Most of the research is very preliminary, but some of it is promising in unexpected ways. Here's a roundup of some of the less publicized, but intriguing, nutritional therapy news.

Asthma: Can Vitamin C Help?

A way to breathe easier.

Researchers from the John B. Pierce Foundation Laboratory in New Haven, Connecticut, have found that vitamin C may dilate your swollen bronchial tubes.

How? By causing an increase in the production of prostanoids—your body's own bronchial-tube dilating agents. According to James S. Douglas, Ph.D., a pharmacologist involved in the study, a 500-milligram dose of vitamin C increases prostanoids a small but significant amount. These results may also explain why asthma incidence is greater among those with a dietary deficiency of vitamin C, he says.

Bedsores: A Nutritional Prescription

Elderly patients who suffer from bedsores may find relief with nutritional supplementation, say doctors from Our Lady of Mercy Medical Center in New York City. They found that hospitalized older patients became more susceptible to bedsores as their nutritional status deteriorated. To improve this situation, the patients were given at least 2,000 calories per day, including carbohydrates, protein, trace minerals and vitamins. Nutritional supplementation improved the bedsores in 11 of 12 patients, say the doctors. What's more, when the sores healed, the patients were found to have greatly improved nutritional status.

In 11 out of 12 patients, bedsores improved.

Cancer:
Vitamin C Teams Up with Drug

What do you get if you combine vitamin C with the toxic drug acetyl acrolein? You get a new, nontoxic drug that has a "marked ability" to stimulate or restore your own natural immunity. It's called Nafocare, and researcher Robert Veltri, Ph.D., of the National Foundation for Cancer Research in Philadelphia, thinks it may have real potential in the fight against cancer and other diseases where immunity is compromised.

Can vitamin C help a drug fight cancer?

"Most cancer drugs work by destroying the cells' DNA," Dr. Veltri says. "Unfortunately, it kills the DNA in normal cells right along with the cancerous ones."

Nafocare doesn't work directly on individual cells. It enhances the body's immune response, which in turn kills the tumor just like it would any foreign substance in the body.

"Right now, we are about to begin to test the substance on human cancer patients," says Dr. Veltri, "and hope to get FDA approval soon."

Can Vitamin E Prevent Hair Loss in Cancer Chemotherapy?

Hair loss as a result of chemotherapy may be prevented if vitamin E is given in advance of the drug, according to Lee Wood, M.D., of Covina, California. Of the 16 patients he treated with vitamin E, 11 had

Cancer patients lose less hair than usual.

only slight or moderate loss of hair. Of the 5 who did suffer complete hair loss, says Dr. Wood, 3 had taken the vitamin less than 72 hours before the first dose of the drug. In the future, Dr. Wood plans to give the vitamin E five to seven days before chemotherapy is begun (*New England Journal of Medicine*).

Celiac Disease:
The Selenium Connection

British researchers think it's no coincidence that victims of celiac disease (a chronic intestinal disorder caused by intolerance to wheat gluten) have a high incidence of cancer along with a low body level of selenium.

Selenium: a force against free radicals.

Selenium is a component of an enzyme responsible for preventing the buildup of free radicals and lipid peroxides—chemicals that have the potential to damage cell membranes and increase the risk of malignancy. When the researchers compared the selenium levels of 16 celiac patients with 32 healthy volunteers, the celiac patients' were far lower.

There are two possible explanations for this, say the scientists. First, the gluten-free diet may not contain enough selenium. Second, selenium is absorbed primarily in the duodenum, a portion of the small intestine which, in celiac patients, is abnormal (*British Medical Journal*).

Colds:
A Link with Zinc Lozenges?

A group of researchers associated with the University of Texas at Austin may have stumbled upon a remedy that licks cold symptoms. It's zinc gluconate tablets, the same ones available as nutritional supplements. But instead of swallowing them whole, you suck them like lozenges or cough drops.

The researchers discovered this possible use for zinc from a child being treated for acute leukemia who also suffered from frequent colds. One day at the onset of a new cold, she refused to swallow the zinc gluconate tablet that was being given to improve her immunity and dissolved it in her mouth instead. "Within several hours," say the researchers, "her cold disappeared without further treatment."

Did the zinc lozenges make the difference?

The researchers decided it was worth testing the zinc against a placebo (dummy pill) in a group of patients suffering from colds. After seven days, 86 percent of the zinc-treated group had no symptoms compared with only 46 percent of the group taking the placebo.

The doctors speculate that the zinc attacks the cold viruses living in the throat and keeps them from reproducing, so the sooner the germs are zapped, the better. And they suggest the treatment (one lozenge every two hours during the day) be continued until a few hours after the last symptom has gone, since the antiviral effect of zinc may be reversible. Since such a cumulative dose (from 100 to 200 milligrams) of zinc daily is normally considered excessive, the doctors caution that this treatment be used only seven days or less. In that way there's no danger of toxicity, they say, because zinc is "generally regarded as noncumulative and nontoxic when briefly ingested" (*Antimicrobial Agents and Chemotherapy*).

Zinc may attack cold viruses.

Deafness: A Vitamin D Deficiency?

Nutritional help for hearing problems? Possibly. Dr. Gerald B. Brookes, a London ear, nose and throat specialist, has linked one form of deafness with a vitamin D deficiency.

It has to do with the cochlea, the snail-shaped bone inside the ear, considered to be the essential organ of hearing. A lack of vitamin D is thought to cause a demineralization of the tiny bone, which leads to progressive cochlear deafness.

So far, Dr. Brookes says, he has studied 22 patients with the disorder and all of them had low or borderline vitamin D levels. But he's only just begun to evaluate treatment with calciferol, a synthetic vitamin D metabolite. He has found that 4 out of 6 people taking calciferol have had some improvement in their hearing.

A possible cause of some types of deafness: vitamin D deficiency.

Because treatment is generally "harmless and cheap," Dr. Brookes recommends screening for vitamin D deficiency in patients with certain types of progressive deafness (*Journal of the American Medical Association*).

Dialysis Dementia from a Biotin Deficiency?

As if having kidney failure isn't bad enough, people on long-term dialysis often develop an additional burden to cope with. It's called "dialysis dementia," and it leaves its sufferers with dizziness, restless legs, memory loss, even psychosis. Worst of all, the disorder is progressive, leading to total disability.

Until just a few years ago, doctors had no idea what caused the problem nor how to correct it. Now a group of Greek researchers has changed forever that bleak outlook. They discovered that long-term dialysis patients often become deficient in an essential nutrient—biotin. It's easy to see why, say the doctors. "The dietary restriction routinely imposed in such patients decreases the intake of biotin." And the various supplementary vitamins given to them were found to be "completely biotin free."

The doctors decided to try ten milligrams of biotin daily on nine dialysis patients with dialysis dementia. "Within three months," say the researchers, "there was a marked improvement in all patients" in respect to disorientation, loss of memory, restless legs and more. One of the patients, who had been unable to even stand up, improved so much after six months of treatment that he now walks several miles each day, unassisted, and has for the past two years.

Daily doses of biotin relieved symptoms of "dialysis dementia."

Naturally, the doctors urge routine biotin supplementation for all dialysis patients (*Nephron*).

Lupus: A Need for Vitamin A?

Scientists are finally tuning in to the effects of nutrition on the body's immune system—your own natural defense against disease. That's especially true with autoimmune diseases, the ones that cause your body to turn against itself.

At the University of California at Davis, researchers are working with animals susceptible to a disease similar to systemic lupus erythematosus (SLE), an autoimmune disease that often affects young women.

The researchers suspected that a vitamin A deficiency might reduce the production of autoantibodies (the ones that attack your own cells). To test their theory, they fed lab animals a normal diet, until there were clinical signs of the disease. Then they were put on a vitamin A-deficient diet.

Testing the vitamin A theory on animals.

Far from improving their condition, the vitamin A deficiency accelerated it. These results have implications for human patients with SLE, say the researchers, since "vitamin A deficiency is one of the most common nutritional deficiencies throughout the world and occurs even in developed nations. On the basis of these results, a lupus patient who was A deficient might experience significant acceleration of the disease process.

Lupus patients: Ask your doctor about the vitamin A connection.

"Patients with lupus should not try to adjust their intake of vitamin A until further studies have been done or at the suggestion of their doctor" (*Journal of Immunology*).

Wilson's Disease:
Zinc May Replace Penicillamine

For those who have Wilson's disease, a rare hereditary disorder involving abnormal copper metabolism, therapy has always centered around the drug penicillamine. And it worked well to "decopper" the patients and reduce symptoms of copper toxicity—muscle tremors, psychotic behavior and cirrhosis of the liver.

So what's the problem, you say? Drug toxicity. Penicillamine causes severe side effects in about 30 percent of the people who take it. The good news, however, is that now there appears to be a safe, easily tolerated alternative. According to doctors from universities in Michigan, oral zinc therapy worked well to rid the body of excess copper in all five patients they treated. Although more research is needed, the doctors say that "eventually it may be desirable to switch even those patients who tolerate penicillamine to zinc therapy," since the only adverse effect of zinc is some stomach upset in an occasional patient (*Annals of Internal Medicine*).

People with Wilson's disease, however, should *not* switch to zinc without consulting their physician.

Zinc seemed to rid the body of excess copper in Wilson's disease patients.

Chapter 55

How to Take Vitamins and Minerals Safely

T o many, vitamins are as harmless as a kiss on the cheek. They are those tiny tablets or capsules that they take regularly to compensate for what may be lacking in an unbalanced diet.

Things can get a bit out of hand, however. After a report in the morning newspaper that vitamin X may prevent cancer, or a spot on the evening news that a certain mineral may help you live to be 100, some people are tempted to add larger doses to their daily routine.

The problem comes as the dosages start to inch upward. Without realizing it, you could unintentionally be close to a megadose level, which should be taken only under a physician's direction. There's increasing evidence that too much of some nutrients may be harmful. The fat-soluble vitamins that can accumulate in the body, such as vitamins A and D, are particularly suspect.

Caution: Don't be tempted to overdose on vitamins.

Too much vitamin A or D can hurt you.

Heed the Vitamin Safety Zone

If you take supplements, your goal is to stay within the vitamin safety zone, that range beginning at the U.S. Recommended Daily Allowance (USRDA) and ending "at a level that is still safe and well below the toxicity level," says John Hathcock, Ph.D., a vitamin-toxicity expert with the U.S. Food and Drug Administration's (FDA) experimental nutritional section.

It's not easy for a vitamin-consuming public to decide where to draw the line between safe and excessive micrograms, milligrams or international units. "There are no officially established limits for maximum doses. We've spent a lot of time debating and establishing the USRDAs at the low end, but no one's set suggested guidelines for the other end," says Dr. Hathcock.

The best source of vitamins and minerals: food.

The simplest and safest solution is to rely on food for most of your essential nutrients. "Nature has helped us out tremendously by giving our bodies the ability to get almost all the necessary vitamins and minerals we need from logical food consumption," says nutrition researcher Virginia Vivian, Ph.D., of Ohio State University. "Granted, you may need extra amounts of some nutrients, but a multiple vitamin will usually do."

That's easier said than done, however, for some people. Research has shown that many people either don't eat enough or do not eat balanced meals. Then there are people with medical conditions, pregnant women, the elderly and others who may have increased needs for specific nutrients.

Right or wrong, many people take supplements.

Which is why so many people turn to supplements. An FDA survey shows that about 40 percent of the general population take supplements daily, with women taking more than men. Among the elderly, surveys show that between 66 and 72 percent take supplements.

Avoid Megadoses

It's also estimated that 5 to 10 percent of the people who take supplements ingest megadoses, defined by some researchers as ten times the USRDA or more, of certain vitamins and minerals. In light of this, some nutrition experts have stopped trying to tell people that they don't need vitamins and instead have started advising them how to supplement wisely.

If you're wondering whether your personal vitamin program falls within safe bounds, the answer's not easily had. "There are no reference guides or tables you can check to see what levels of vitamins trigger harmful effects," says Paul Saltman, Ph.D., a professor of biology doing research in nutrition at the University of California at San Diego. "That's because the danger levels vary from person to person and depend on factors such as weight, health status, metabolism, diet, nutritional status, the form of the nutrient and how often you take it. The safest approach is to accept the fact that there is no scientific evidence that massive doses have any benefits."

There's no evidence that megadoses work.

Guidelines for Sensible Supplement Use

You may wish to check the following list of the more common vitamins and minerals to see where your dosages fit in. The "maximum" levels are approximations compiled from discussions with experts and surveys of the latest available data. These numbers should be viewed as general guidelines only, intended to help you make sure you're safe. This does *not* necessarily mean that it's appropriate or advisable to increase your intake to these limits. Also keep in mind that all metabolisms are not created equal. Although the most current information may suggest that a vitamin is relatively harmless, some people with unusual metabolic traits may react adversely to even the safest nutrient.

When considering your current total intake, don't neglect to add in the amounts in your multiple, if you take one each day, and the nutrients from food. In other words, if you're taking a vitamin A supplement, don't think that's all the A you're getting. It's in your meals and probably in your multiple.

Calculating your total intake.

Vitamin A

Scientists have a keen, new interest in this fat-soluble vitamin because of its link to cancer prevention. It speeds healing, aids vision and fights infection and skin diseases. It's also highly toxic in large doses because vitamin A accumulates in organ tissues, primarily the liver. Headaches, blurred vision, nausea, hearing loss, itchy eyes, aching bones or skin sores are signs that you may be taking too much. *USRDA: 5,000 international units; MAXIMUM: 25,000 international units.*

Beta-carotene may be safer than vitamin A.

(Beta-carotene, a carotenoid that offers many of the same benefits as vitamin A, appears to be safer than A in large doses. "So far, it looks relatively harmless, and you should consider taking it instead of the riskier vitamin A," says Dr. Saltman. Be aware, however, that large doses of vitamin E can interfere with beta-carotene absorption.)

Thiamine (Vitamin B$_1$) and Riboflavin (Vitamin B$_2$)

There are very few reports of people experiencing adverse effects from either of these two B vitamins, partly because there's little if any evidence that large doses offer health benefits. *USRDA FOR B$_1$: 1.5 milligrams; USRDA FOR B$_2$: 1.7 milligrams; MAXIMUM FOR EACH: 25 milligrams.*

Niacin

A possible way to lower cholesterol.

Studies have shown that this B vitamin may play a role in lowering cholesterol and triglyceride levels. But some people who take large doses in the form of nicotinic acid may experience niacin flush—a burning, itching, tingling sensation usually in the face, neck, arms, and upper chest that may persist for half an hour or longer. Doses large enough to trigger this reaction may also cause reddening of the skin, nausea, headaches, cramps, diarrhea and feelings of faintness. *USRDA: 20 milligrams; MAXIMUM: 50 milligrams.*

Vitamin B$_6$ (Pyridoxine)

Many women went running for this member of the B-complex family after reports that it helps ease premenstrual stress symptoms. "More research is needed to confirm that claim, but we have established that large doses can cause nerve damage," says Dr. Saltman. Numbness of the feet or hands may be a sign to reduce your intake. *USRDA: 2 milligrams; MAXIMUM: 50 milligrams.*

Do not take too much B$_6$.

Vitamin B$_{12}$

Vitamin B$_{12}$ is vital to healthy blood and a normal nervous system, but there's little scientific evidence that massive doses will either harm or help. *USRDA: 6 micrograms; MAXIMUM: 25 micrograms.*

Vitamin B$_{12}$: Large doses don't help.

Pantothenate

There is no known toxicity level, but caution should still be exercised, since "we're just beginning to explore the effects of megadoses of some of these vitamins," says Dr. Saltman. *USRDA: 10 milligrams; MAXIMUM: 50 milligrams.*

Vitamin C (Ascorbic Acid)

Surveys continue to show that ascorbic acid is the most popular vitamin supplement, dominating the nutritional supermarket for the past decade. Claims that it helps fight cancer, boosts immunity against colds and infections, speeds the healing of wounds and aids in combating cardiovascular disease have made it one of the most megadosed vitamins. Although it's water soluble, and excesses are usually excreted, large doses have been known to cause diarrhea and abdominal cramps in some people. Too much vitamin C may also interfere with certain medical tests, such as checking sugar levels in diabetics or looking for blood in stools. *USRDA: 60 milligrams; MAXIMUM: 500 to 1,000 milligrams.*

Excessive doses of C may hurt you.

(The need for ascorbic acid varies from one person to the next. Exposure to illness, tobacco smoke, pollutants, certain drugs, burns, trauma, surgery, alcohol and other stressors may increase the need. So may pregnancy and aging. Some nutritional researchers now regard the USRDA as too low for optimal health.)

Vitamin D

Taking too much vitamin D can be dangerous.

Another fat-soluble vitamin that can accumulate in your body, vitamin D is usually obtained from sunshine. It's a crucial link in the process that helps calcium strengthen bones and is essential for women in their osteoporosis-prone years. People who live in regions where winters are long and exposure to sunlight is infrequent may need to take supplemental vitamin D. Muscle weakness, joint pain, headaches, nausea and vomiting may be signs that you should reduce your dosage. *USRDA: 400 international units; MAXIMUM: 400 international units.*

(If you drink a quart of vitamin D-enriched milk daily or get out in the sun year-round, you may not need D supplementation.)

Vitamin E

Signs of too much vitamin E.

Many people take vitamin E for its possible usefulness as an antioxidant, allegedly preventing premature aging or damage to body cells. "But in excessively large doses, vitamin E can upset the balance of other fat-soluble vitamins, and it can interfere with the functions of vitamins A and K," says Dr. Vivian. Nausea, gastric problems or muscle weakness may be signs of too much. *USRDA: 30 international units; MAXIMUM: 600 international units.*

Calcium

Excessive doses of calcium may cause kidney stones in some people.

More and more scientific investigations are suggesting that calcium may help slow osteoporosis, the disease of weakened, brittle bones. It also appears that postmenopausal women need more than the USRDA because their bodies' natural calcium-absorbing abilities decrease with age. Large doses may cause kidney stones in people prone to stone formation. *USRDA: 1,000 milligrams; MAXIMUM: 1,500 milligrams.*

Chromium and Selenium

The USRDAs for these two trace minerals have yet to be set. *SUGGESTED RANGE FOR EACH: 50 to 200 micrograms; RECOMMENDED MAXIMUM FOR EACH: 100 micrograms.*

Iron

This mineral is enormously important to human health, preventing and curing iron-deficiency anemia. Iron supplements are widely used in the United States, but reports of iron overload are rare. In those cases where too much is taken, nausea, abdominal cramping, constipation and diarrhea can result. *USRDA: 18 milligrams; MAXIMUM: 30 milligrams.*

(Iron supplemental needs will vary. Women who are on low-calorie diets or who are pregnant or nursing, vegetarians, and the elderly, who often have poor dietary habits, for instance, may have increased needs.)

Do you need more iron?

Magnesium

Although there's little evidence of harm from moderately large doses of this mineral, caution is urged, since scientists are just beginning to study its effects in large doses. *USRDA: 400 milligrams; MAXIMUM: 400 milligrams.*

Zinc

The noticeable side effects of too much zinc can include nausea, vomiting and diarrhea. Yet, it's the unseen that may be of more concern. High doses of zinc can create a copper deficiency, a condition that has been shown to increase levels of LDL cholesterol (the kind that causes coronary heart disease) in laboratory animals. To be safe, the ratio of zinc to copper should be about 10:1. If, for instance, your multiple contains 20 milligrams of zinc, it should also have 2 milligrams of copper. *USRDA: 15 milligrams; MAXIMUM: 30 milligrams.*

Balancing zinc and copper.

Don't Stop Cold Turkey

If you suspect that you're taking too much of a vitamin or mineral, don't stop completely. "Cut back to about half of your current dosage," says Dr. Vivian. "Your body has adjusted itself to handle a massive dose, so if you stop altogether, it could trigger a deficiency."

As a general rule, Dr. Saltman concludes, it's best to stay below five times the USRDA for minerals and vitamins.

For advice on supplements, see your doctor or a registered dietitian.

If you're thinking about increasing the dosage of some nutrients or are just curious about your present vitamin regimen, consult your doctor or a registered dietitian. This is especially important if you have an illness such as diabetes or high blood pressure, since large doses of some supplements can interfere with the function of medications.

"It's a multifaceted issue. It's not as simple as popping the top off a bottle and swallowing a few pills," says Dr. Saltman. "The most positive step that people can take is to realize that there is a real potential for harm when taking megadoses of some vitamins and minerals."

Do you really need supplements?

And before you use supplements, ask the key question: Do I really need them? Most nutrition experts say supplementation is rarely necessary. Many people think otherwise. Only your body knows for sure. So before you supplement, find out from your doctor, a nutritionist or your personal analysis of your own diet whether you really require extra nutrients.

Part **VI**

BETTER NUTRITION FOR THE STAGES OF YOUR LIFE

Getting Ready to Eat for Two

The kind of nourishment you're getting (or not getting) today may help (or harm) the baby you may be carrying tomorrow. Studies have shown that the stores of fat, protein and other nutrients that are called upon for fetal nourishment during pregnancy are built up over the years.

We also know now that the fetus is profoundly affected by what and how much the mother eats. And the most critical effects often occur in the early weeks of fetal development—even before you know you're pregnant.

"Sometimes all it takes is a gradual modification of your own nutritional habits to give the fetus the best chance at healthy development," says David Paige, M.D., professor of maternal and child health at the Department of Public Health, Johns Hopkins Hospital. So start taking inventory of your current food habits, and let your health-care provider in on your pregnancy plans.

Here are some changes to make today to guard against fetal damage and to ensure yourself a healthy baby (while it's still but a twinkle in your eye).

Your unborn baby depends on *you* for nutrients.

Aim for Your Ideal Weight before Conception

"Pregnancy is not the time to worry about pounds," says Dr. Paige. In fact, most physicians today agree that maternal weight gain has more effect on the development of a healthy baby than anything else. So when you do get pregnant, you'll likely be instructed to "eat to appetite" and to gain weight—an average of 28 pounds or so. (But you can take the worry out of weight gain during pregnancy if you breastfeed after your baby is born—it will help you lose pounds faster.)

So lose weight gradually before conceiving. Don't crash diet. "Women should not enter pregnancy with depleted body stores," says Roy Pitkin, M.D., professor and head of nutrition, Department of Obstetrics and Gynecology, University of Iowa. That also means underweight women should gain weight prior to pregnancy.

Gradual weight loss is better than crash dieting if you want to slim down before pregnancy.

Wean Yourself from Wine and Spirits

The National Institute on Alcohol Abuse and Alcoholism says you should abstain altogether. But many doctors continue to suggest limiting drinks to one or two a day. "There's no known safe drinking level, so play it safe during pregnancy—don't drink," says Dr. Pitkin. And now—before pregnancy—is a great time to start discovering nonalcoholic ways to quench your thirst, socialize or entertain.

Cut Caffeine Consumption

Start brewing a weaker cup of coffee. Caffeine crosses the placenta and reaches the fetus. While caffeine may or may not cause birth defects, the U.S. Food and Drug Administration (FDA) warns pregnant women to eliminate or limit caffeine-containing products such as cola, tea, chocolate and common cold remedies.

If you consume caffeine, so will your unborn baby.

What's more, caffeine can suppress your appetite and rob you of sleep—both pregnancy no-nos. So it's better that you go through the caffeine-withdrawal jitters now. And urge the father-to-be to cut caffeine, too. Studies have shown that "reproductive loss" occurred when the man's caffeine intake was high before conception.

To get going in the morning—and keep going— look for other breakfast boosters (like cheesy eggs) that pack plenty of protein, a nutrient you'll need once you are pregnant anyway.

Rev Up Your Nutrient Intake

Everything you eat counts when you're pregnant, but certain nutrients are especially critical.

Iron. Like many women, you probably have an iron-deficient diet. After you conceive, you will need even more iron to keep your blood rich for the baby. But even vegetarians can build up iron stores by eating plenty of prunes, leafy green vegetables, dried beans and blackstrap molasses. Enhance iron absorption by eating those foods along with foods containing vitamin C.

Make sure you're getting enough iron in your diet.

Calcium. Before you're pregnant, you'll need about 1,000 milligrams of this mineral per day to ward off osteoporosis, a bone-loss condition. After you get pregnant, be certain to get 1,200 milligrams per day for the proper development of your baby's bones and teeth. Start cultivating a taste for calcium-rich foods, such as milk, tofu, yogurt, cheese, broccoli and almonds.

When you're pregnant, your need for calcium increases.

Folate. A deficiency during pregnancy could mean your unborn baby may develop neural tube defects. Start eating more wheat germ, brewer's yeast and raw spinach now.

Vitamin B$_6$. The Pill robs you of this nutrient, which some medical people say can combat cramping and swelling during pregnancy. Use a barrier method of birth control for three months prior to conception, and increase your B$_6$ supply by eating bananas, wheat germ and poultry.

In general, don't take vitamin megadoses if you plan a pregnancy. Large doses of some vitamins, like A and D, have resulted in fetal defects.

Stick to Several Small Meals

**During pregnancy, skip-
ping meals is a no-no.**

Meal skipping is strictly forbidden during pregnancy, so you might as well get into the habit of eating regularly. Eating minimeals throughout the day will help you to stabilize your blood sugar and to maintain your energy and weight both before pregnancy and after delivery. During pregnancy, eating several small meals a day will help you gain the weight you need and prevent morning sickness.

What Pregnant Women Should Know about Nutrients and Birth Defects

Before the sleeping potion thalidomide wrought its infamous fetal deformities, before rubella was found to work dark changes in the unborn, before researchers showed that alcohol and cigarettes were the enemies of the fetus, people believed that the womb was a kind of fortress. Babies, they thought, huddled there, shielded from the harm originating beyond the placental walls.

But we learned the hard way that the walls are thin and that the life inside often responds readily to forces from outside, whether they're good or evil.

The fetus is more vulnerable than we once thought.

And we're still learning. Right now, there's a race on among scientists to identify and deal with such forces, and there's plenty of evidence—especially in the area of nutrition—that the effort is paying off.

Vitamins and Minerals May Prevent Birth Defects

Researchers have known for decades that malnourished women often give birth to deformed infants, and doctors and laymen alike have vaguely acknowledged the importance of prenatal nutrition ("You're eating for two now"). But it's only recently that research has started to focus heavily on specific nutrients in the expectant mother's diet. So far the data coming in are incomplete, but some of the latest results hold out a tantalizing prospect: the prevention and treatment of many birth defects with vitamins and minerals.

Fetal health is critically linked to its mother's nutrition.

"We don't yet fully understand the biochemical impact of certain nutrients on fetal deformities. But it's clear that each is crucial," says Thomas Brewer, M.D., a San Francisco obstetrician and author of *Metabolic Toxemia of Late Pregnancy*. "The challenge is to convince the medical profession and pregnant women that a balanced diet of protein, carbohydrates, fats, vitamins and minerals, including a moderate amount of salt, is necessary. The biochemistry behind this remains an exciting academic problem."

The sense of urgency here is understandable. In this country the rate of birth defects is about 7 percent of all births—amounting to a quarter of a million babies born each year with mental or physical abnormalities. And in 60 to 70 percent of these cases, medical people don't have the slightest idea what the cause is. If the nutrient approach pans out—and lots of researchers think it will—a whole new front could open up in the conflict between science and the "accidents" of birth.

Battling Parental Nightmares

The most intriguing news of the nutrient connection comes from Great Britain. There, R. W. Smithells, M.B., of the University of Leeds, and his colleagues have been amassing evidence that vitamins and minerals may be able to prevent a class of birth deformities known as neural tube defects (NTD).

These relatively common malformations (which include spina bifida) are the embodiment of parents' nightmares—fetal vertebrae fail to fuse and the spinal cord protrudes through the gap, or the head is too small, or the brain is missing, or there's some other neural calamity. NTD children usually must endure lifelong handicaps. Some can't walk. Some can't control their bowels or bladder. And many must repeatedly submit to surgery to correct congenital errors.

Early on, Dr. Smithells realized that whatever caused NTD (and there may be several factors), the mother's nutrition probably played a major role. After all, he noted, circumstantial evidence suggests that women who have the worst diets seem to have the greatest chance of delivering a baby with an NTD, and women with low levels of certain nutrients appear more likely to have babies with defects in the central nervous system.

So the question was—and a radical query indeed—could supplementing a woman's diet with specific nutrients lower her chances of having an NTD baby? To find out, Dr. Smithells and his associates gave a daily multivitamin/mineral supplement to 454 women who had already delivered at least one NTD infant (and who were therefore at higher risk for delivering another) and who planned to become pregnant again. Since NTDs develop near conception, the women took the supplements from at least 28 days before conception to the time of the second missed period. The investigators compared the pregnancy outcome of this group to that of 519 women taking no supplements at all, who also had had one or more NTD babies.

A study of women who were at high risk.

The results are still reverberating in the medical world. The rate of NTD births among the unsupplemented women was 4.7 percent. But the rate among those taking the vitamins and minerals was only 0.7 percent, about one-seventh as high (*Lancet*). The researchers concluded, "The presumptive evidence of a protective effect of vitamin supplementation remains very strong."

For those concerned about neural tube defects, some startling data.

But if nutrients administered in moderate amounts do alter the congenital throw of the dice, how do they do it? The most favored explanation is that women prone to deliver NTD babies suffer from vitamin or mineral deficiencies or the inability to properly metabolize certain nutrients.

Dr. Smithells's hunch was that the key nutrient in his supplement formula was folate, or folic acid, which was supplied at a level of 360 micrograms. Another group of researchers has already found that supplementing high-risk women with only folate reduces their risk of having NTD babies. (Of course,

Dr. Smithells: The likely birth-defect preventive is folate.

pregnant women should not consider use of folate supplements without the consent of their physician.)

There could be more than one active agent in the formula, of course, so Dr. Smithells and his colleagues are still looking.

Nutrients against Cleft Lip

Such compelling study results are bound to prompt a few scientific minds to ponder a most attractive possibility: If it's true that supplements can work against one class of birth defects, maybe they can make war on a related class.

Dr. M. Tolarova of the Institute of Experimental Medicine in Prague has suggested just that. It wouldn't be surprising, says Dr. Tolarova, if supplementing women who've delivered babies with cleft (split) lips could reduce the chances of the deformities recurring. After all, NTD and cleft lips (inaccurately and unkindly labeled harelips) are physiologically related.

Can supplements prevent cleft lips?

At any rate, a trio of early studies has hinted at the idea, and Dr. Tolarova has done some testing, too. The researcher first selected women who had given birth to cleft-lip babies but had no other family history of mouth or facial clefts. Then the women were given supplements (similar to Dr. Smithells's formula) to take daily from at least three months before conception to the end of the first trimester of pregnancy. For comparison, a group of unsupplemented women with a similar cleft-lip history was also chosen.

When all the women had delivered and the results were tabulated, the numbers seemed just as impressive as the NTD data.

"In 85 pregnancies, fully supplemented," says Dr. Tolarova, "there was just one recurrence [of cleft lip]. Acting as control, 212 pregnancies, not supplemented, ended in 15 recurrences." Which means that the women who took the vitamins and minerals had one-seventh the risk of bearing cleft-lip children as the unsupplemented women (*Lancet*).

Folate Deficiency Implicated
in Some Premature Births

Women who experience a lifetime of poor nutrition are at high risk of delivering premature babies. The consequences of that can be devastating. According to the experts, it's the most significant contributor to infant mortality, and even the babies who do survive—especially the really tiny ones—often have some residual defects.

Besides that, the medical costs are staggering—up to $100,000 for 30 to 60 days in the preemie nursery. That's why research that helps uncover the specific factors that cause these problems is so important.

Now a group of doctors from the University of Mississippi Medical Center in Jackson may have isolated one of the contributors—a deficiency of folate, a B vitamin. Of the women they studied (85 percent of whom were poor and black), the doctors found that 32 percent giving birth to premature babies were folate deficient. By comparison, only 6 percent of those having full-term babies were deficient.

The researchers say that folate deficiency may be a factor in as many as one-third of the preterm deliveries in the patients they studied (*American Journal of Clinical Nutrition*).

"Folate deficiency may not be recognized as much as it should be," adds James Carter, M.D., chairman and professor, Department of Nutrition at Tulane University School of Public Health in New Orleans. "Sometimes it's masked by an iron deficiency, which is most common and easy to diagnose.

"Clearly, it would help to increase the amount of folate in the diet with foods such as broccoli, liver, spinach, cabbage, romaine lettuce and black-eyed peas—all good sources.

"Still," says Dr. Carter, "it would be wrong to give the impression that you can correct the problem of low-birth-weight babies that simply. Black women in particular have a high incidence of this problem because they themselves were often raised on a marginal diet or were low-birth-weight babies themselves. It may take a full generation to bring their reproductive performance up to what we see in affluent white women."

A Catastrophic Deficiency

The zinc link to birth defects.

There is, however, an even more heavily researched nutrient link with birth defects: zinc. For at least 15 years, scientists have been scrutinizing the effect that zinc deficiencies have on birth defects, and the evidence has been consistently provocative.

First came reports that pregnant rats deficient in zinc gave birth to offspring with a variety of abnormalities. Then there was word that people in Egypt and Iran have widespread zinc deficiencies, as well as high rates of birth defects involving the central nervous system. Later, researchers established a similar relationship in Turkey.

Lowell E. Sever, Ph.D., formerly of the University of Washington School of Public Health in Seattle, was one of the first to identify the zinc/malformation phenomenon in the Near East and has since surveyed the full spectrum of the research.

A zinc deficiency in pregnancy may threaten the unborn child.

"Data support the idea that a lack of zinc in pregnancy may precipitate human birth abnormalities," he says. "And none of the investigations suggest that moderate levels of dietary zinc are in any way harmful."

But can the research tell women precisely what zinc intakes may be protective? "Not yet," says Dr. Sever. "All we know so far is that under normal circumstances the Recommended Dietary Allowance [RDA] for a pregnant woman—20 milligrams per day—should be enough."

Vitamin Therapy for Birth Defects

Some rare successes: reversing birth defects with vitamins.

Fortunately, beyond the safety net of prevention, there's treatment. To be sure, treating abnormalities in fetuses is still highly experimental and far less prevalent than preventive measures. And certainly many congenital mistakes simply can't be corrected. But the work goes on, and vitamins are a small part of it.

At Yale University School of Medicine in New Haven, Connecticut, Maurice Mahoney, M.D., has treated a potentially lethal birth defect with high doses of vitamin B_{12}. The defect is called methylmalonic acidemia, a rare metabolic disorder.

"In this abnormality, there's a blockage of vitamin B_{12} in the fetus's system," Dr. Mahoney says. "The vitamin is prevented from facilitating the metabolism of certain amino acids, and that allows other acids to increase in the fetus's bloodstream. An infant born with such a problem will be lethargic, unable to feed properly, even semicomatose. Ultimately, he will become severely retarded or die if treatment is not started shortly after birth."

Dr. Mahoney overcomes the blockage by supplementing the expectant mother with B_{12} as soon as the diagnosis is made (at about 16 or 17 weeks).

"We administer the vitamin either orally or intramuscularly," he says. "It crosses the placenta to the fetus and causes a very sharp decline in methylmalonic acids in the blood. If we continue therapy until delivery, the baby will be virtually normal." When last contacted, Dr. Mahoney said his success record was 100 percent.

With vitamin B_{12}, 100 percent success.

The story is much the same with a similar fetal disorder called multiple carboxylase deficiency. It, too, is marked by faulty metabolism—failure to break down amino acids and carbohydrates with a resulting buildup of acids in the blood and cells. And it, too, leaves newborns lingering between retardation and death. The stabilizing influence this time, however, is biotin, another B vitamin.

Saving babies with biotin.

"We administer the biotin the same way we do the B_{12}," says Dr. Mahoney. "And the result is similar—fairly rapid normalization of the metabolism."

All of which intimates that in pregnancy, getting enough to eat and shunning alcohol and cigarettes are a big part of the battle against birth defects.

Remember, however, that you should never take any supplements during pregnancy without first checking with your doctor.

Chapter 58

How to Avoid Dieters' Deficiencies

A re you losing vitamins and minerals as well as pounds? Maybe you'd better count nutrients along with calories.

Researchers have found that immune system response drops in people on very low-calorie diets, says Peter Lindner, M.D., director of continuing medical education for the American Society of Bariatric Physicians (obesity specialists). "In one study, the researchers were interested in the changes in disease-fighting white blood cells when exposed to vaccine. What they found was that the immune response was reduced in those individuals on improperly administered ultralow-calorie diets, making them more subject to infection. That is probably one of the most dangerous aspects of very low-calorie diets."

Starvation Diets Are Dangerous

If you're a dieter—and surveys show two out of three people are—there's a very good chance you may be endangering your health, warns Dr. Lindner. You may be able to take nutrition for granted when you're eating like a horse, but it becomes critical when you start eating like a bird.

"A good balanced diet in the higher caloric range probably gives you all the vitamins and minerals you need. It gives you some leeway to play with," says the physician. "Drop it down to 800 or 1,000 calories, and everything counts."

In fact, according to the Food and Nutrition Board of the National Academy of Sciences—which sets our Recommended Dietary Allowances (RDAs)—it is difficult to get adequate nutrition on diets that provide less than 1,800 to 2,000 calories. Most popular reducing diets call for 1,200 or less.

Are you getting enough calories?

It's hard enough to juggle the four food groups into a nutritionally balanced diet when you've got a few thousand calories to work with. Dieters have a tougher task. They have to concoct three healthful meals with roughly half the calories they're used to consuming. And they start out with a handicap—they don't know beans about nutrition.

Following a diet guide may not help. Many of the popular diet plans are full of dubious nutritional advice. And most dieters know only enough to plan a 1,200-calorie menu down to the last morsel. But knowing calories isn't enough. You can create three low-calorie meals a day without ever straying from the candy counter.

The Problem with Weight-Loss Diets

Perhaps the most important thing to remember when you're counting calories is that it's the nutritional value of the calorie that counts. If you don't know the value of a calorie, you don't know what you're missing.

Count nutritional value, not just calories.

But Paul LaChance, Ph.D., does. Dr. LaChance, professor of nutrition and food science at Rutgers University, evaluated the nutritional content of 11 published weight-loss diets. He chose the 11 because they ran the gamut of popular weight-reducing plans—from high protein/low carbohydrate to low protein/high carbohydrate, with variations in between. They carried such familiar names as Scarsdale, Stillman, Atkins and the Beverly Hills Diet.

Using the RDAs as a frame of reference, Dr. LaChance and his associate, dietitian Michele C.

Popular diets get a bad report card.

Fisher, R.D., Ph.D., found that most of the diets were low in thiamine (B_1), vitamin B_6, vitamin B_{12}, calcium, iron, zinc and magnesium. Thiamine, vitamins B_6 and B_{12} and magnesium were often at levels less than 70 percent of the RDA. One, the Beverly Hills Diet, supplied less than 70 percent of the RDAs for more than half of the vitamins and minerals the researchers evaluated, and it was so low in protein they predicted it would lead to a serious protein deficiency over a long period of time.

And there's the rub. Most diets are protracted, if not forever. "Most people stay on a diet for a long time. After all, weight loss doesn't occur overnight," says Dr. LaChance. "If a diet lasts only two weeks, the vitamin and mineral loss is not going to be significant. As far as I'm concerned, women are dieting all the time and may have other risk factors—smoking, contraceptive pill use—that can affect nutrient metabolism. For them, the loss can be very significant."

In fact, researchers studying otherwise healthy men found that even without those extra risk factors, a prolonged low-calorie diet had a damaging effect on their health. One group, which had previously eaten more than 3,000 calories daily, ate about half that for a period of six months. Even though they were eating more calories than prescribed by most reducing diets, the men suffered from depression, anemia, edema, slowing of heartbeat and loss of sex drive. They also tired easily and lacked endurance.

Fasting can be hazardous to your health.

Some weight-loss regimens, specifically those that are mainly protein, can lead to a potentially serious condition called acidosis, which also can occur on fasting diets. In one study, people fed a diet of solely protein and fat lost about two pounds a day— along with large amounts of nitrogen and salt in their urine. They suffered from the symptoms of acidosis, which can include weakness, malaise, headache and heart arrhythmias.

Acidosis can be remedied by adding as little as about three ounces of carbohydrate to the diet.

Needless to say, bizarre diets that rely heavily on one food—such as grapefruit—are going to be nutritionally bankrupt. Very low-calorie liquid diets can be deadly.

Women's Nutritional Needs May Exceed Supply

Women are always going to have to pay extra attention to the nutrient content of their diets because of their increased needs for certain nutrients. "For women it's hard enough to get things like calcium and iron," says Cindy Rubin, a clinical nutritionist formerly with the obesity research group at the University of Pennsylvania.

Women generally need more iron and calcium than men.

"Many women are going to have to supplement their diets with calcium and iron," says noted weight and fitness expert Gabe Mirkin, M.D., who ordinarily doesn't advocate dietary supplements. "One out of four women between 12 and 50 is iron deficient."

Are you getting enough iron and calcium?

Though an iron deficiency may eventually lead to anemia, it has its own immediate health consequences. "When you're iron deficient, even though you're not anemic," says Dr. Mirkin, "you can't clear lactic acid as rapidly as normal from your bloodstream, so you tire earlier at work and play."

"The problem with calcium is that it's scarce except in milk products—the first thing many dieters cut out. Unless you choose skim milk, dairy products can be high in fat and calories," says Dr. Lindner. "It's difficult to get adequate calcium without milk unless you want to eat sardines, small bones and all."

How food is prepared may also affect a dieter's nutrition. "If you're eating a salad that was tossed three days ago, vitamins are lost simply by exposure," says Dr. Lindner. "If food is cooked too much, you can lose more. Especially at risk are the water-soluble vitamins, such as C and the B vitamins."

How cooking can destroy vitamins.

One of those B vitamins is folate. Women are particularly at risk of developing anemia when they aren't taking in enough folate, which is found in leafy greens. A form of anemia occurs when there isn't enough folate in the body to produce red blood cells. Folate deficiency also has been pinpointed as a factor in an often-precancerous condition called cervical dysplasia.

Another risk of low-calorie diets: zinc deficiency.

Studies have also shown that low-calorie and starvation diets can lead to an excessive loss of zinc, possibly as a result of tissue breakdown. Researchers at the Veterans Administration Hospital in Hines, Illinois, found that weight-loss diets between 600 and 1,240 calories can be zinc deficient, depending on the type and source of dietary protein from which the zinc is derived. Diets that derive most of their protein from red meat tend to supply more zinc than those that rely on chicken, fish, milk products and eggs, which are, unfortunately, the main protein sources of many low-calorie diets.

Tips for the Diet-Wise

If it all sounds discouraging, rest assured that the obesity experts understand—and have more than one solution to a dieter's nutritional dilemma.

Solving the dieter's nutritional dilemma.

Use a supplement to help fill the gap. If you don't feel you can add red meat to your diet or if time and money constraints make it impossible to eat only freshly prepared foods, you can take supplements. "Theoretically, it's not necessary to supplement your diet," says Dr. Lindner, "but realistically, most people don't have the knowledge or the time to do it right. Especially if you're a woman, a standard multiple vitamin that contains iron, B_6, folacin [folate] and zinc along with a calcium supplement should help you make sure you're getting all of the 26 micronutrients you need."

Learn the value of a calorie. You know there's a big nutritional difference between a 200-calorie candy bar and a 200-calorie protein salad. But even so-called diet foods aren't created equal. "Choose nutrient-dense foods," suggests Cindy Rubin. "For instance, eat broccoli as opposed to lettuce. Both are low in calories, but lettuce is mainly water. You're not getting the heavy doses of vitamin A that you get in broccoli."

Go for variety. Not only is it the spice of life but it also improves your chances of getting all the vitamins and minerals you need.

Plan your diet menu from the four basic food groups. "Each of the major categories represents certain vitamins and minerals," says Dr. Mirkin. "Grains and cereals, for example, give you E and the B vitamins. Fruits and vegetables supply C and A. If you take in at least 1,500 calories a day and distribute your calories over the four food groups, you'll probably be taking in the nutrients you need."

Eat more calories. This may come as a surprise, but by eating more, naturally, you're more likely to meet your nutritional needs. But will you lose weight? Yes, say the experts, as long as you burn up some of those calories through exercise.

In his book *Getting Thin*, Dr. Mirkin advises eating 1,500 calories a day—and using an hour of exercise to burn off 300.

There are some unique advantages to this plan. Aside from losing weight healthfully, you'll stimulate your metabolism to burn even more calories. "You see, diets don't work," says Dr. Mirkin. "When you go on a diet, your metabolism slows down. When you're lying in bed, not even moving, you burn 60 calories an hour. If you're on a diet, you burn only 50. If you exercise, you burn 70—without even moving. Exercise speeds up your metabolism, not to mention suppressing your appetite."

Dr. Mirkin recommends picking two sports—aerobic dancing and biking, for instance—and working up slowly to an hour of each on alternating days. "I specify two sports because it takes you 48 hours to

Not all calories are created equal.

How to eat well and still lose weight.

Why older people need exercise.

recover, and you should rotate the stressors on your body," he says.

Older people especially need exercise as an integral part of any diet plan. "The two have to be together," says Dr. LaChance. "When you're young, your metabolism is higher, and you can get away with more. When you get older, your body changes. Your metabolism slows, your lean body mass goes down and your propensity for adipose [fat] tissue goes up. You lower your need for calories, so if you don't add exercise, you get fat."

The Exerciser's
Guide to
Vitamins and Minerals

L egend has it that the ancient Greek wrestler
Milo of Croton killed a bull with a single blow
and ate it in just one day, thereby setting the tone for
the millions of athletes who came after him, whose
training tables would be a smorgasbord of nutrition
fads.

Milo reputedly built his prodigious strength by
eating 20 pounds of meat a day. And, until about a
decade ago, everyone from the high school track star
to the mile-a-day jogger thought the magic potion was
a slab of marbled steak at every meal. Once they
discovered carbohydrate loading, it was goodbye
beef and hello pasta. In fact, athletes have always
been the first to pounce on the "perfect" elixir, which
could make them the biggest, the fastest, the strongest, the . . . (fill in your favorite superlative). Athletes
sang the praises of bee pollen, glorified ginseng and
gulped down handfuls of vitamins and minerals as if
they were candy.

How to Achieve
Your Personal Best

But does any of this wishful eating do any good?
Separating nutrition fact from fancy is not as easy as it
seems. There's been more agreement among warring
factions in the Middle East than among nutritionists
and fitness experts talking about the special needs of
the physically active. Should you load up on potas-

sium-rich foods? Should you take supplemental vitamin C? Are you sweating away more zinc and riboflavin than you're getting in your diet? In answer, authorities' voices rise like a discordant choir.

If you aren't planning to challenge Navratilova at Wimbledon or break records at the Boston Marathon, the controversy surrounding performance boosting can remain academic. But what if you are looking for a way to improve your personal best—or at least not lose ground while you're getting fit? Is there some nutritional fine-tuning you might be doing?

Doing some nutritional fine-tuning.

Though some of it is contradictory, the evidence indicates you might, particularly if you are a woman or a vegetarian, if you are losing weight or eating a poor diet. Your nutritional needs may be altered by exercise, especially if you are training hard or involved in an endurance sport like marathon running.

The first thing you may have to do is eat more. Most nutrition experts agree that the diet that meets the needs of a sedentary individual is not adequate for a person involved in vigorous physical activity. So if your three-mile-a-week run has whetted your appetite for half-marathons, you will probably have to adjust your diet to include more foods with high energy concentration. That means calories.

Advice for the physically active: Eat more.

If you're a recent convert to physical fitness, that probably sounds ominously like the first step on the road to fat. But when was the last time you saw a fat marathoner? Long-distance runners monitored along a 312-mile course in Hawaii ate an average of 4,800 calories a day. ("They were eating their way through 312 miles," commented one researcher.) Had they not been averaging over 16 miles a day on this runner's holiday, they would have gone home like a flotilla of blimps. But because they were running, they were using—as fuel—every last calorie they ate.

More calories but not more fat.

In Search of a Good Diet

"High-mileage runners—greater than 60 miles per week—need not worry about excessive calorie intake. If their diet is well balanced and contains a variety of foods, they will be receiving the necessary vitamins and minerals," says Rudolph Dressendorfer, Ph.D., professor of physical education at the California PolyTechnic State University in San Luis Obispo, California.

Many nutrition specialists believe that the proverbial "good mixed diet" is high-octane fuel for the exerciser. But others aren't so sure the average jogger or tennis player is so scrupulous about his three squares a day. Jack Cooperman, Ph.D., director of nutrition at the New York Medical College, believes marginal B-vitamin deficiencies are epidemic among the otherwise health-conscious because of dieting and meal skipping. Two University of Missouri researchers, testing the iron, zinc and copper intakes of women track team members, discovered nearly half of them consumed less than two-thirds of the Recommended Dietary Allowance (RDA) for iron and zinc in diets that were generally poor.

Is the average jogger really getting enough vitamins and minerals?

One thing science seems clear on is that dietary deficiencies can impair athletic performance. Studies have shown that when thiamine (B_1), a B vitamin found mainly in high-carbohydrate foods, is added to a thiamine-deficient diet, muscular endurance is enhanced in a very short time. Researchers also found that people whose diets are lacking sufficient amounts of vitamin C grow fatigued more quickly than those who have higher intakes.

Add exercise to a nutrient-deficient diet and you could run—or bike or walk—right into trouble. Unfortunately, research on the nutritional requirements of ardent exercisers is as sparse as a toddler's vocabulary—but there is enough to signal a few dietary warnings.

Nutritional deficiencies + exercise = trouble.

Watch Your Iron Intake

If you are involved in an endurance sport and are a woman and/or a vegetarian, you should pay close attention to your iron intake. Doug Clement, M.D., co-director of the University of British Columbia's Sports Medicine Clinic, believes "the vast majority" of female runners and a quarter of male runners have what he terms a nonanemic ferritin deficiency. Ferritin is an iron compound, and its levels are a sensitive gauge of the body's iron stores. A deficiency may result in a runner's failure to improve with training, Dr. Clement says.

The most prominent victim of ferritin deficiency is Olympic marathoner Alberto Salazar, who in just two years went from setting records to straggling in dead last. Dr. Clement, a college running teammate of Salazar's coach, diagnosed the troubled runner long-distance. Tests later confirmed his diagnosis, and Salazar was placed on an iron-enriched diet. He showed improvement, enough to qualify for an Olympic berth, a feat his previous performances had placed in doubt.

Alberto Salazar learned about iron deficiency the hard way.

Iron can be easily lost through sweat, urine, feces and, in women, menstrual flow. Studies also indicate runners can actually break iron-laden red blood cells when the thin-skinned soles of their feet batter relentlessly on hard surfaces. Red blood cells have been found in runners' urine.

It's easy to lose too much iron.

"As a result of one study we've done, we suspect runners are not absorbing iron from their diets as well as they should," says Dr. Clement. "One speculated factor is their decreased transit time. Runners generally have more active bowels, decreasing the time between intake and exit, so the iron isn't in the body long enough to be absorbed properly."

At greatest risk are active vegetarians—because iron is not as readily absorbed from plant sources—and women, whose need for iron is almost twice as great as men's. Women should get 18 milligrams of iron a day, and Dr. Clement believes running and other equally strenuous sports add 6 to 8 milligrams to that requirement. The average woman gets only about 10 to 12 milligrams a day.

At risk for iron deficiency: women and vegetarians.

One study of women in an aerobics class at the University of Illinois, conducted by Scott Blum and Adria Sherman, Ph.D., of the Department of Foods and Nutrition, found that the women's ferritin levels dropped after only six weeks, though not into the deficient range.

There is some evidence, however, that performance can suffer in the absence of full-blown anemia, particularly when there is a depletion of tissue iron.

Getting More Iron in the Active Person's Diet

How does a fitness buff make sure the iron in his or her diet is sufficient—short of becoming a ravaging meat eater?

Nancy Clark, a nutritionist with Sports Medicine Resource and the author of *The Athlete's Kitchen,* offers some helpful advice.

Include a food rich in vitamin C with meals. Vitamin C has been shown to make iron more absorbable. In one study, a glass of orange juice increased the amount of iron absorbed from an iron-enriched breakfast cereal by 250 percent.

Cook with cast iron rather than aluminum or stainless steel. Frying scrambled eggs in a cast-iron pan can increase iron content threefold. Simmering a half cup of spaghetti sauce for three hours in a cast-iron pot can raise iron from 3 milligrams to 88 milligrams.

Try to eat breads, cereals and pastas that have been iron fortified. A quick look at the label will tell you.

Avoid drinking coffee and tea with meals. These beverages can reduce iron absorption by as much as 50 percent. A glass of wine with a meal, on the other hand, can boost your iron absorption by as much as 300 percent.

Several iron-containing proteins in the muscle play a key role in energy metabolism.

Minerals Lost in Sweat

There is far from a consensus on the effects of mineral loss in exercise, but add a few more to the list of nutrients to monitor. Potassium, magnesium and zinc are lost in sweat, though losses vary widely from one person to the next.

Are you suffering from "mineral blues"?

A nutrition expert and a runner himself, Gabe Mirkin, M.D., coauthor of the *Sportsmedicine Book*, says exercisers who feel weak and tired may be suffering from "the mineral blues," a deficiency of potassium and magnesium inside muscle cells. When Dr. Mirkin, who ran 100 miles a month, suddenly found that running a quarter-mile "felt like a marathon," he had his blood tested. He learned that he was potassium deficient, something he remedied with copious quantities of fruit juices. (Other potassium-rich foods include all vegetables, molasses, wheat germ, soybeans, pecans and walnuts.)

You can lose potassium by working out in hot, humid weather.

Researchers at the University of Florida in Gainesville found that experienced long-distance runners training in hot, humid weather needed more than the recommended amount of 2.6 grams of potassium to maintain potassium balance, even if they were accustomed to the heat. In fact, if they were sweating profusely, they needed at least 3 grams. Runners who were not acclimatized had even greater sweat losses and so may have been losing even more potassium.

A loss of magnesium through sweat can bring on fatigue and muscle cramps because of the role the mineral plays in controlling muscle contraction and regulating the conversion of carbohydrates to energy. A French doctor perked up a soccer team plagued by chronic fatigue by giving them magnesium supplements, though you might choose to defend against magnesium loss by eating more nuts, dairy products, soybeans and green leafy vegetables.

Studies on marathon runners show that zinc levels tend to decrease with hard training, though just how that might affect performance is not known. "Very few studies have looked at the effects of plasma-level deficiencies on performance," says Dr. Dressendorfer, who has been studying the mineral needs of marathoners. In one of his early studies, about 23 percent of his marathoner subjects had zinc levels in the extreme lower limit of normal. At the time he speculated that endurance athletes might need to increase their zinc intake when training. He found in a subsequent study, however, that even over long distances, a well-balanced, high-calorie diet kept zinc and other mineral levels in normal ranges.

Are marathoners risking zinc deficiencies?

"If people are exercising hard and not losing weight, they are probably getting enough calories, vitamins and minerals. But," he cautions, "people who are losing weight might not be getting enough calories or enough of the right vitamins and minerals, either. And vegetarians have to be especially careful in order to get vitamins and minerals like zinc and iron, which are found in higher quantities in animal sources."

Getting Your B's

So should women, who may be sweating away more than minerals. In that valuable perspiration may be riboflavin (B_2), one of the B vitamins that helps the body convert food into energy. Several studies done at Cornell University led researchers to suggest that the Recommended Dietary Allowance for active women is too low. Daphne Roe, Ph.D., and her associates found that the more active a woman is, the more riboflavin she requires. The RDA for riboflavin is 1.2 milligrams a day, or 0.6 milligrams for every 1,000 calories consumed. According to Dr. Roe's research, a young woman exercising regularly should be taking in 1.2 milligrams for every 1,000 calories she eats, or almost double the RDA.

Sweating away riboflavin.

When you're active, your body needs more thiamine.

The need for thiamine increases in proportion to how much energy you expend, at about 0.5 milligrams per 1,000 calories consumed. Fortunately, it's readily available in the high-carbohydrate diets many athletes have adopted. Like riboflavin, thiamine is a part of the body's food-to-fuel system—it helps the body use sugar—so it's no surprise there's additional need when the body is revved up by exercise.

In the same way, the body seems to call up its stores of vitamin B_6 when it goes into high gear. Scientists at Oregon State University studying teenage cross-country runners and cyclists found B_6 levels rose after their subjects worked out. Since there was no extra B_6 in their diets and the body cannot manufacture its own, the researchers theorized that the vitamin was being mobilized from the tissues to meet the body's need. There is also some indication that B_6 may play a role in increasing muscle endurance.

The B's work as a team.

You'll find B_6 plentiful in foods like wheat germ, beans, bananas, lentils, soybeans and chicken. But, according to one source, getting a lot of one B vitamin is virtually worthless if you aren't getting sufficient amounts of the other B vitamins in your diet, because these nutrients operate as a team.

Researchers are still studying possible increased requirements for vitamins C and E, sodium and some of the trace minerals, but early results are ambiguous. Though we may know more about good training table fare than Milo of Croton, science still hasn't filled in all the gaps on the menu.

Chapter 60

Boosting Your Brainpower

Water lilies double in area every 24 hours. At the beginning of the summer, there is one water lily on a lake. It takes 60 days for the lake to become covered with water lilies. On what day is the lake half covered?

How does your mind work when you read a brainteaser like this? Is it tickled pink—or tormented to tears? Is it too tired to tackle the task? Do you spend time puzzling over an answer, or lose interest if it doesn't jump right out at you? Do you logically begin counting lily pads from day one? Or, without much apparent effort, does your mind leap to the solution? If the lake is totally covered on day 60, it must be half covered on . . . why, day 59, of course. Why didn't I think of that?

Teasing your brain.

We all have days when our thinking is fuzzy, when our logic defies reason, or when we can't for the life of us remember some name or fact that was so familiar just the day before. On days like those, you might want to trade in your gray matter for a new, improved model with rechargeable batteries and a software system that lets you discover the unknown secrets of the universe in one easy lesson.

Unfortunately, we have to make do with what Mother Nature has given us. Luckily, that's usually more than adequate. But it doesn't mean we can't make better use of the brainpower we do have. Here are some ways to do just that.

Poor Posture, Poor Thinking?

Ever feel like you just can't think straight? Check to see if your posture is putting a crimp on the blood supply to your brain, says E. Fritz Schmerl, M.D., teacher of gerontology at Chabot College, Hayward, California.

Why fuzzy thinking and bad posture go together.

"The brain needs up to 30 times more blood than other organs," Dr. Schmerl says. "But allowing your upper body to sag—with rounded shoulders, head hung over and chin jutting outward—can create kinks in the spine that squeeze the two arteries passing through the spinal column to the brain, causing an inadequate blood supply." The result? "Fuzzy thinking and forgetfulness, especially as we age," says Dr. Schmerl.

Hunched-over posture can contribute to strokelike symptoms, known as transient ischemic attacks, which are brief blackout periods. Worse yet, disturbances in the blood flow of the pinched artery might cause a buildup of fatty deposits that can cause partial blockage, according to Dr. Schmerl.

"It's important to get a head start on proper alignment while you're young," Dr. Schmerl says. "Poor posture is a hard habit to break when you're older. Be consciously on guard to prevent this process by holding yourself straight, with your head back and your chin in," he says.

Iron-Poor Intellect

The brain needs large amounts of oxygen to function effectively, and the only way it can get it is through iron-packed red blood cells, says Don M. Tucker, Ph.D., associate professor of psychology at the University of Oregon at Eugene.

Some studies show that children who have iron-deficiency anemia have short attention spans and trouble learning new material. They also know that boosting iron intake reverses these problems.

And Dr. Tucker's research shows that adults can suffer from related problems with alertness and memory when their iron levels are in the "low but normal" range. In one study, for instance, the higher the blood iron levels, the greater the word fluency. (Volunteers were asked to come up with as many words as they could that begin with "Q" and end with "L.") In another, in adults over age 60, blood iron levels were one of the more important measures in determining whether or not the person had normal brain-wave patterns.

Are you too iron-poor to think straight?

"Getting enough oxygen to the brain is certainly part of its function, but we think iron also influences brain chemicals and pathways," Dr. Tucker says. "We know now that iron is heavily concentrated in a part of the reticular activating system. This area of the brain turns the brain on, so to speak. It maintains alertness. So we can't help but think that iron plays an important role in awareness and alertness."

How iron turns the brain on.

Aerobic Aptitude

Exercise makes people feel good and can help lift depression. Now researchers are finding it also builds mental "muscles" and may postpone aging's effects on the brain.

Researchers in Utah recently found that reaction time, short-term memory and the ability to reason all greatly improved in a group of out-of-shape people aged 55 to 70 who were put on a four-month program of brisk walking. They were better able to remember sequences of numbers, for instance, or to use abstract thinking to correctly match numbers and symbols.

Exercise boosted the thinking power of elderly people.

"I was surprised at the amount of improvement we saw," says Robert Dustman, Ph.D., of the Salt Lake City Veterans Administration Hospital. "We expected to see some results in some people, but we didn't think it would be across the board."

Aerobic exercise makes the body better at transporting oxygen to all its organs, "so we are assuming that the brain benefits by receiving more oxygen," Dr. Dustman says. Those who showed the most improvement (their scores rose by 27 percent) had walked long and hard enough to be aerobically fit.

Stay Stimulated

Keep your thinking
sharp with mental
exercise.

Mental gymnastics may do as much as physical exercise to keep our brains healthy. In fact, there's evidence that the brain may actually increase in size when it's regularly "stretched" out.

Being in an environment that makes you use your brain helps keep your thinking sharp and efficient, says Marion C. Diamond, Ph.D., a professor in the University of California's Department of Physiology and Anatomy. Boredom, on the other hand, can cause restlessness, depression and a lack of fulfillment, all of which can interfere with thinking at your best.

Can a stimulating envi-
ronment make you
smarter?

Dr. Diamond has studied the effects of an enriched environment on the brain cells of young rats. After a month-long stay in a roomy cage that included playmates and plenty of gizmos to fiddle around with, rats' brains actually showed an increased thickness in the outer layers of the cerebral cortex, which represents an increase in the dendrites. "The rats' brains became heavier and more chemically active," says Dr. Diamond. The rats also went on to run a maze better than those that hadn't been in the enriched environment. "So they became better learners, too," she says. "I've seen the same results raising my children and teaching my students. The greater the exposure, the more adaptable they are to facing other problems."

Keeping yourself stimulated should be a lifetime pursuit, Dr. Diamond says. "Keep dreaming and satisfying those dreams. Keep looking forward, and each time you come to a lull, decide what new thing you want to do with your life, the new people you want to meet, how you're going to help people. Make changes, and make each change a new beginning."

Is Lecithin a Brain Booster?

Many of the foods touted as "brain foods"—fish, for instance, and liver and eggs—contain choline, a substance some researchers think may help preserve the brain's ability to reason, learn and remember.

Researchers at Ohio State University, for instance, found that mice fed a diet heavy in choline-rich lecithin or one of lecithin's "brain-active" ingredients, phosphatidylcholine, had much better memory retention than mice on regular diets. They took much longer to go into a back room in their cages where they had received a mild electric shock, meaning they hadn't forgotten their unpleasant experience.

Is lecithin brain food?

What's more, their brain cells, examined under a microscope, showed fewer of the expected signs of aging, says Ronald Mervis, Ph.D., of Ohio State University's Brain Aging and Neuronal Plasticity Research Group.

"Normally, as the brain ages, its cell membranes become more rigid with fatty deposits and lose their ability to take in and release brain chemicals and to relay messages," Dr. Mervis says. This can cause memory loss and confused thinking.

As part of the deterioration process, aging brain cells also tend to lose dendritic spines, the chemical receptor areas that are vitally important in passing along information. Having too few dendritic spines is like having a bad phone connection. Messages get distorted and lost. But older mice that were fed lecithin had the same number of dendritic spines as much younger mice.

Lecithin-fed older mice had brains similar to those of younger mice.

"Despite the differences between mice and men, there are, nevertheless, remarkable similarities in the structure of their nerve cells," says Dr. Mervis. "I believe lecithin could help to repress or delay similar problems in man, although we have yet to verify that."

"B" Smart

The brain seems to have a special need for the B vitamins. Memory loss, disorientation, hallucination, depression, lack of coordination and personality changes can occur with B-complex deficiencies.

Without enough B vitamins, your brain malfunctions.

Alcoholics, for instance, who sometimes develop thiamine (B_1) deficiencies, have problems with short-term memory. They may remember in detail that little café in Paris 20 years ago, but not what they had for supper the previous night. Thiamine-deficient mice have trouble balancing on a tightrope, a skill that's normally a snap for them.

Elderly people with B_{12} deficiencies had poor memories and thinking skills.

B_{12} deficiencies have been linked with poor memory and an inability to concentrate. Researchers at the University of New Mexico School of Medicine in Albuquerque found that people age 60 or older with even a mild B_{12} deficiency had poor memories and abstract thinking skills. (They had trouble repeating a short story and matching symbols with numbers.) "I think it's likely that in older people, subclinical deficiencies can indeed lead to less-than-optimal mental performance," says James Goodwin, M.D., one of the study's researchers.

Thiamine is needed to produce and use one of the brain's major chemical messengers, acetylcholine, says Gary E. Gibson, Ph.D., a thiamine researcher at the Cornell-Burke Rehabilitation Hospital, White Plains, New York. And since the B-complex vitamins are chemically related and may perform some similar functions, it's possible that others are also involved in brain chemical actions, Dr. Gibson says.

Clear Away Mind "Clutter"

Strong emotions can short-circuit your thinking.

How well your brain performs often hinges on your emotional state. Anxiety, with its turmoil of thoughts and rush of adrenaline, can enhance memory in some rare moments, but more often it dulls it. Physical tension all too often means mental confusion, as anyone who's ever botched a crucial job interview or important exam can tell you. A state of calm alertness, on the other hand, can help you think and learn at your best, says Stanford University psychiatry professor Jerome Yesavage, M.D.

Dr. Yesavage studied two groups of elderly people. Both were taught what's known as mnemonic technique to improve their ability to recall names and faces. (They associated a prominent feature of the face with a fanciful, visual image of the name. If the name were Yesavage and the person had a distinctive chin, for instance, the image might be of a savage grabbing the person's chin.)

But members of one group also learned a technique to relax their bodies before using the memory trick. They went on to recall 25 percent more faces and names than the group that wasn't taught to relax.

With relaxation, their memories improved dramatically.

"Anxiety and worry actually clutter your thoughts and decrease your thinking ability," Dr. Yesavage says. "We talk about processing capacity, which is the amount of information someone can be actively thinking about at any one time. The brain can handle only a certain amount of information at once, so if half its capacity is being used for anxiety and rumination, it can't be used for learning or remembering. It's being wasted. Getting rid of anxiety opens up more space in the brain to work on the task at hand," he says.

Convincing someone *not* to worry isn't an easy task, but worry goes hand in hand with physical tension, according to Dr. Yesavage: "Ease the physical tension and the mind follows." Calming music, deep breathing exercises, meditation, yoga, biofeedback and progressive relaxation training all help to soothe the body and free the mind.

Think You Can

Telling yourself you just weren't born smart, that you can never remember things, or that you're too old to learn are good ways to sabotage your true intellectual potential, say David Lewis, Ph.D., and James Greene, authors of *Thinking Better*. Such negative thoughts "put your brain behind bars." They keep you

Positive thinking helps you reach your intellectual potential.

from pursuing knowledge and learning better ways to remember. They can push you into a mental rut as you age.

Feeling good about your ability to learn is important to intellectual functioning, and it's one of the first things to be tackled at Mankind Research Unlimited, a Silver Spring, Maryland, "superlearning" center that has turned high school dropouts into gifted learners and blind people into computer programmers.

"We tell people who don't think they can learn that they really have a lot more brain than they think and that they can learn to use more of it than they ever thought possible," says director Carl Schleicher, Ph.D.

The power of positive images.

His learning program uses a number of different techniques—listening to stately baroque music, visualizing a quiet, private getaway place for thinking, and breathing deeply to create an aura of relaxed awareness. Then, the student receives suggestions—that he *will* do better, that he *can* learn. He begins to picture himself doing that successfully, and his successes in real life are praised. He may also use creative imagery to bolster a sagging self-image. An insecure scientist might practice imagining himself in the role of a successful professional in his own field—Albert Einstein, let's say, or, if he prefers a neater-looking appearance, Robert Oppenheimer.

"Limits on learning are self-imposed," says Dr. Schleicher. Make the sky your limit by keeping your thinking powers fit.

Chapter 61

Natural Sparks
to Get Your
Energy Sizzling

Richard Curtis may have done what hitherto has been thought impossible. He may have discovered a perpetual-motion machine: himself.

In the morning he teaches creative writing and journalism at a private boys' school in Connecticut. In the afternoon, he's a chimney sweep—The Sultan of Soot, as he's listed in the Yellow Pages. At night, he grades papers, books chimney-cleaning appointments and attends committee meetings. In his spare time, he is a competitive rower and coach, a writer (one book published, two more on the way), and he's teaching himself to play the piano.

In short, Richard Curtis usually wrings 20 waking hours out of each day, sleeping catnap-style for only about 4. It's a schedule that would leave most of us with eyelids permanently at half-mast, but Richard Curtis says he never runs out of energy.

Wringing 20 waking hours out of each day.

"I love it," he says. "I keep discovering something else that fascinates me. I never stop to think if I have the energy for it. When you love something, it creates its own energy. In fact, your energy level can depend on how much you love life in general. I mean, if you're at a good party, you don't leave when it's still going great."

High-Energy Living
Is Not Just for a Lucky Few

There are some who would say Richard Curtis is a genetic anomaly, a man who moves to the ticking of a different clock. And they would be right—in part. "We all come with different energy levels," says Charles Kuntzleman, Ed.D., author of *Maximum Personal Energy.* "Some people have God-given high-level energy even though they do everything wrong, just as some people are born beautiful and some are born average."

How to beat your genetic programming.

It's true that Richard Curtis is the recipient of some genetic good fortune. But that's not his only edge. He improves on what nature gave him by leading a full, active life, doing things he loves. He has a good reason to get up in the morning and a good reason not to be in such a hurry to go to bed at night.

Fourteen Ways to Boost Your Energy Levels

Like Richard Curtis, you can beat your genetic programming, too. You may not be able to go from a shuffle to a sprint, but you can quicken your step. And you can start right now.

Decide what you want to do—then do it.

1. Lead the active life. It's the best lesson you can learn from Richard Curtis: Energy begets energy. Don't give in to boredom and malaise. Get up and do something you really want to do, even if you think you're too tired to do it. You'll be amazed at how much energy you really have. "Love is energy, being creative is energy, health is energy," says Harold H. Bloomfield, M.D., author of *The Holistic Way to Health and Happiness.* "The more good things you do for yourself, the more energetic you're going to be." In fact, the very act of *doing* can help you shake the ennui that made you tired in the first place.

How to rev up by working out.

2. Get physical. A regular aerobic workout, one that gets your pulse rate galloping, won't poop you out. It will actually pump you up. You'll have more oxygen-carrying hemoglobin in your red blood cells. Your heart will eject more blood with each beat, so it has to work less to circulate it through your body.

Your skeletal muscles will gain a greater capacity to use oxygen, and your muscle cells will be better able to burn fats as fuel. With your trained muscles able to use oxygen more efficiently, your breathing rate drops, so you won't get winded so easily. In fact, your whole body will work so efficiently you'll have even more energy to expend. Not only that, studies have shown that regular exercise can help you beat stress, one of life's biggest energy zappers.

3. Take a minibreak. When your motor's about to die on the expressway, you rev it up. When you're about to die at your desk at quarter of three in the afternoon, you've got to put a figurative pedal to the metal. Get up! Remind your body that it's awake. Do a few tension-relieving exercises, advises Dr. Kuntzleman. Shrug your shoulders, roll your head or, better yet, do a lap around the office, the building or the block.

Stretch away tension.

4. Know thyself. Schedule tough jobs for when you're at your energy peak. If you're full of spit and polish in the morning, don't tackle the Great American Novel at 10:00 P.M., after a busy day at the office. If you're a night owl, don't set your alarm for an early start on refinishing the kitchen cabinets. Listen to the ticking of your own biological clock, say the experts. Otherwise, you'll wind up fatigued from all that swimming upstream.

5. Lose weight. Picture yourself climbing two flights of stairs with a bowling ball under each arm. It would be a lot easier without them, wouldn't it? If you're overweight, you're doing roughly the equivalent every time you exert yourself. "Physically carrying 30 to 40 extra pounds is going to make you more fatigued," says Dr. Kuntzleman.

Get rid of the bowling balls.

That's just common sense. But obesity loads you with a weight of a different kind. "It can wear you out psychologically, too," he says. "It affects your perception of yourself, making you self-conscious, which is energy draining. You're always mentally defending yourself: 'Hey, I'm okay, my waistline is just a little large.' "

6. Check your iron levels. Your body uses iron to help manufacture hemoglobin, a protein in red blood cells that carries oxygen to all your tissues and cells. Deprived of that oxygen, your cells—and you—will soon be running on empty. Menstruating women and people over 65 are particularly prone to iron deficiency, which, even before it becomes full-blown anemia, can lead to chronic, foot-dragging fatigue. Iron is abundant in meats, especially beef liver, and to a lesser extent in foods like sunflower seeds, broccoli, apricots, almonds and raisins.

Replace potassium and magnesium.

7. Grab a handful of nuts. If you're feeling fatigued, especially after a strenuous exercise program, you may have what one medical expert calls "the mineral blues"—a deficiency of potassium and magnesium in muscle cells. Both minerals can be lost through sweat. When stores drop below normal, even a mild deficiency can bring on fatigue. Both potassium and magnesium are abundant in nuts and soybeans. You'll also find potassium plentiful in fruits and vegetables and magnesium in grains.

Is a vitamin C deficiency slowing you down?

8. Take C and see. Several medical studies have suggested that people whose diets are lacking in vitamin C grow fatigued more quickly than those whose C intakes are high. There's a bonus with C. It also helps increase your absorption of dietary iron, sometimes as much as 300 percent. But don't pop C—or any other nutrient supplement for that matter—expecting it to act like a pep pill. It will only have its energizing effect if your lack of energy is the result of a nutrient lack. Besides, food is the best source of any nutrient.

9. Eat a light lunch. It's 2:00 in the afternoon and you and the pile of work on your desk have slid into a mirror-image slump. What happened? You might review your lunch menu. If you ate a heavy meal, you're the victim of postprandial dip, characterized by a drop in body temperature, blood sugar, work efficiency and mood. In many countries, lunch is followed by a siesta. If you can't get a daily nap written into your benefit package, most experts advise eating a light meal—raw veggies or salads—at noon.

10. Eat a good breakfast. Depending on how much you toss and turn, you can use up 500 to 600 calories getting a good night's sleep. Even if you don't wake up hungry, your body has still been depleted of the vitamins and minerals that give you the energy to tackle a brand-new day. If you don't eat breakfast, warns Max M. Novich, M.D., coauthor of *The High-Energy Diet for Dynamic Living,* you're likely to "drag along" all morning, feeling tired, headachy and with a touch of low blood sugar.

Why skipping breakfast is a drag.

11. Make upbeat friends. Did you ever get trapped in a conversation with a chronic griper? As each complaint drones into your consciousness, you feel yourself turning to lead, cell by cell. Unhappy, unpleasant people are downers who sap your energy. You can't avoid them entirely, short of taking up residence in a cave. The next best thing is to make them the minority in your circle of acquaintances. Fill your life with energetic, upbeat people, and you'll be known by the company you keep. "People who love, have fun and care give you good feelings about yourself and your energy levels," says Dr. Kuntzleman.

12. Get enough B's. If you have even a marginal deficiency of B-complex vitamins, you could find yourself with a case of the blahs. The B's work together to help convert proteins, carbohydrates and fats into fuel. Without them, you're out of gas.

Beating the blahs with adequate B vitamins.

13. Give yourself something to look forward to. Anticipation of good things to come can give you a burst of energy that can very nearly rouse you out of a coma. That sense of excitement is like "an amphetamine response," says Michael Liebowitz, M.D., author of *The Chemistry of Love.* "When we are looking forward to things, especially when pursuing a valued goal, we liven up, have more energy and concentrate better."

14. Get away from it all. You'll learn the secret of this energy booster when you get back from it.

Vacations put your life in a new context.

Taking a vacation—whether it's skiing in the Alps or boating on the local lake—is a sure-fire way to recharge.

"The reason is pretty simple," says ball-of-fire Richard Curtis, who explored the vacation phenomenon in his book *Taking Off.* "Getting away from it all gets you out of your rut. Putting some distance between yourself and whatever you're working on makes you feel relaxed. In addition to physically separating yourself from your problems, you're opening yourself up to other things. Essentially you're taking your mind off one thing and putting it on something else. When you come back, you've gotten yourself into the mode of seeing new things. You begin to see your life in a new context, and that's invigorating."

Chapter 62

On the Mend
with Better Nutrition

One minute, Kathleen Lynch was the picture of good health and vitality. The next, the 27-year-old Delaware woman was as close to death as she'd ever been in her life. While stopped by the side of a road to fix a flat tire on her car, she was hit by a car. The impact left her head "looking like hamburger," as she puts it.

Thanks to her youth and good health and a diet emphasizing protein, fresh fruit, vegetables and whole grains, Kathleen is alive and well today.

The only evidence of her injury is a thin scar across her forehead. Doctors had said she would require three months in the hospital to recover. She was discharged in 16 days. "They were all amazed at how quickly I recovered, but none of the doctors wanted to believe it had anything to do with nutrition," Mrs. Lynch says. "My husband and I happen to believe that it had everything to do with nutrition."

So, apparently, do some researchers, who call trauma "the forgotten disease" simply because relatively little attention has been focused on the care and nutrition of the millions of people each year who suffer from auto accidents, burns, falls, head injuries, gunshot wounds and chainsaw accidents.

Out of the hospital in just 16 days: a story about nutrition.

The care and feeding of trauma patients.

"Emergency Rations" for Accident Victims

Certainly, important work has been done to help victims of trauma survive the crucial first few hours after injury occurs, says Ronald Birkhahn, Ph.D., associate professor of surgery and director of trauma studies at the Medical College of Ohio in Toledo.

"Helicopters, emergency medical teams, fluid therapy, antibiotics—all help the patient survive," he says. But after the excitement dies down, guess who is left to virtually fend for himself?

Vitamins and minerals are critical to survival.

"They've got him out of the emergency room, got him stabilized, and they say, well, now, he is going to recover," Dr. Birkhahn says. "But the patient doesn't recover. He ends up getting infected, his muscles waste away, and he dies, not from the initial injury but from malnutrition. That's the problem we're working on solving."

And solving it has not been easy, for a body in trauma acts much differently than a healthy body.

Faced with any severe injury, the body goes into a true emergency state. "Real trauma makes your body mobilize everything it's got in an effort to survive," says Sheldon V. Pollack, M.D., associate professor of medicine and chief of chemosurgery at Duke University School of Medicine, Durham, North Carolina. Dr. Pollack has a special interest in nutrition and wound healing.

Why you need top-notch nutrition when you're injured.

The body's energy requirements go up 25 to 100 percent higher than normal, and it immediately starts breaking down protein in the muscles to provide itself with the energy it needs to repair damaged tissues and to maintain essential organs like the heart, liver, kidneys and brain, Dr. Pollack says.

The body's stores of vitamins and minerals are mobilized, used and quickly excreted. Vitamins C, B-complex and A, zinc and calcium pour out of the body as a result of trauma. What it all adds up to is a body that's in desperate need of all the nutritional help it can get. But researchers have found extra amounts of some nutrients to be particularly crucial to repairing body tissues, preventing infection and counteracting some of the stress of trauma.

Rebuilding Broken Bodies with Protein

Absolutely essential for rebuilding body tissue is protein, which contains the amino acids needed for the body's growth and maintenance. Normally, the body breaks down protein from foods into amino acids, then reassembles them as body tissue. In intravenous or tube feeding, the proteins are already broken down into amino acids.

Certain amino acids may help alleviate the muscle wasting and tissue loss seen in trauma victims. Some may also help speed wound healing.

Can certain amino acids help rescue trauma patients?

"There have been some hypotheses that three essential amino acids, what we call branched-chain amino acids—leucine, isoleucine and valine—will help reduce the loss of body protein, because those are the three amino acids that are primarily being used for energy for the muscles," Dr. Birkhahn says.

Another amino acid, arginine, also seems to help save body tissue and to have immunity-stimulating benefits. Researchers at Sinai Hospital in Baltimore, for instance, found that adding arginine to the diets of injured rats significantly increased the rate at which reparative connective tissue, called collagen, was deposited in the wound. And once healed, wounds were more likely to stay healed.

In rats, arginine speeded up wound healing.

Arginine also minimized the quick weight loss that comes with trauma. It apparently gave the rats' immune systems a boost, increasing the weight of the thymus, a gland behind the breastbone that produces infection-fighting white blood cells. Normally, this gland tends to shrink when faced with severe trauma (*American Journal of Clinical Nutrition*).

The significance of this study, says Adrian Barbul, M.D., Sinai's assistant surgeon-in-chief, is that arginine accelerated wound-healing time beyond what is considered its normal rate. That certainly could be good news for trauma patients.

Vitamin C
Hastens Wound Healing

For injuries, the body
needs more vitamin C.

Faced with trauma, the body's stores of vitamin C are rapidly depleted. Possibly as part of the effect of being mobilized to fight injury, vitamin C goes directly to the site of the injury. This means a deficiency can appear in a matter of days, and at a time when C is needed most. In studies of postsurgical patients, blood levels dropped sharply even in patients receiving 500 milligrams a day. Doctors using vitamin C in trauma recommend that patients get doses much higher than the Recommended Dietary Allowance (RDA).

Many studies have shown that vitamin C is essential for the formation of wound-repairing collagen tissue. Vitamin C's role in bolstering the immune system is also well researched. It has been shown to increase the activity of white blood cells and to stimulate the immune response of cells under attack.

Can vitamin C benefit
burn victims?

New ways to benefit from vitamin C are still being discovered. Researchers at the New Jersey Medical School in Newark found that vitamin C helped lessen the degree of severity of burns in mice. Starting 30 minutes after being burned, the mice were given either 12.5 or 25 milligrams of vitamin C twice a day for five days. The burns of the mice in the group receiving no vitamin C were judged to be almost twice as bad as those receiving the larger amount of the vitamin. And in both supplemented groups, vitamin C kept the burns from progressing from second to third degree (*Clinical Research*).

Burn Victims Need Vitamin A

Using vitamin A to fight
trauma.

Vitamin A also plays a major role in the body's ability to fight back in the face of disaster. Body levels of vitamin A have been found to drop sharply one to three days after trauma, especially in burn victims. Enormous amounts—up to 300,000 international

units a day—have been found to be required to restore blood levels to normal. (The RDA is 4,000 international units for women and 5,000 international units
for men.) Surprisingly enough, there have been no
reports of toxicity in patients taking these large
amounts under medical supervision—although no
more than 25,000 international units should be taken
without supervision.

"When the body is injured, through infection,
physical injury, burns, disease, whatever, the immune
mechanism will begin to fail," says Merrill S. Chernov,
M.D., a Phoenix surgeon who has done research with
vitamin A and burn victims.

"For some reason, vitamin A will get the immune
mechanism activated again. Vitamin A stimulates
what we call the intercellular killing power of the
white blood cells, which are the most important
means of protection in the human body. The white
blood cells not only destroy bacteria in the blood, but
in burn patients they may engulf bacteria that are
invading through the burnt skin."

Dr. Chernov also found that vitamin A prevents
what are known as stress ulcers. In fact, it does such a
good job that it's now fairly common to see it used
preventively in burn centers.

**Burn victims taking vita-
min A had fewer stress
ulcers.**

Stress ulcers are multiple superficial ulcers that
often develop in the stomachs of people who have
been burned or severely injured. They can cause
heavy bleeding, require surgery and jeopardize a patient's chances of recovery.

Dr. Chernov studied 35 severely stressed patients—those with burns over more than 25 percent of
the body or major injury to two or more organs. He
divided them into two groups. One group received
10,000 to 400,000 international units of vitamin A a
day; the other received no supplemental vitamin A.
Evidence of stress ulcers was found in 15 of the 22
patients who did not receive vitamin A, and bleeding
was serious in 14. But stress ulcers occurred in only 2
of the 14 patients treated with vitamin A.

"Vitamin A apparently stimulates the production of mucous cells lining the stomach," Dr. Chernov says. "These cells have a very short life—only 36 hours—so the stomach is one of the first body organs to be affected in the event of serious trauma. The cells die, and the body can't manufacture new ones because it is under too much stress. Vitamin A makes these cells grow and stimulates their mucous production. The mucus protects the stomach from its own acid, and the ulcers are prevented."

Vitamin E, Too, Speeds Healing

Vitamin E has its own special function in burn and wound healing. It may indirectly help speed the healing of wounds when found in the company of vitamin A.

"Vitamin E may protect vitamin A from oxidation [breakdown] in the digestive tract and in the wound, making more vitamin A available," Dr. Pollack says.

And because it somewhat delays the formation of collagen, applying vitamin E to a wound or burn may help produce a thin, flexible scar. This effect is particularly welcome in cosmetic surgery, Dr. Pollack says, where a delicate scar line is desirable. Vitamin E also may help prevent wounds from contracting too much as they heal, which can be a crippling consequence of severe burns.

Vitamin E and cosmetic surgery.

Don't Forget Zinc and Calcium

People suffering from severe injuries, burns or extensive abdominal surgery can rapidly become deficient in zinc, which will slow the rate at which wounds heal, says Augusta Askari, Ph.D., assistant professor in the Department of Surgery at the Medical College of Ohio. Dr. Askari's specialty is the role of trace minerals in the nutrition of trauma victims.

"Zinc is an essential nutrient," she says. "The body requires zinc to make the protein it uses to repair damaged tissue. The need for zinc increases greatly when the body needs to heal itself."

Just how much more zinc the injured body needs is something Dr. Askari would like to find out. "You can't just give a lot of zinc," she says. The reason is that zinc competes with other minerals that are important in healing, including copper, which is needed for the formation of blood vessels. Excess zinc can also retard bone healing because it interferes with the body's ability to use calcium.

The body uses zinc in damage control.

Broken bones can mean double trouble if you are not getting enough calcium in your diet to heal them properly. Being immobilized with an injury can cause a patient to lose up to 1.1 percent of his bone mass in just one week.

Mending bones with calcium.

If you're not getting enough calcium in your diet to heal a fractured bone, your body will dissolve this mineral from your other bones to use to mend the broken one. The result is that you'll have less calcium in *all* your bones, which could lead to more fractures, says Joseph Lane, M.D., professor of orthopedics at Cornell University Medical School and chief of orthopedics at Memorial Sloan-Kettering Cancer Center in New York City.

Many people with bone fractures show signs of having been calcium deficient long before their break, Dr. Lane says. "Many have metabolic bone diseases like osteoporosis, associated with a chronic calcium deficiency," he says. "Often, it's not until a fracture occurs that the deficiency is recognized, and sometimes not even then.

Broken bones may signal a calcium deficiency.

"Anyone with a fracture, young or old, should be getting at least their RDA of calcium, and a little bit more," he says. Women past menopause should be taking 1,500 milligrams of calcium a day.

Chapter 63

Let's Put "Recovery" on the Menu

When you think of malnutrition, does your mind conjure up images of hungry children in faraway places like Africa or Asia? After all, it's not very likely that you'd ever experience such a thing firsthand. Unless you happen to spend a couple of weeks in a hospital, that is.

"Roughly half the patients in some general hospital wards have been found to exhibit protein calorie malnutrition," says Marion Nestle, Ph.D., formerly associate dean, School of Medicine, University of California, San Francisco. "That observation has been repeated in at least ten studies, ranging from general medical and surgical patients to pediatric patients and residents in nursing homes. And the longer someone is in a hospital, the higher the risk for malnutrition."

Malnutrition: It happens in hospitals.

Malnutrition Where You Least Expect It

According to a study by Roland L. Weinsier, M.D., Dr.P.H., and co-workers at the University of Alabama, a large proportion of patients hospitalized for two weeks or longer have a high likelihood of malnutrition. And the study took place in a teaching hospital, where you'd expect the care to be the very best (*American Journal of Clinical Nutrition*).

"Protein calorie malnutrition is basically starvation," explains Dr. Nestle. "It refers to the loss of muscle mass and body protein that occurs when people just don't have enough to eat.

"Starvation affects every organ system and every metabolic process. The effects we're most concerned about in hospitals or nursing homes are the effects on the immune system. People who have been starving are well known to be more susceptible to infection. In fact, the major cause of death in hunger strikers or people who have been fasting is pneumonia, because their resistance to infection has gone down.

Starving under medical care.

"In addition, people often lose their appetite during an infection. They don't want to eat or can't eat. So you get into a cycle where the infection makes the malnutrition worse, and the malnutrition makes the immune response worse."

A Woeful Lack of Vitamins and Minerals

Of course, vitamin and mineral deficiencies accompany starvation. But they can happen on their own, too. Researchers in Colorado, for instance, found diminished iron stores in 40 percent of nursing home patients studied. And the incidence of iron lack was greater for nursing home patients than for residents of private homes. Iron deficiency is dangerous because it can cause anemia. "Whether the cause of a given deficiency is nutritional or pathological, nutritional intervention is a crucial part of programs designed for comprehensive care of the elderly," say the researchers (*American Journal of Clinical Nutrition*).

Risking nutrient deficiencies in nursing homes.

A study in Ireland found vitamin D deficiency to be common among the elderly and found lower vitamin D levels in institutionalized people than in individuals living at home. Part of the problem was that more of the institutionalized people were confined indoors. Without exposure to the sun, their bodies could not produce enough vitamin D, and their dietary intake was inadequate. Low levels of vitamin D, say the re-

A not-so-rare problem among the elderly: vitamin D deficiency.

searchers, predispose to the development of osteomalacia, a bone disease. And a broken bone is the last
thing an elderly person needs. "The value of increased vitamin D intake, either by direct supplementation or augmented fortification of foodstuffs with
vitamin D, is manifest," they say (*American Journal of
Clinical Nutrition*).

Why is malnutrition so rampant in hospitals and
nursing homes? It's a multifaceted problem. "The
main reason why patients in hospitals are malnourished is because they're sick," says Dr. Nestle. "Cancer, surgery, infection—any severe illness or injury is
stressful to the body and raises the nutrient requirements."

There are other reasons, too. Someone recovering from gastrointestinal surgery, for instance, may
not be able to eat. And certain diseases can cause
nutrient deficiencies. So can drugs that induce an-

**Reasons for hospital
malnutrition.**

Good Nutrition
Adds Power to Flu Shots

Good nutrition can help prevent flu, even if
you've had a flu shot. Researchers in Canada
gave flu vaccine to 30 malnourished elderly
patients and then divided them into two
groups. The first group learned to eat more
nutritiously and received supplements. The
second group got no dietary improvement or
supplementation. Four weeks after the flu
shot, the nutritionally boosted patients had
significantly more antibodies to flu virus than
those whose nutrition wasn't improved.

"The correction of . . . undernutrition in
the elderly may be expected to improve immune responses," say the researchers, "and
perhaps result in better protective immunity"
(*British Medical Journal*).

orexia or interfere with absorption, utilization or excretion of nutrients.

"There's a whole slew of drugs that can make you develop a vitamin deficiency," says Herman Baker, Ph.D., professor of preventive medicine and medicine at the New Jersey Medical School. "Levodopa, a drug used in the treatment of parkinsonism, for instance, interferes with vitamin B_6. Anticonvulsants, barbiturates, anticoagulants, diuretics, tranquilizers and prolonged use of antibiotics can all interfere with vitamins. The problem is of particular concern among the elderly because about 25 percent of all prescriptions in the United States go to the elderly."

But the aged are at risk for other reasons, too. "The elderly don't absorb enough vitamins out of their food," explains Dr. Baker. "They suffer from a chronic hypovitaminemia [low levels of vitamins in the blood], usually involving the B vitamins. It's a subclinical vitamin deficiency, which means there are no clinical signs. But it's very debilitating because it doesn't permit them to feel well, concentrate or function properly, and it has a dire effect on their ability to resist disease and infection. That can be very deleterious, especially at an old age." You can see why nutritional problems might become magnified in nursing homes, where people tend to be older and more seriously ill.

Not absorbing enough vitamins and minerals.

Many Meals Go Untouched

But how can someone actually *starve* in a hospital or nursing home? "Patients in hospitals don't want to eat because they don't feel like it," explains Dr. Nestle. "People in hospitals are just not ravenously hungry." Add to that the fact that many patients find institutional food tasteless, bland and uninteresting, plus poorly prepared and frequently cold, and you can see why people don't eat as well as they should.

Why is institutional food so bad? "The economics of hospital food are very important," explains Dr.

Why many patients shun hospital food.

Nestle. "Hospitals are paid for these days by fixed room charges. Food is part of that charge. So the object of the game from the hospital director's point of view is to keep the cost of the food to a minimum, in order to keep the fixed room charge as low as possible." The reason institutional food is so bad is that everybody's trying to keep costs down.

Not getting a chance to eat.

Another reason people don't eat in hospitals is that they frequently don't get the chance. "When people have tests over and over again, they can miss meals," says Alice L. Tobias, Ed.D., R.D., director of the nutrition program at Herbert H. Lehman College of the City University of New York. "Someone must go out of their way to make sure a replacement meal is delivered.

"In addition, patients might not eat enough if they don't see foods they like. In cities, for instance, some hospitals may cater to one ethnic group and some of the patients may be in another. That's why I think the selective menu (with a number of choices) is very important. But it's not available everywhere."

Vitamins and Minerals Not on the Menu

Does hospital food have enough nutrients?

But even if patients eat a normal amount of food, they may not get what they need. John P. Sheehan, M.D., then at the Cleveland Clinic, found that meals in two different hospitals provided only 200 to 300 milligrams of magnesium daily; the Recommended Dietary Allowance (RDA) is 300 to 350 milligrams. Dr. Sheehan identified 35 magnesium-deficient patients over an 18-month period. The deficiencies went unnoticed because the symptoms—depression, sleepiness and weakness—were attributed to old age or illness.

Another study of hospital food by researchers at Washington State University turned up thiamine (B_1), riboflavin (B_2) and vitamin C values low enough that the researchers "suggest that it may be advisable to consider vitamin supplementation for hospital patients, especially those on restricted diets or with limited appetites, whose needs may not be met by institutional foods" (*Journal of the American Dietetic Association*).

Should hospital patients take supplements?

And when researchers at the Veterans Administration Hospital in Washington, D.C., analyzed meals for zinc content, they found that the regular hospital diet provided 97 percent of the RDA for zinc, while the vegetarian diet provided 81 percent and the renal (kidney-patient) diet provided only 49 percent of the allowance! "In view of the osteomalacia problems apparent in kidney disease and experimental evidence that zinc may be involved in bone metabolism, the zinc intake of renal patients should be more carefully monitored," they say.

"The allowances assume that the individual is healthy.... [However] many hospital patients undergo alterations in zinc metabolism and may require more dietary zinc than healthy individuals. Yet [the] regular diet did not provide any extra zinc beyond the recommended allowances" (*Journal of the American Dietetic Association*).

Unfortunately, doctors are still largely unaware of the problem. "In the hospital, when you're dealing with someone who's acutely ill, and you're the physician, then your main concern is to take care of that illness," says Dr. Nestle. "Because of this, sometimes the doctor forgets about nutrition. Similarly, in a nursing home you might be most concerned about keeping the patient clean or infection free and not pay attention to the total amount of food that's being taken in."

Why some doctors forget about nutrition.

"Although the terms *iatrogenic* and *hospital-induced* have been used in connection with malnutrition, they do not imply malicious intent or callous disregard for a patient's welfare," explain Dr. Weinsier and his colleagues. "Nevertheless, malnutrition does occur as a result of what the physician does or does not do. To a considerable extent, physician-induced malnutrition is caused by emphasis on some complex modern treatment program, while fundamental principles of nutrition remain in the background.... Whatever the cause may be, the result is the same: Many patients fail to receive the full benefit of existing nutritional knowledge" (*Alabama Journal of Medical Sciences*).

Overlooking the clues to bad nutrition.

In a survey of nutritional practices in two teaching hospitals in New York City, Dr. Tobias and a coworker reported discouraging findings. In the 67 patients studied, nutritional problems were common. But nutritional status was not adequately assessed by the physician or dietitian, and often the patients' nutritional problems went untreated. Many of the clues suggestive of nutritional problems—alcoholism, gastrointestinal problems, kidney disease, excessive weight loss—often went unheeded.

Nutrition should be an integral part of medical care.

"This preliminary survey provides evidence that many basic principles of nutrition are neglected in the diagnosis and care of hospital inpatients," say the researchers. "Major omissions include the failure to obtain a dietary history when indicated, to provide specific dietary management and appropriate vitamin and mineral supplementation in a variety of clinical situations, to record height and weight, and to give nutritional counseling" (*Journal of the American Dietetic Association*).

What You Can Do to Prevent Hospital Malnutrition

When someone you know enters a hospital or nursing home, you like to take comfort in the fact that they're in good hands. But it's becoming clear that it's dangerous to assume they'll be given adequate nutritional care. So what can you do?

"A blood test is of prime importance in the elderly to detect marginal vitamin deficiencies as well as acute vitamin deficiencies where there are clinical signs," says Dr. Baker. "The best thing to do is find out what they're deficient in and see that they're treated, without waiting for clinical signs to appear."

"If you have a family member in the hospital who's not eating, it's important that you go feed him [or her]," recommends Dr. Tobias. "If it's a hospital that has a selective menu, make sure it's filled out, so he gets what he likes. Speak to the dietitian who has responsibility for that patient. Describe his likes and dislikes, ethnic background, cultural patterns, food allergies, food intolerances, his previous diet and any medical conditions the staff might not know about. If he's on a special diet, don't bring in food unless you check with the nutritionist to make sure it's not contraindicated."

How to make sure you're properly nourished in the hospital.

If he's not on a special diet, though, food from home might be just what the patient ordered. "If the patient can eat and has relatives or friends who are willing to bring more interesting foods—that should be encouraged," says Dr. Nestle. "I really believe in patients taking responsibility for their own illness. Sometimes they can't, but maybe their relatives can. Or their friends can.

An alternative to hospital food: bringing food from home.

"I think it's very important to ask for a nutritional assessment if somebody's going to be in the hospital for a long period of time. Get an estimation of their requirements, and then discuss with the physician how those nutrients will be supplied. Then monitor to make sure that it's being done," she says.

"Some of the major teaching hospitals are now using nutrition support teams," Dr. Tobias says. "It's a sophisticated team consisting of a registered dietitian, a physician, possibly a pharmacist, a nurse and a technician. They screen to find patients at risk of nutritional deficiencies, perform tests to determine their status and make sure they're given what they need. It's a relatively new concept, though, and in a hospital with a staff of two dietitians, you're not going to find somebody trained in that area."

A new approach to nutrition in hospitals.

The dawning of nutritional awareness.

Awareness of nutritional considerations is coming slowly to doctors. According to Dr. Weinsier and his colleagues, "Hospital-associated malnutrition is being disclosed with a heretofore unexpected high frequency.... This fact changes the mistaken impression that hospital malnutrition is overrated and reserved for the unfortunate few who have malignant disease. Conversely, too often patients had been expected to tolerate illness well and to recuperate rapidly without regard for the importance of nutritional support. It is now realized that conventional forms of medical and surgical therapy may not be sufficient: that antibiotics do not replace host defenses, that sterile gauzes and sutures do not heal wounds, and that even the most sophisticated life-support systems, when applied out of the context of adequate nutritional support, will neither sustain nor revitalize the malnourished patient."

Can We Defeat the Aging Factor with Diet?

The Aging Scenario. It is as familiar and predictable as the outcome of a John Wayne movie. It is human planned obsolescence. At a certain age—different for each of us—we begin to run down. Our hair drains of its color, our skin sags like melted candle wax, our hands gnarl and ache. In time, we build a battlement of medicine bottles to repel the illnesses that attack us like a ravaging horde. In the end, the invaders win.

But there are scientists who challenge the inevitabilities of aging, who believe that anywhere along the line, this scenario can be rewritten, often by something as simple as diet. And they have set about to do it. They have begun by taking the eraser ends of their pencils to one of the most critical manifestations of human aging—the decline of the immune system.

Revitalizing a declining immune system.

Keeping Your Immune System Young

A hundred years ago, scientists discovered an interesting phenomenon. As people grew older, their organ weights changed. The lungs, liver and brain weigh slightly less in an 80-year-old than they do in a 20-year-old. And the thymus actually shrinks to a mere fraction of its original size.

It was only about 20 years ago that that phenomenon went from interesting to significant. That was

Looking for a mechanism of aging.

The thymus: base camp for an army of white knights.

when scientists learned the function of the thymus, a flat, pinkish gray, two-lobed gland that nestles behind the sternum and lungs high in the chest. Put simply, the thymus distributes and nourishes (with its hormones) white blood cells, called lymphocytes, that act as the body's army against disease.

The thymus appears to be the command headquarters for an army of cells known as T-lymphocytes, which, when they meet a foreign invader like a virus or cancer cell, can be stimulated to divide into larger, active cells that react with the invader and kill it. At the same time, the T-cells seem to stimulate other parts of the immune system into action: the macrophages, PacMan-like scavengers that literally gobble up the enemy (known as antigens), and B-cells, which the T-cells encourage to produce antibodies against the antigen.

If your immune system is working at its optimum, right now the T-cells in your body could be leading a battle against cancer or infection without your even knowing it.

In aging, the thymus, at its maximum when we are teenagers, shrinks markedly, leaving us with less of the nourishing thymic hormones and fewer young T-cells to replenish our aged army. The aged T-cells decline in their ability to reproduce and stimulate the B-cells to produce antibodies. "As a unifying concept, what is happening is that the control of the immune system begins to decline with age," states William Adler, M.D., chief of the clinical immunology section, Gerontology Research Center, National Institute of Aging, Baltimore.

The Role of Diet

This shrinking of the thymus and resultant decline in T-cell function is believed to be largely responsible for the increasing illness and death rates among the elderly, particularly for cancer and infection, which until now have been considered simply part of the aging process.

Fortunately, that assumption has been called into question. "There is at least a distinct possibility that some illness and abnormalities we are seeing in the immune response in the elderly may not be a part of the normal aging process, that there are environmental factors, particularly diet, that may have a causal role to play," says Ranjit Kumar Chandra, M.D., of the Health Sciences Center, Memorial University of Newfoundland, and the Department of Immunology at the Dr. Charles A. Janeway Child Health Center in Newfoundland.

A bright possibility: To some extent, the aging process may be controllable.

In 1984, Dr. Chandra organized an international conference on nutrition, immunity and illness in the elderly, drawing scientists from North America, Europe, Scandinavia and even Japan to St. Johns, Newfoundland, to discuss the possibilities for intervening in the process that leaves the elderly so vulnerable to disease.

One prime area of research involves the thymic hormones. Researcher William Ershler, M.D., now at the University of Wisconsin, has studied the effects of the thymic hormone thymosin on human lymphocytes in the test tube. When he added a dose of thymosin to test tubes containing white blood cells of aged subjects who had received shots for tetanus and influenza, the cells of the elderly were stimulated to produce a normal amount of antibodies, something they were unable to do before. Dr. Ershler says he hopes to test thymosins outside the test tube in elderly people inoculated against flu. But it may be some time before thymosins become the treatment of choice for the aging immune system.

Boosting immunity with thymic hormones.

Zinc Is Critical to Peak Immunity

Another area of immune research focuses on zinc. The thymus is chock-full of zinc, which is essential to both protein synthesis and cell division. And the efficient working of the immune system depends on the rapid proliferation of cells.

Zinc was the answer to a paradox that confronted Robert Good, M.D., Ph.D., professor and chairman of the Department of Pediatrics at the University of South Florida, St. Petersburg campus, and physician-in-chief of All Children's Hospital. In his fieldwork among malnourished children, he and his colleagues noted that malnutrition was accompanied by a profound decline in immunity. Children whose calories and protein were restricted were far more susceptible to disease and infection. Yet, in well-known laboratory studies, the restriction of protein and calories in animals prolonged their lives.

Correcting an immune problem with zinc.

What Dr. Good discovered was that it was neither the protein nor calorie deprivation that caused the drop in immunological function, but the lack of zinc. And other researchers have found that it is possible to correct the immunological malfunction just by giving the children zinc, before correcting anything else, says Dr. Good.

Dr. Chandra, who has also done extensive field research on immunodeficiency among malnourished children, tested the immune response in a group of elderly people whose diets were supplemented with zinc for six weeks.

A test for disease resistance that many fail.

He gave them a skin test, injecting a variety of antigens largely derived from bacteria and molds into the superficial layers of their skin. In a normal, healthy person, at least one of the spots should show a swollen, inflamed reaction in about two days, meaning the lymphocytes are proliferating and the immune system has swung into action. It is not unusual for many elderly people to show no reaction to the skin test, indicating their immune systems are not mobilized to fight a threatening disease. Not surprisingly, this lack of reaction is a fairly accurate predictor of death. "Those elderly individuals who are found to be anergic [nonreactive] often die in the next three to five years," says Dr. Chandra.

But zinc may be able to change those odds. In Dr. Chandra's zinc-supplemented group, at least half increased their number of responses to the skin test, indicating there was some new life in their immune systems.

Boosting immune power in the elderly with zinc.

A Little Zinc Goes a Long Way

More recent research strengthens the case for zinc. A group of scientists in Italy has discovered that at least one of the thymic hormones, called FTS, is not so much affected by the shrinking of the thymus as it is by the kind of marginal zinc deficiencies so prevalent among the elderly.

They noticed that children with Down's syndrome and elderly people had a similar lack of active circulating FTS and zinc. The finding intrigued them because Down's syndrome children "show at an early age normal subjective factors of aging, such as auto-immunity, an increase in leukemia, the graying of hair, and cataracts," says researcher Claudio Franceschi, M.D., professor of immunology at the University of Padua, Italy.

That led him to consider the possibility that the shrinking thymus was taking the blame for a failure of the FTS hormone. "The glands work," says the researcher, "but produce inactive molecules." Blood samples taken from the two groups turned up a substance that was capable of inhibiting the activity of FTS in the test tube. When zinc was added to the culture, it induced concentrations of FTS comparable to those of normal, healthy young people.

Can zinc make the thymus gland young again?

What Dr. Franceschi and his colleagues believe is that FTS is biologically bound to zinc and needs it to be active and effective. Dr. Franceschi speculates that this inhibitory factor found in the blood samples was FTS hormone not bound to zinc. "When we added zinc, the hormone was able to bind itself to the zinc molecules to become active," he says.

But the clinical results speak more than the test-tube studies. When the Down's syndrome children were given relatively small amounts of zinc as a dietary supplement (1 milligram per kilogram [22 pounds] of body weight), the results were remarkable. "Though it's difficult to measure," says Dr. Franceschi, "the children had less infections and lost fewer days of school. We think this is directly related to the zinc."

Vitamins E and C Boost Immunity

But zinc isn't the only nutrient under investigation. Several researchers are probing the effects of vitamin E on the aging immune system. One of them is Simin Meydani, a scientist with a unique pedigree—she is a veterinarian with a Ph.D. in human nutrition. Dr. Meydani, a consultant at the U.S. Department of Agriculture's Human Nutrition Center at Tufts University in Boston, tested vitamin E on immune responsiveness in aged mice.

In mice, vitamin E boosted immune response.

"We supplemented aged mice with vitamin E and compared the effects by measuring different parameters of immune response," she explains. The supplemented mice showed an improvement in their responses to skin tests, similar to those given by Dr. Chandra to his elderly human subjects. And in the test tube, lymphocyte proliferation was significantly improved by vitamin E supplementation.

And Dr. Meydani thinks she and her colleagues obtained those results because vitamin E inhibits substances called prostaglandins, which can significantly influence the effectiveness of the immune system. "Prostaglandins derive from polyunsaturated fatty acids and, though they're not hormones, they act like hormones. They have a lot of different functions. In the immune system, they generally have an inhibitory effect, and vitamin E appears to inhibit the synthesis of prostaglandins," she explains.

Another group of scientists in Belgium tested the effects of another potential immunity booster, vitamin C, in a group of healthy volunteers over 70. One group was treated for a month with intramuscular injections of 500 milligrams of vitamin C—many times the Recommended Dietary Allowance—while the other group was treated with a placebo injection of saline solution.

Can vitamin C boost immunity in the elderly?

The group that received the vitamin C had better skin test responses to tuberculin antigens and, in the test tube, their lymphocytes were more active when exposed to a stimulatory substance. One of the reasons for the results may be the role vitamin C plays in helping thymic hormones in their job of changing immature, inactive T-lymphocytes into cells ready to battle disease, the researchers suggest (*Gerontology*).

Vitamins and Minerals for Lifelong Resistance

The practical implications of this exciting research are obvious. It could mean a major reediting of the aging scenario. It is particularly important now because the world's population is graying.

"In the year 2020 the proportion of the elderly will increase to at least 15 percent of the population of North America and Europe," says Dr. Chandra. "Even at present, though they constitute only about 10 percent of the population, they use up at least one-third of the health-care dollars, perhaps more. If we can make any dent in the illness of this age group, we are likely to save a considerable amount of health-care costs. My own feeling is that if we can identify those individuals who have nutritional problems that lead to immune deficiencies and can correct those nutritional problems, we can expect an improvement in immunity and also, hopefully, a reduction in illness."

Nutrition and the graying of the world's population.

Chapter 65

More Good News on Nutrition and Aging

So you've left dissipated youth and its wild excesses behind. You've reached whatever the current generation considers middle age—anywhere from 40 to 60. You're on top of the hill, enjoying the view, and you want to be able to stay there a good long time. You want the second half of your life to be as healthy and active as possible.

Slowing "old age" in the middle years.

Your concerns are shared by scientists exploring the connection between aging and nutrition. These researchers, several of whom presented their work at the Bristol-Myers/Tufts University Symposium on Nutrition and Aging in 1985, are discovering that many diseases traditionally associated with aging are strongly influenced by other factors, especially poor nutrition. They're looking at the possibility of increased nutrient needs for older adults. And they're seeing that any good nutritional program intended to lighten the load of old age is best started during middle age—before you head down the hill.

A Diet for the Sunset Years

It's well known that older people are at higher risk for developing low nutrient levels, even when they're healthy, educated and well off.

Why older people are at risk for nutrient deficiencies.

One reason for this is simply a matter of numbers, says Walter Mertz, M.D., director of the U.S. Department of Agriculture's (USDA) Human Nutrition Research Center in Beltsville, Maryland. "As they age, people eat less and less, until at about age 70 they're getting 20 percent fewer calories than they were at age 40. Their average calorie intake becomes too low to meet the Recommended Dietary Allowance [RDA] for a number of nutrients." Combine this with less-than-ideal food choices and you're setting the stage for the marginal intakes found among older adults for calcium, B complex, vitamins C and A, zinc, iron, copper, chromium, even protein.

Minerals for Young Bones

Dr. Mertz is particularly interested in pinpointing the consequences of chronic marginal intakes of trace minerals like zinc, copper, chromium and silicon (an element proved necessary for animals but not humans).

Zinc, copper and silicon, for instance, are important in maintaining bone tissue. Dr. Mertz would like to see if people with osteoporosis are deficient in these trace elements. "We must get away from focusing just on calcium while we ignore other nutrients involved in osteoporosis," he says. "This condition may be the result of multiple deficiencies and requires a total nutritional approach."

Osteoporosis: Is it caused by multiple deficiencies?

While supplements may help, they aren't always the answer, Dr. Mertz says. "The ideal solution would be to increase your activity level as much as you can, to boost your appetite and food intake," he says.

A Bone Builder in Milk and Sunshine

People with osteoporosis may also have osteomalacia, says Michael F. Holick, M.D., Ph.D., director of the Vitamin D and Bone Metabolism Laboratory at the USDA Human Nutrition Research Center on Aging at Tufts University in Boston.

Osteomalacia is a vitamin D-deficiency disease that keeps bone tissue from mineralizing and becoming hard. It's common in northern Europe, where milk

"Soft bones disease": It may be more common than you think.

is not fortified with vitamin D. It was thought uncommon in the United States, but that's not what Dr. Holick found when he collaborated in a survey of patients coming into Massachusetts General Hospital with hip fractures. "We found 40 percent were vitamin D deficient, and 30 percent had clear signs of osteomalacia," he says.

Getting this vitamin's maximum RDA of 400 international units is sufficient, Dr. Holick says. That's the amount found in most multivitamin tablets, or in four eight-ounce glasses of fortified milk. Another source of vitamin D is sunlight. (Vitamin D is made in the skin on exposure to sunlight, but this ability decreases with age.) Wearing a sunscreen of an SPF of 8 or more will block vitamin D production, so Dr. Holick suggests waiting 10 to 30 minutes (but before sunburning occurs) before applying.

How to get enough daily vitamin D.

Vitamins That Keep Your Skin Young

But you don't have to trade off osteoporosis for skin cancer, insists Barbara Gilchrest, M.D., chairman of the dermatology department at Boston University's School of Medicine.

Like other organs in the body, the skin's function declines as we age. It becomes dry, wrinkled and takes longer to heal. But that decline may be more a matter of diet and exposure to sunlight than to passing years, Dr. Gilchrest says.

Slow down aging skin.

"Diet and exposure to sun probably cause most of the changes we think of as aging. We know the sun can damage cell membranes and genetic structure and that diet can exert positive or negative effects on the skin."

Dr. Gilchrest discovered one positive nutritional effect using beta-carotene, a form of vitamin A found in green, yellow and orange vegetables. She grew human skin cells in culture, some with and some without beta-carotene. Then she exposed the cells to increasingly strong amounts of harmful sunlight. At the first two exposures (equivalent to moderate sunburn), the cells receiving the beta-carotene showed significantly fewer signs of damage than the cells without beta-carotene. "They grew normally and looked better," Dr. Gilchrest says. "In fact, they looked just like the control cells, which had received no radiation at all." At the highest level of exposure, the cells did show some damage but still not as much as those without beta-carotene.

Can beta-carotene protect you from harmful radiation?

It would be premature to translate this finding into recommendations for people, Dr. Gilchrest says. "Beta-carotene does seem to protect cells from damage, but I can't tell you how many carrots a day you should be eating." At least not yet.

As Goes the Skin, So Goes the Body

Skin might provide an easy-to-observe model for testing theories of nutrient protection for other parts of the body, Dr. Gilchrest says. "There's evidence that damage similar to the type sunlight causes to the skin is produced inside the body by some foods, chemicals and everyday metabolic reactions." Exposure to these things can cause the formation of errant molecules called free radicals, which damage body parts just as surely as they rust iron or spoil food. In fact, one "theory" of aging contends that the process is a buildup of free-radical damage to body tissues.

The theory of chemically induced aging.

That's probably not the whole story, but it's a place to start, at least when you are looking at possible nutritional intervention, says Jeffrey B. Blumberg, Ph.D., associate professor of nutrition at Tufts and acting associate director at the USDA Human Nutrition Research Center on Aging at Tufts.

"We know that animals deficient in antioxidants like vitamins E, C and A and selenium develop cell damage similar to that seen with aging," Dr. Blumberg says. "But in experiments where animals are given supplemental antioxidants, it's not clearly shown that these nutrients alter the basic aging rate. That is, it's not clear that they extend the maximum life span of the animals, although they do seem to increase the average life span because they reduce the incidence of early death from diseases like cancer."

The Power of Vitamin E

As pieces of the aging puzzle come together, though, evidence seems to indicate an increased need for certain antioxidants in some tissues. Dr. Blumberg's work so far has focused mostly on the cells of the immune system and their interaction with vitamin E.

With age, the immune system slows, leaving the body more open to infection. Important to the immune response are white blood cells known as lymphocytes. When the body senses a "foreign invader" like a bacterial infection, the lymphocytes proliferate in great numbers, then move in to destroy the bacteria. This process is slower in old than in young animals. But Dr. Blumberg found that old animals given supplemental vitamin E had a significant boost in the proliferation and activity of lymphocytes. He's now doing an experiment to see if the same thing happens in humans.

"We are giving 800 international units a day of vitamin E to healthy elderly volunteers to see whether the animal results we found are matched in humans. We'll be measuring a number of immune-response parameters, including lymphocyte proliferation," he says.

One thing Dr. Blumberg noticed in his lymphocyte study were changes in body balance of an important group of biochemicals called prostaglandins. These chemicals influence many functions in the body, including blood clotting, the production of neurotransmitters and the production of the body's own free-radical "quenchers." The balance of prostaglandins changes to an apparently less-favorable mix as we age, and Dr. Blumberg believes that this may be an important mechanism in the development of age-related declines in function. If he's right, it could mean that vitamin E's effect is pervasive throughout the body and that it could influence a number of aging-related conditions—kidney failure, cataracts, atherosclerosis, and even some nervous system and brain functions.

He's found, for instance, that the cerebellum and brain stem have high metabolic needs for vitamin E. Among other things, these two regions of the brain control reflexes. One of the first symptoms of vitamin E deficiency is the loss of reflex response. Could older people be losing their reflexes because of low vitamin E intake? Dr. Blumberg would love to find out.

Could vitamin E slow the progress of age-related conditions?

With further study, there may well be recommendations for the increased intake of antioxidants as we age, Dr. Blumberg says. "But there's a certain irony in talking about higher doses when we know that many older people are not getting even the RDA of these vitamins and minerals."

Older People Do Not Always Absorb Nutrients

Eating well does not guarantee that you are absorbing the nutrients you need, and that's especially true for older people, says Robert M. Russell, M.D., associate professor of medicine at Tufts and associate director of the USDA Human Nutrition Research Center on Aging.

Nutrients may be less readily absorbed because stomach-acid secretion slows down in many older people. In 20 percent it becomes a potential problem, according to Dr. Russell. It changes the acid content of the small bowel, where most nutrients are ab-

Poor absorption can spell trouble.

sorbed, and it prevents foods from breaking down into particles small enough to be absorbed through the lining of the bowel. It can inhibit absorption of iron, calcium and folate, and affect the bacteria in the bowel that produce vitamin B_{12}.

Unfortunately, the condition is usually symptomless. "Like high blood pressure, it's silent, with no particular discomfort," Dr. Russell says. Severe cases are discovered when the person develops pernicious anemia, a vitamin B_{12}-deficiency disease. Less serious cases are picked up by accident.

Diagnosing absorption problems.

"We know it is a prevalent condition," Dr. Russell says. "What we are trying to pin down right now is just how important this condition is to diagnose because of possible long-term nutritional effects."

The "cure" may be simple: More of whatever nutrients are being affected by this condition.

No Magic Potion—Yet

"People are always looking for it, but there simply is no single magic bullet or fountain of youth to let us stay young forever," Dr. Blumberg says. Healthy lifestyle and nutrition habits are currently about as close to the magic bullet as we can get. Some of those habits are "negatives"—don't smoke, don't overeat or eat too much fat, don't drink and drive. Others are dos—the positive, active things we can do to stay active and healthy as long as possible. Among those, researchers would list regular exercise, staying mentally active and, of course, good nutrition. "No area has greater potential for improving people's health and well-being," Dr. Blumberg says.

The real "fountain of youth" is a set of health habits anyone can adopt.

Part **VII**

COOKING
AND EATING
FOR MAXIMUM
NUTRITION

Chapter 66

The Top 25 Superfoods

There was a time when the phrase *health food* conjured up the image of a monastic meal with all the lip-smacking lusciousness of grass and moon dust.

Today, healthy foods have taken on a whole new mainstream meaning. No longer esoteric edibles available only in health food stores, they are foods fresh from the supermarket and produce stand, superfoods that medical researchers believe really may make us healthy.

Their evidence? Healthy people like the Eskimos, whose snacks of whale blubber should make them prime candidates for heart disease before the age of 40, but whose fish diet actually seems to protect their hearts from harm; Italy's Neapolitans, whose high-fiber, low-fat natural foods keep them fit; the Seventh-Day Adventists, a group composed largely of vegetarians, who serve up a menu for long life.

Diets that make a difference.

There's evidence from the laboratory, too. As reported elsewhere in this book, there is a substance in cabbage and its clan that actually may "trap" cancer-causing agents in your body before they do any harm. Plain old carrots, rich in beta-carotene, can decrease your risk of lung cancer. And something called a protease inhibitor, which is found in seeds, beans and rice, may actually be an antidote to the cancer-causing effects of a high-fat diet.

Some foods may reduce your risk of cancer.

Raiding Nature's Pantry for Health-Building Foods

Like medical researchers, we turned to the laboratory and to healthy people when we put together our own well-balanced menu of superfoods. We also filled in with some of the foods nature endowed with a cornucopia of nutrients, such as liver, oysters and green and red peppers. To make shopping easier, we included foods that, with perhaps one exception, you can find in any supermarket. And now we offer them to you with a toast: To your health!

Amaranth: A Versatile Source of Iron and Magnesium

A new grain with big benefits.

You might not find this little-known grain on your market shelves—yet. Amaranth is a food of the future. It is literally manna to the millions of malnourished people of the Third World because it is remarkably high in protein and lysine, an essential amino acid— far higher than any other cereal grain. It also contains significant amounts of iron and magnesium. And it's versatile. You can use its leaves in salad and its seeds for breakfast cereal, snacks or flour for baking.

B's from Bananas

The banana disputes the old theory that if something tastes good, it can't be good for you. Bananas are a great-tasting source of potassium, vitamin B_6 and biotin, another B vitamin. A medium-size banana contains about 100 calories, making it a delicious snack or dessert for dieters.

Beans Have Magnesium and B Vitamins

Why beans may improve your health.

If you don't know about beans, consider this: In several tests on patients with high blood lipids (a risk factor for heart disease), a bean diet brought down cholesterol and triglyceride levels significantly, with no serious side effects. Beans are also high in magnesium, a good heart mineral, and the B vitamins thiamine (B_1), B_6 and riboflavin (B_2). They're also an excellent nonmeat source of iron.

Bran's Many Benefits

One researcher calls wheat bran "the gold standard" against which the other brans, like oat and corn, are measured. Well, these days the other two are measuring up just fine. In a study of the effect of bran on constipation, corn bran was found to be therapeutically superior to wheat bran, probably because corn bran is 92 percent fiber compared to wheat bran's 52 percent fiber. Another group of researchers, at the University of Texas Health Science Center, also found in a feeding study with rats that corn bran cereal, even though it contained sucrose, helped prevent cavities.

And oat bran has been found to lower cholesterol as much as 13 percent in studies that were done by James Anderson, M.D., and his associates at the Veterans Administration Medical Center in Lexington, Kentucky.

Oat bran—a powerful cholesterol fighter.

Cabbage and Its Clan

Include broccoli, brussels sprouts and cauliflower in this happy family. They all figure prominently in the anticancer diet prescribed by the National Academy of Sciences a few years ago. They all appear to have some cancer-fighting properties, including vitamin A. And three cooked stalks of broccoli have all the Recommended Dietary Allowance (RDA) of vitamin A and five times the RDA of vitamin C, another cancer fighter, as well as calcium and potassium. Cabbage, brussels sprouts and cauliflower contain a substance that has been shown to "trap" certain carcinogens before they do any damage to the body. University of Minnesota researcher Lee Wattenberg, M.D., found that these vegetables enhance a natural detoxification system in the small intestine that keeps the carcinogen away from susceptible tissues.

Carrots: Raw Material for Vitamin A

Carrot power.

Carrots are very high in beta-carotene, a precursor of vitamin A that is associated with a decreased risk of cancer. Carrots are high in fiber and low in calories, and crunching on carrots tones and strengthens the gums.

Citrus Fruits Shine on Health

Can an orange a day keep cancer away?

A group of Florida researchers noticed an interesting statistic. Residents of southeastern Florida, many of whom have backyard citrus trees, have a lower incidence of colon and rectal cancers than people in the northern parts of the nation. The scientists at Florida Atlantic University in Boca Raton believe the secret is in the fruit. They say the vitamins A, C and E and pectin fiber have a synergistic effect that may prevent cancer.

Fish Is So Fine

Holy mackerel! Would you believe you could lower your blood pressure and cholesterol and triglyceride levels by eating mackerel and salmon? Researchers worldwide have discovered that certain types of fish—those containing eicosapentanoic acid (EPA), a fatty acid—protect against heart disease. They were tipped off by the healthy hearts of Greenland Eskimos, whose diets were otherwise high in fat. Apparently, it's a special kind of fat, which researchers at the Oregon Health Sciences University say may be "metabolically unique" and useful in controlling other fats that can clog the bloodstream.

Garlic and Onions: The Good-for-You Duo

Science probes the health benefits of garlic and onions.

These two may be bad for your breath, but they're wonderful for the rest of you. A spate of studies found these two odoriferous roots can lower cholesterol, and their oils inhibit tumor growth in the laboratory. Onions have been used to slow down platelet aggregation, or clumping, which can lead to deadly blood clots.

Herbs and Spices Add Zip to Food

Before you throw away your saltshaker and sugar bowl, consider refilling them—with herbs and spices. They're actually more flavorful substitutes. A couple of dashes of curry powder on fresh roasted nuts or popcorn, and you'll never miss the salt. And as for sweets, a panel of tasters for the American Spice Trade Association gave rave reviews to desserts and beverages flavored with spices instead of sugar and other sweeteners. They even loved blueberry short-cake sweetened with fruit juice and cinnamon, as well as creamy custard with reduced sugar and a surprising bay leaf added for sweetness.

Kale, Spinach and the Leafy Greens

Your mother—and the National Academy of Sciences—insisted that you eat your leafy green vegetables. Here's why you should: Greens like spinach contain chlorophyll, a substance that helps plants turn sunlight into food. Chlorophyll also has been found to lower the tendency of cancer-causing agents to cause genetic damage to your body's cells. Spinach and other greens also contain significant amounts of vitamin A and calcium, although their oxalic acid content can change calcium into an indigestible compound in the body. Kale, on the other hand, has far more calcium than oxalic acid, so it's a good source of this bone-strengthening mineral.

The health-promoting power of leafy greens.

Liver: A Storehouse of Vitamins and Minerals

Usually found smothered in another superfood, onions, beef liver contains almost every nutrient going. It's rich in iron, zinc, copper, vitamins A, E, K, thiamine, riboflavin, biotin, folate, B_{12}, choline and inositol. Who can ask for anything more?

Is liver nature's multi-vitamin?

Melons Make the Grade

Cantaloupes and honeydews are low-calorie treats or high-energy breakfast sources of vitamin C.

One cup of cubed honeydew, for example, has only 60 calories but supplies more than half the RDA of vitamin C.

Nuts Are Chock-full of Zinc

You can consume a considerable portion of your minimum daily requirement of zinc during an afternoon snack if you're snacking on nuts. Nuts, especially cashews and almonds, are very high in this trace mineral that's so necessary for cell growth. But don't go nutty with nuts. Zinc, notwithstanding, you're also munching a handful of calories, so enjoy them in moderation.

Oysters for Minerals

Zinc and your sex life.

Legend has it that oysters are an aphrodisiac. We don't make any claims for that, but oysters are high in zinc, which is shown to be necessary for proper prostate and sexual functioning and sperm motility. Oysters are also rich in calcium, iron, copper and iodine. But a word of caution that we rarely give about anything else: Don't eat them raw. If they're not cooked, oysters tend to pick up bacteria that can make you ill.

Peppers Supply C

Which has more vitamin C, an orange or a pepper? Better bet on the pepper. One of these gorgeous green beauties contains more vitamin C than an orange. And an amazing thing happens when peppers age. They turn red—and fill up with a good supply of vitamin A.

Poultry Fills the Bill

Poultry—loaded with vitamins, minerals and protein.

Let's talk turkey—and chicken, while we're at it. They're low in calories, low in fat and high in essential nutrients and taste. An average half a chicken breast contains 26.7 grams of protein, just 3.1 grams of fat and only 142 calories. With that you get a side order of vitamin A, riboflavin and niacin, not to mention iron. A chicken drumstick contains only 76 calories and 2.5 grams of fat. Turkey is equally good news. Three ounces of light meat without skin totals 119 calories, 26 grams of protein and 1 gram of fat, with respectable amounts of B vitamins.

Seeds Yield Zinc

High in zinc and protein, seeds (such as pumpkin, sunflower and sesame) also contain something called a protease inhibitor, which seems to help protect us against cancer. Protease inhibitors have been shown to prevent liver, mammary and colon cancer in cancer-prone laboratory animals.

Why seeds aren't just for the birds.

Soup Keeps You Trim

It's not only good food but it's the food that makes you eat less. A study that analyzed the food diaries of 90 patients determined that those who ate soup more than four times a week ate fewer calories a day and lost more weight than those who didn't eat as much soup. In fact, the researchers found, a soup meal contained an average of 54.5 percent fewer calories than a nonsoup meal.

Soybeans Stand In for Meat

They're good protein—as good as animal sources, say nutritionists at the Massachusetts Institute of Technology. They lower cholesterol, say researchers at Washington University School of Medicine. And there's some indication that soybeans are cancer fighters. Like seeds, soybeans contain protease inhibitors. And soybean products like tofu (bean curd) and miso (soybean paste) tested by researchers in Tokyo seemed to inhibit potential carcinogens called nitrosamines in the stomach.

How soybeans may fight cancer and heart disease.

Sprouts Add C—and More

They're more than just a grassy accoutrement to salads and sandwiches. Studies show that the ascorbic acid (vitamin C) in some sprouted seeds and beans increases 19- to 86-fold after germination!

Mung bean sprouts are especially high in magnesium and calcium. But the best news concerns the wheat sprout. It's been shown to inhibit the genetic damage to cells caused by some cancer-causing agents.

Sweet Potatoes: Rich in A

This superfood is a sleeper that deserves to appear on the dinner table at times other than Thanksgiving and Christmas. Besides being tastier than white potatoes (which are not related), they're high in vitamin A, the substance that makes carrots such a potent cancer fighter. Sweet potatoes are also low in calories. One five-inch potato contains only 148 calories.

Sweet potatoes—low-calorie cancer fighters.

Wheat Germ Is More than Just Breakfast Fare

The B vitamin thiamine is abundant in only a few foods. But one of them is wheat germ, which is also rich in vitamin B_6. This versatile food was once relegated to the breakfast table but is now being used in everything from breads to salads.

Yogurt: A Valuable Source of Calcium

African Masai warriors eat large portions of fermented cow's milk daily, which makes their already low cholesterol levels drop even lower. In the United States, fermented cow's milk is marketed as yogurt and appears to have a similar effect on American cholesterol levels. When 26 people in a study at Vanderbilt University went on a diet of whole- and skim-milk yogurt, their cholesterol levels dropped significantly. Rich in calcium and all the nutrients in a glass of milk, yogurt is also easier to digest for people who are intolerant to plain milk.

Lowering your cholesterol with yogurt.

Chapter 67

Healthy
Gourmet Foods

I f a friend offered to treat you to a delicious gourmet meal, would you feel cheated if the menu
didn't include a tempter like huîtres à la crème
(creamed oysters) but featured such fare as steamed
squash instead? "That's gourmet?" you might ask dis-
appointedly.

You bet your brioche it is.

"Gourmet" doesn't have to mean high-fat, high-
calorie, hard-to-get food. You can find a whole new
menu of healthful, exciting foods as easily as reaching
past the tomatoes and other typical fare at the supermarket or perusing the bins and baskets at ethnic
markets or specialty stores.

The new world of low-fat gourmet foods.

Guilt-Free
Gourmet Pleasures

From main dishes to beverages, you'll discover
items that lend themselves to healthier preparation
methods—items that are higher in nutrients, lower in
calories and as palate pleasing as the more expensive
traditional gourmet cuisine.

The path to healthy, pal-ate-pleasing cuisine.

So to sate your adventurous appetite and still
respect your body, head to the kitchen with the unusual foods and recipes suggested here.

Most large supermarkets and grocery stores
should carry the healthful gourmet foods that follow.

Arugula, Mâche, Radicchio and Vitamin A

These greens make a salad snappier and, with only a minimal amount of calories, give the go-ahead for an all-you-can-eat serving. Each green has a distinctive taste and is a good source of vitamin A.

Arugula's pungent, peppery taste intensifies into a fiery tingle as the narrow, pointed leaves grow larger.

Mâche, or lamb's lettuce, has a sweet, hazelnut taste. The spoon-shaped, blue-green leaves are firm and chewy with an agreeable texture.

Radicchio (*Ra-DEECK-i-o*) is appealingly bitter, with vivid red, baseball-size heads. It also contains vitamin C.

Belgian Endive: More Versatile than It Looks

This versatile vegetable can be braised and served with meats, tossed into salads (a great partner for radicchio) or rolled up and filled with low-calorie cheese, spread or a scallion dip. Three and a half ounces of the creamy, ivory petals have just 15 calories and provide good roughage. Avoid brown-tipped petals, as the taste will be too bitter.

Boniato: Another "Sweet" Potato

This South American version of the sweet potato has a brown-red skin and very sweet flesh. The boniato is excellent baked, boiled, steamed or even creamed like pumpkin for pie filling. (Health bonus: It is a delicious source of fiber and no additional sweetener is needed.)

Café au Lait with a Calcium Bonus

If you're looking for ways to cut down on caffeine, add one part hot skim milk to one part strongly brewed, decaffeinated coffee. Skim milk spares you the fat and calories of cream, and it adds calcium. The decaffeinated coffee spares your nerves. The taste is smooth and rich.

Fava Beans Supply Iron and Potassium

Favas pleasantly blend the taste of lima beans and peas, and they contain comparable amounts of iron, potassium and protein.

When bought fresh, favas have green skins covering their plump, 1½-inch-long, kidney-shaped beans. Canned favas are often skinless and a pale mustard color. Young beans are excellent simmered, steamed or stir-fried, while older beans are best for stewing.

A change-of-pace loaded with minerals.

Mashed favas mixed with olive oil and garlic are a popular first course in Italy. Middle-Eastern cultures star the fava in a healthful dish called fool (fa-hool), where the beans are mashed, laced with lemon juice and garlic and eaten with pita bread.

Cornish Game Hens Are Leaner than Chicken

Here's a novel alternative to chicken. Cornish game hens are so small that a whole hen serves only one or two people. With its neutral taste, the meat takes well to marinades. When stuffed, Cornish game hens complement the flavor of the filling. Nutritionally, you get slightly less fat than with chicken.

Even lower in fat than chicken.

Flatbreads: Low Salt and Crunchy

Beautifully textured and hearty in flavor, flatbreads are more like crackers than bread. They're made from whole grain flours such as wheat, rye, barley or a combination of all three. Some are sprinkled with seeds or herbs, and some are fortified with bran.

The makings of high-fiber snacks or hors d'oeuvres.

Check package labels for nutritional information; some brands are high in fiber and low in salt and calories. All flatbreads are low in fat.

Create healthy hors d'oeuvres by pairing flatbreads with cheeses, fruits, vegetables or thinly sliced smoked fish. An herbed chicken salad with flatbread makes a great casual lunch.

Flavored Carbonated Waters "Taste" Crisp

Flavored sparkling seltzer or mineral waters refresh you without added sugar, salt or calories—only a tingle of lemon, lime or orange essence is added. The taste is clean and crisp.

Adding a splash of good health.

Try mixing a flavored water with fruit juice or punch to "mellow out" the juice's sweet taste. To concoct a nonalcoholic Sparkling Sunrise, for example, pour chilled apple juice into a tall, fluted glass, leaving about an inch of space at the top. Pour in about ¾ inch of chilled sparkling mineral water (any flavor), and let it settle. Add a splash of grenadine, which will slowly sink to the bottom of the glass, creating a layered effect. Garnish with a nasturtium bloom or sprig of mint.

Goat's-Milk Cheese: A Low-Fat Source of Calcium

From French imported to American farmers' country-fresh own, goat cheese is becoming one of the most sought-after gourmet items.

High in taste, low in fat.

Until now, the nutritional makeup of goat cheese was unknown. Five Samples analysed for this book, however, revealed that the rich, savory cheese has a lot more going for it than great taste. In addition to being an excellent source of calcium, goat cheese turns out to be lower in fat than many other cheeses.

A serving of goat cheese, in general, delivers between 40 and 50 percent of its calories from fat, depending on whether it is an aged, imported, soft or semisoft version. This is comparable to creamed cottage cheese. By contrast, you're faced with 74 percent calories from fat in cow's milk cheddar, and 67 percent calories from fat in ricotta cheese.

Gourmet Pastas: Two Foods in One

The new "specialty" pastas add excitement and variety to recipes. Vegetables like spinach, tomatoes, corn, Jerusalem artichokes and mung beans enhance the flavor of the noodles and may give them festive coloring. Garlic, basil and other herbs can also be added to the pasta flour. In moderation, pasta serves up just minimal amounts of fat and sodium. An average serving (one cup) contains approximately 192 calories, rectifying the "fattening food" reputation pasta has had.

Kabocha Squash: A "New" Source of Vitamin A

This Japanese squash is a good source of vitamin A. Its orange flesh has a bland, slightly honeyish taste and is delicious steamed or baked with a light sprinkle of spices. These short, fat squashes vary in appearance—ranging from pale orange on the outside to striped with green and white.

A squash of a different color.

Mussels: An Iron Source from the Sea

Beautiful, blue-black shells enclose these highly flavorful bivalves. They're available in fish stores year-round on the East Coast and from November through April on the West Coast. Mussels now being cultivated in Maine are clean, sand free, uniform in size and very tasty.

Mussels, which are a better source of iron than sirloin, should be bought fresh from a reputable source and cooked well. Pull off the ropelike beard that hangs out of the shell, then prepare the mussels in the same way as clams. Their outstanding flavor can suffice without any sauces or butters at all. Tossing some lemon juice and herbs like basil and garlic into the water during steaming will add a little lift to their taste.

Cooking up the iron-rich mussel.

Papaya Packs A and C

What looks like a large green pear with bumpy skin is actually a sweet, fragrant papaya, whose creamy orange flesh packs lots of vitamins A and C.

The fruit is smooth and soft in texture and can be

used as a dessert or a tossed-salad ingredient. When eaten alone, papaya needs no sweetener.

Papaya stores a surprise inside: soft little BB-like black seeds that are very crunchy and flavorful. Rinse them, place them in a jar with vinegar, refrigerate and then sprinkle them over a salad or grind them to flavor dressings and marinades. Papayas that are ready to eat are slightly soft to the touch and have a flowery scent at the stem end.

Sapsago Cheese: Grated for Goodness

A little of this hard, low-fat cheese goes a long, flavorful way. Made from slightly sour, skimmed cow's milk, it is not a cheese-and-crackers cheese—the sharp, pungent, herby taste makes it suitable for grating. (Hot pasta welcomes a judicious dusting of sapsago. And a salad comes alive with a sprinkling.) This cheese is packaged into four-inch cones. The greenish tint comes from Alpine clover.

Mango: A Vitamin A Powerhouse

A fragrant, tropical fruit, the mango is shaped like a rather flat football with rounded ends and a mottled green to rosy rind. (The skin is not edible.) The pale, orange-pink flesh has a very smooth texture. A huge stone nestled in the center makes cutting the fruit into attractive slices nearly impossible, and as a result the most popular uses of mangoes are in beverages, purees and sorbets.

For a low-calorie treat, mix mango, yogurt and vanilla with a touch of honey, then freeze.

Mangoes pack lots of vitamin A and are good sources of vitamin C. Three and a half ounces contain just 65 calories.

Skirt Steak, with Removable Fat

Skirt steak appears to be very fatty when you see it in grocery stores, but the fat isn't marbled throughout. It is on the outside, so you can easily cut it off.

When skirt steak is thinly sliced and served in Mexican or Chinese dishes, you end up eating less meat than usual, because the accompanying vegetables "will fill you up."

In search of a good, lean steak.

Skirt steak adopts the taste of a marinade very well, prompting less use of oil and salt.

Oils Add Savor to Veggies and Salads

Gourmet-variety oils such as chili, hazelnut, walnut and sesame taste great and are very aromatic. With the exception of chili oil, they have a short shelf life and should be bought in small amounts. All are low in saturated fat. Their biggest health boon is their prominent flavor. You'll use less and won't be tempted to add salty enhancers, thereby cutting your intake of both fat and sodium.

Red-chili oil is hot! Popular in Szechuan and Hunan cooking, it's made by either steeping chilies in the oil or adding chili extract.

Hazelnut and walnut oils look like regular oil, but they can complement flavors very well—for example, chop walnut pieces into a salad drizzled with walnut-oil vinaigrette for a layering of tastes.

Layering on the taste.

Sesame oil is extremely nutty and is available in light, dark and spicy-hot versions.

Spaghetti Squash's Hidden Delights

Inside this oval, yellow squash waits delightful, stringy flesh that, when fluffed out with a fork, becomes true "vegetable pasta"! The delicate, slightly sweet, low-calorie strands can be used instead of noodles in spaghetti-type Italian recipes. Or chill them and toss into a green salad.

The texture of the strands is bumpy, so sauce clings well. You may wish to use a special sauce—perhaps with a yogurt base—to perk up the squash flavor.

Serving up tasty squash "noodles."

For an attractive presentation, bake, boil or steam the squash. Then cut it in half, fluff the strands, add sauce and put the "noodles" back into the hollow shell to serve.

Split Salmon Gets High Marks

This nutritious fish should probably be featured on your menu quite often. It's very high in a substance called eicosapentanoic acid (EPA), which has been linked with reducing the risk of heart disease.

The term *split* refers to the way the fish is cut down the middle. That lets you open it up flat for easier cooking.

Yard-Long Beans Feature Fiber

Long on taste, high in fiber.

The name is a slight size exaggeration, as the actual length of yard-long beans is only about a foot and a half. The Chinese feel the beans shouldn't be cut but simply steamed enough to tenderize the skin, stir-fried and then served as an elegant "edible nest" along with fish, meat, poultry or seafood. Fiber is one of this bean's nutritional benefits.

Some Not-So-Common Specialties

Specialty stores or ethnic markets will feature these foods that are slightly harder to find.

Basmati Rice Soaks Up Surrounding Flavor

Basmati rice has little taste of its own, but it does have an enticing, buttered-popcorn aroma. The rice absorbs flavors around it (try cumin and coriander).

The aromatic grains are thin and fragile. Look for the brown type (the bran has not been removed), which is higher in fiber than white (branless) Basmati.

Nopalito Adds A and C to Salads

You'll recognize this unusual vegetable (also called nopal) as a cactus! After the spiky cover is cut off, the insides resemble soft cucumber. In fact, salads get the same lift from nopalitos that cucumbers give. This tangy vegetable is a source of vitamins A and C.

Pheasant: A Lean and Flavorful Bird

Pheasant is mild, not overwhelming or gamy, which makes it good for herbing and spicing. Young pheasant is prime for roasting; older pheasants are better in stews. A hen pheasant is more tender than the male. You'll get lean meat from this bird.

Low-fat meat for stews or roasting.

Redfish and Amberjack: Tasty, Flaky and Low Fat

These meaty, nonoily fish are extremely popular in Cajun cooking.

Redfish is one of the lower-fat fish, having only 2.5 grams of fat per 3½-ounce raw fillet. It is usually featured in the tasty Cajun recipe Blackened Redfish.

Amberjack, although it doesn't have the chic image of redfish, is still a low-fat fish and is flakier than redfish.

Yellow Finnish Potatoes for Still More C

Nature has already "buttered" these potatoes for you! A creamy, buttery taste actually does permeate this potato, so there's no need to heap on golden globs of extra fat. They're best steamed in a regular vegetable steamer, not baked. (Small potatoes can be steamed whole, while larger potatoes should be sliced or cubed.) Try them in any nonbaked recipe calling for white potatoes. Or top a steamed potato with plain yogurt and chopped scallions. Yellow Finnish potatoes are a good source of vitamin C.

Self-buttered potatoes with lots of C.

A Portfolio of Healthful Gourmet Recipes

Here are a week's worth of dinner recipes to help you introduce healthful gourmet foods to your menus.

BELGIAN ENDIVE
WITH WALNUT VINAIGRETTE

This makes a vivid salad, first course or lunch dish. You may use mâche and arugula in addition to or instead of radicchio. And although you may eat this salad in a conventional manner, it's more fun to use the radicchio petals as scoops for the endive and other ingredients.

- 2 small heads radicchio
- 2 heads Belgian endive
- ¼ cup chopped walnuts
- ¼ cup crumbled blue cheese
- 3 tablespoons minced scallions
   (green part only)
- 2 tablespoons rice vinegar
- 1 tablespoon French walnut oil
- ½ teaspoon French-style mustard

Separate the radicchio and endive into petals. Arrange radicchio on four individual plates, then place endive petals in daisy patterns on top of radicchio. Sprinkle with walnuts, cheese and scallions, so each endive petal contains a bit of each.

In a small bowl, whisk together vinegar, oil and mustard. Drizzle over salads.

Yield: 4 servings

HERB-STEAMED MUSSELS
WITH BASMATI RICE PILAF

You may substitute clams for the mussels, but the cooking time will be slightly longer.

  2 teaspoons olive oil
  1 cup chopped Spanish onions
  3 cloves garlic, minced
  1 cup Basmati rice
  2 tablespoons minced fresh oregano
  2 cups chicken stock
24 mussels, scrubbed and beards removed
  1 medium carrot, cut into julienne strips
  1 cup snow peas

Heat oil in a 14-inch paella pan (or other slope-sided pan). Add onions and garlic; sauté for 5 minutes. Add rice and oregano; sauté for 3 minutes. Add stock and bring to a boil. Reduce heat and simmer for 5 minutes.

Add mussels and carrots. Cover pan loosely with foil. When mussels begin to open, add snow peas. Cover and simmer until mussels are fully open, about 6 minutes. Discard any mussels that don't open. Serve immediately.

Yield: 4 servings

YARD-LONG BEANS WITH OYSTER SAUCE

The Chinese consider it bad luck to cut these beans, so they eat them bite by bite, using chopsticks to hold the bean as they eat.

 5 dried shiitake mushrooms
   (1 to 2 inches each)
 1 slice gingerroot
 ¾ pound yard-long beans
 2 tablespoons oyster sauce
 1 tablespoon rice vinegar
 1 teaspoon cornstarch
 2 teaspoons oil
 2 cloves garlic
   dash of sesame oil
 1 tablespoon sesame seeds

Rinse mushrooms and remove stems. Soak in very hot water for 15 to 20 minutes, or until soft. (Weigh mushrooms down if they float.)

Place about an inch of water in a large saucepan. Add ginger. Cover. Bring to a boil. Place beans in a steamer basket, then add to pan. Cover and steam for 2 or 3 minutes. Remove pan from heat and let stand for 3 minutes. Remove beans and set aside.

Drain mushrooms, then pat dry and cut into slivers. Combine oyster sauce, vinegar and cornstarch in a small bowl and stir until smooth. Set aside.

Heat a wok over medium-high heat. Add oil and garlic and stir for about 30 seconds, then discard garlic. Quickly add beans and mushrooms. Stir-fry for 2 minutes. Make a space in the bottom of the wok and add the oyster sauce mixture. Stir quickly until thick (be careful not to burn the sauce). Toss beans and mushrooms to coat with sauce. Sprinkle with a little sesame oil and toss again. Remove from wok and arrange on a round platter in a nest shape. Sprinkle with sesame seeds.

Yield: 4 servings

APRICOT-STUFFED CORNISH GAME HENS

- 1 cup apple juice
- 1 cup apricot nectar
- ½ teaspoon crushed star anise (about 2 stars)
- ½ teaspoon crushed cardamom seeds
- ½ teaspoon ground ginger
- 5 whole black peppercorns
- 2 teaspoons low-sodium soy sauce
- 4 Cornish game hens
- 1½ cups chicken stock
- ½ cup wild rice
- 1 bay leaf
- ⅓ cup minced onions
- ¼ cup chopped dried apricots
- 2 tablespoons coarsely chopped pine nuts

In a large, deep dish, combine juice, nectar, anise, cardamom, ginger, peppercorns and soy sauce. Place hens in dish, then cover and marinate overnight.

In a 1-quart saucepan, combine stock, rice and bay leaf. Bring to a boil, then reduce heat, cover and simmer for about 40 minutes, or until liquid is absorbed and rice is tender. Set aside.

Remove hens from marinade and set aside, reserving marinade.

In a 2-quart saucepan, cook onions in 1 or 2 tablespoons of marinade until wilted. Add apricots, pine nuts and cooked rice. Heat through, adding more marinade if mixture becomes too dry.

Preheat oven to 350°F.

Spoon stuffing into body cavities of hens. Set in a lightly oiled baking pan. Bake for 1 hour, basting occasionally with marinade. If hens appear to be getting too brown, cover with foil.

Yield: 8 servings

SIZZLING FAJITAS

1 skirt steak (1 pound)
¼ cup lime juice
1 teaspoon olive oil
1 tablespoon minced fresh coriander
¾ teaspoon ground cumin
¼ teaspoon dried oregano, crushed
1 clove garlic, minced
  freshly ground black pepper, to taste
½ cup thinly sliced onions
1 cup seeded, diced tomatoes
1 lime
6 flour tortillas, warmed
1 ripe avocado, chopped
  lime wedges
3 chili peppers, cut into thin strips
1 cup canned nopalitos (optional)

Trim fat from steak. Cut meat into ¼-inch slices, cutting across the grain and slightly on the bias.

In a large bowl, combine lime juice, oil, coriander, cumin, oregano, garlic and pepper. Add meat strips. Cover and let stand for 2 hours, stirring occasionally.

With tongs, remove meat strips from marinade. Place meat in a single layer on a broiler pan and broil about 5 inches from heat for 5 to 7 minutes, or until lightly browned, turning once during cooking.

Coat a large nonstick skillet with vegetable spray. Add onions and cook for 3 or 4 minutes, or until crisp-tender. Add tomatoes and cook, stirring occasionally, for 1 or 2 minutes, or until just heated.

Combine meat and vegetables in a heated cast-iron skillet or platter. Cut lime in half and squeeze juice over meat and vegetables. Serve as filling for tortillas, along with avocado, lime wedges, chilies and nopalitos, if used.

Yield: 6 servings

PASTA WITH SALMON AND SUN-DRIED TOMATOES

  1 cup water
  1 tablespoon rice vinegar
  1 bay leaf
  ½ pound salmon fillets
  ¾ cup low-fat cottage cheese
  2 tablespoons skim milk
     freshly grated nutmeg
  ½ pound spinach pasta, cooked
12 sun-dried tomatoes, sliced (about ⅔ cup)
  1 tablespoon grated locatelli cheese

In a large skillet, combine water, vinegar and bay leaf. Bring to a boil. Reduce heat to very low, add salmon and cover pan. Cook for 4 to 6 minutes, or until salmon is opaque pink. Remove salmon with a large slotted spoon or spatula and let cool. Gently pulling against the grain, separate fish into 1-inch chunks. Set aside.

In a blender or food processor, combine cottage cheese, milk and a pinch of nutmeg. Process until smooth.

In a large warmed bowl, toss together pasta, tomatoes, locatelli and half of cottage cheese mixture. Add salmon and remaining cheese mixture and gently toss together.

Yield: 4 servings

SOUP OF PHEASANT, PORCINI AND TRUFFLES

Make this soup a day ahead to heighten its delicate flavors. If pheasant isn't available, substitute dark chicken meat.

¼ cup dried porcini mushrooms
1 teaspoon margarine or butter
¾ cup minced onions
3 cups chicken stock
¼ cup grated carrots
1½ tablespoons minced celery leaves
1 tablespoon red wine vinegar
1 teaspoon mushroom ketchup (optional)*
¾ cup cooked pheasant, shredded
1 white Piemonte truffle, finely minced with a razor blade

Soak mushrooms in enough water to cover for about 20 minutes. Drain, reserving the soaking water. Remove any stems and mince mushrooms.

In a 3-quart saucepan, melt margarine or butter. Add onions and sauté until rich brown, about 10 to 15 minutes. Add stock, carrots, celery, vinegar, ketchup, if used, mushrooms and soaking liquid. Bring to a boil, then reduce heat and simmer for 15 minutes. Add pheasant and truffle and cook for 15 minutes.

If not serving immediately, let soup cool to room temperature before refrigerating. When ready to serve, heat slowly.

Yield: 4 servings

*Mushroom ketchup is available in oriental food markets.

The Fruits and Vegetables Your Mother Never Mentioned

I f the advice you've been hearing lately from groups bent on preventing heart disease and cancer sounds suspiciously like something your mother once said, there's a reason for that. The scientific community has confirmed mom's age-old command to eat more fruits and vegetables. Study after study of large populations has indicated that people who eat more of these foods suffer less coronary problems, stroke and cancer.

Reasons to eat your veggies.

Fruits and vegetables tend to be low in fat and salt and high in fiber and vitamins A and C—all traits that contribute to their disease-preventive status.

So you've started including more of those foods in your diet. At restaurants, you'll order a salad instead of pâté; at home, you end more meals with an apple instead of chocolate cream pie. But let's face it, the same old salad greens, apples, oranges and bananas get a little boring after a while.

There are alternatives. These days, it's not unusual for supermarkets to stock not one but three, four or five different kinds of fresh peppers, half a dozen or more varieties of squash and a dizzying array of tubers, cabbages and tropical fruits. During the summer, roadside produce stands and farmers' markets offer lots of variety. If you live in a large city, you might also try ethnic markets, such as Italian, Hispanic and oriental, where novel foodstuffs often are featured.

Out-of-the-ordinary but nutrient-rich fruits and vegetables.

Nutritious Additions to Your Shopping Bag

Whether you're shopping for unusual fruits and vegetables or you're just seeing more of them on restaurant menus, here's a brief rundown on some that are growing in popularity.

Bok choy. A Chinese chard or cabbage that resembles celery, bok choy has good, fresh flavor and crunch, and it's high in vitamin A. Steam for about 10 minutes, stir-fry, or add it to other dishes. It complements the flavor and texture of many foods, including beef and seafood. It can be found at Chinese markets or as a popular ingredient in Chinese restaurant food.

A new source of vitamin A.

Boysenberries. These are large, soft berries with a purplish black cast, large seeds and an excellent tart flavor. They are a good source of vitamin C and are available in local markets.

Crenshaw melon. A hybrid variety of muskmelon with a yellow skin and salmon-colored flesh, crenshaw melon is high in vitamins A and C. It has a delicate flavor and is available in local markets.

Gooseberries. Similar to currants, gooseberries have translucent skins that vary in color: green, yellow, white, pink or red. There are sweet and tart-tasting varieties. Gooseberries are a good source of fiber and vitamin C and a fair source of vitamin A. They are available in local markets.

Colorful fruits with fiber and vitamins.

Guava. A native of Mexico and South America, guavas are now grown extensively in California, Florida and Hawaii. They are reddish purple on the outside and white on the inside. They are high in fiber and an excellent source of vitamin C. You can cook guavas or eat them raw, and they taste great with pineapples and bananas. They can also be used in pies and tarts. They can be found in various markets.

Jicama. This Mexican potato, whose name is pronounced *he-CA-ma,* is a good source of vitamin C. You can peel and slice it, then dice and toss with salads, or stir-fry, like water chestnuts. It should be available in various markets.

Passion fruit. This tropical fruit (a native of Brazil) is not an aphrodisiac, though it may sound like one. It has a deep, dusty purple color and can look uneven and lumpy when ripe. It's a good source of fiber, however. To eat passion fruit, cut it in half and eat the greenish yellow pulp and seeds with a spoon. Its juice is often used in punch. It can be found in various markets.

Fruit with a punch.

Tamarillo. A New Zealand fruit that's about the size of a kiwi fruit, with bright orange flesh and black seeds, tamarillo is rich in vitamin C. Its texture is similar to a kiwi's, but the taste is more complex, combining sweet and sour flavors. It's eaten fresh without the skin or stewed in a compote. It can be found in various markets.

A New Zealand delight that's high in C.

Chapter 69

Rating Your Refrigerator's "Health Quotient"

There's a housewife in New York who claims she can spot a troubled marriage, a family that pays its bills on time or one in which husband and wife are struggling with their self-esteem—all by studying the art gallery on their refrigerator doors. You know: the Snoopy-shaped magnets and cartoons, the lists and messages, reminders ("Think Thin!"), pictures, calendars, bills and everything else that ends up enshrined in that household Louvre and communications center. If your refrigerator door is an unholy mess, don't worry, she says—that may well be a sign of a happy marriage.

What's in *Your* Refrigerator?

What your refrigerator reveals about your diet.

But if refrigerator doors are revealing, think about what's behind them. The contents of your fridge paint a fairly complete, very up-to-date picture of what your eating habits are really like. Not what you wish or intend them to be, not what they once were, not what they're going to be, but what they are. And since we all foster illusions about ourselves, a cold, objective inspection of your refrigerator's innards might produce some real surprises.

An honest look at your eating habits.

You might find out that much of what you know about nutrition isn't actually making it into practice. Then again, you might discover you've been treating yourself better than you realized. Either way, the point is: How can you expect to improve your eating habits if you're not entirely sure what they are? Which is the point of the following "health consciousness-raising" game.

All you need to play is a pencil and paper, your refrigerator and a pitiless sense of objectivity. All you have to do is open your refrigerator, see what's there and assign a number value (plus or minus) to each kind of food you find. Once you've added up all the pluses and minuses, you'll end up with a total score— your refrigerator's "health quotient," if you will. You will be able to tell from your score whether your "HQ" is terrific, merely great or awful (compared with others who've taken the test).

The rankings have been worked out with the help of a computer, which evaluated a representative "market basket" of foods that might be likely to wind up in your refrigerator. Foods from each of eight different food groups were judged according to the food values (good or bad) that that group is especially noted for. Each dairy product, for example, was ranked according to its protein and fat content, sodium, total calories, riboflavin and calcium; fish were ranked by protein, fat, sodium, vitamin B_6, potassium, iron and niacin; and so on.

Computer rankings based on nutrition.

The rankings have been refined a bit, based on nutritional or healing properties a particular food might have that the computer didn't know about. For example, haddock was bumped up a notch because it's relatively rich in eicosapentanoic acid (EPA), a substance that has been shown to be beneficial to cardiovascular health (but which the computer didn't take into consideration).

How to Keep Score

Please remember that a negative score for a particular food doesn't mean it's a total nutritional loser. It's just a way of giving certain foods a relative weight compared to other foods. Also, the list is not meant to be an exhaustive one. There will be a few things in your fridge that have not been included on the list—just disregard them.

Here are a few other things to remember.

- Try to pick a day when the refrigerator is relatively full, preferably the day you do the week's food shopping.
- Give each type of food only one score. For example, if you have two cartons of skim milk, give yourself five points (not ten). Don't give each carrot three points.
- Count fresh and frozen vegetables the same.
- Disregard condiments such as ketchup, Tabasco sauce, soy sauce and others.
- Count only the contents of your refrigerator (including its freezer compartment). Certainly, what you've got squirreled away in detached freezers and pantry cupboards is a part of your total personal health picture—but that's a different game.

Refrigerator Health Quotient Scorecard

A. Congratulations! You win five points for trying!___

B. Award yourself five points for each of these foods you find:

___ any kind of sprouts	___ red peppers
___ blackberries	___ salmon
___ bran flakes	___ sesame seeds
___ broccoli	___ shrimp
___ cantaloupe	___ skim milk
___ collards	___ strawberries
___ flounder	___ sunflower seeds
___ haddock	___ Swiss chard
___ halibut	___ tahini (sesame
___ kale	butter)
___ liver	___ tofu
___ mangoes	___ trout
___ plain low-fat yogurt	___ wheat germ
___ raspberries	

C. Give yourself three points for each of these foods:

___ acorn squash
___ almonds
___ apricots
___ artichokes
___ avocados
___ beet greens
___ blueberries
___ brussels sprouts
___ buttermilk
___ cabbage
___ carrots
___ cauliflower
___ chicken
___ cod
___ dates
___ endive
___ orange juice
___ grapefruit
___ green peppers
___ homemade or low-
fat salad dressing
___ honeydew
___ kefir
___ lemons

___ lima beans
___ limes
___ mushrooms
___ oranges
___ part-skim mozzarella
___ peaches
___ radishes
___ raw peanuts
___ rhubarb
___ ricotta cheese
___ rockfish
___ romaine lettuce
___ snow peas
___ spinach
___ Swiss or Gruyère
cheese
___ tangerines
___ tuna
___ turkey
___ two percent low-fat
cottage cheese
___ two percent low-fat
milk
___ veal cutlet

D. Give yourself one point for any of these foods:

___ American cheese
___ apples
___ asparagus
___ beef rib
___ beets
___ bottled water
___ Brie cheese
___ butter
___ Camembert cheese
___ celery
___ cheddar cheese
___ chuck steak

___ clams
___ coconut
___ colby cheese
___ crab
___ creamed cottage
cheese
___ cucumbers
___ eggplant
___ eggs
___ figs
___ flank steak
___ fruit yogurt

___ Gouda cheese
___ grapes
___ green snap beans
___ ground beef (regular or lean)
___ half-and-half
___ ham
___ iceberg lettuce
___ lamb loin
___ lamb rib or leg
___ leeks
___ lobster
___ margarine
___ Monterey Jack cheese
___ Muenster cheese
___ mussels
___ oysters
___ Parmesan cheese
___ peanut butter
___ pears
___ pineapple
___ plums
___ pork chops
___ Romano cheese
___ round or sirloin steak

___ rump roast
___ salt-free pickles
___ salt-free spaghetti sauce
___ sardines
___ scallions
___ scallops
___ sweet corn
___ sweet or sour cherries
___ T-bone steak
___ tomatoes
___ turnips
___ unsweetened fruit juice
___ veal breast
___ watermelon
___ whiting
___ whole milk
___ whole wheat bread or any other whole grain product
___ yellow squash
___ zucchini

E. Subtract three points for each of these foods:

___ anchovies
___ beer
___ black or green olives
___ Canadian bacon
___ commercial salad dressing
___ cream cheese
___ fish cakes
___ fish sticks

___ ice milk
___ light or heavy whipping cream
___ mayonnaise
___ pickles
___ sour cream
___ sweetened fruit juices
___ wine

F. Subtract five points for each of these foods:

—— anything with sugar, corn sweeteners or honey listed as first ingredient
—— bacon
—— boiled ham
—— bologna
—— brown-and-serve sausage
—— chicken roll
—— cooked canned ham
—— corned beef
—— cured ham
—— dried beef
—— frozen layer cakes
—— hot dogs
—— ice cream
—— jams and jellies
—— knockwurst
—— liverwurst
—— luncheon meats
—— Polish sausage
—— salami
—— sherbet
—— soda pop
—— spareribs
—— turkey loaf or roll
—— turkey or chicken franks
—— white bread or any other white flour product such as cakes or cookies

Scoring: Here's how your refrigerator's "HQ" stacks up against the rest of the world: 60 or above: excellent; 50–60: superior; 40–50: good; 30–40: fair; 30 and below: needs work. (Can you isolate any particular place to begin?)

Chapter 70

The Good Meats:
A Nutritional
Storehouse

B eef's been on the grill for quite a few years now. "Eat less red meat," medical researchers have said, and we've listened. Fearful of cholesterol and fat, we've switched to more chicken and fish and heaped our salad bowls high.

And—make no mistake—you can eat too much meat. A diet that serves up bacon, sausage, luncheon meats, steaks, chops, hamburgers or hot dogs several times a day is a diet almost certainly too high in fat and too low in fiber to be optimally healthful.

Two sides to the meat story.

But there's another side to the meat story. If you choose the right cuts, prepare the meat properly, and eat it in moderation, meat can be a positively health-building food.

Meat Is More Healthful than You Think

Beef has the same amount of cholesterol as chicken.

Consider, first of all, this question. Which has more cholesterol, beef, chicken or fish? Almost everyone gets that one partially wrong. The answer is that beef and chicken have essentially the same amount of cholesterol—100 milligrams or so—and fish has about 80 milligrams in a four-ounce serving.

Second, the fat and calorie content of various cuts of beef and other meats varies from mammoth to surprisingly modest. Generalizations just don't work. Take a sirloin steak, for instance. Broil a six-ouncer as it comes out of a butcher's case and you've got 476 calories, including lots of fat. But the same cut of steak that weighs six ounces *after* trimming away all the visible fat has only 354 calories, with 26 percent fewer calories from fat.

Even more interesting, certain cuts of beef, such as round and flank steak, are quite lean to begin with. A broiled six-ounce round steak, untrimmed, has 466 calories. But a well-trimmed, broiled six-ounce round steak drops you down to 330 calories and a very respectable fat level.

Don't make the mistake, though, of cooking meat with its fat, then trimming it off at the table. Some of the fat that melts during cooking will actually be absorbed into the meat. So trim before cooking,

Trim fat before, not after, you cook the meat.

Rating the Beef

Cut	Calories	Fat (g.)	Calories from Fat (%)
Eye round	209	7	32
Sirloin	238	10	33
Chuck roast	264	11	39
Rump	236	11	40
T-Bone*	245	12	44
Porterhouse †	249	12	45
Rib eye ‡	257	13	47
Club steak	277	15	48
Flank	278	17	56
Ground beef §	293	19	57

SOURCE: Adapted from *Composition of Foods: Beef Products,* Agriculture Handbook No. 8–13, by Nutrition Monitoring Division (Washington, D.C.: Human Nutrition Information Service, U.S. Department of Agriculture, 1986).

NOTE: Figures are based on a 4-oz. serving, trimmed of visible fat, and cooked. On average, these cuts provide about 33 g. of protein and about 3 mg. of iron, as well as about 93 mg. of cholesterol.

* Strip loin and New York strip are synonyms for this cut.

† Filet mignon and chateaubriand can be included in this cut.

‡ Delmonico and Spencer steak are synonyms for this cut.

§ Extra lean ground sirloin and round, broiled to medium doneness.

then broil on a slotted pan that permits some of the remaining fat to drip away. The result is good, lean, nutritious eating.

And, of course, if you're cooking meat that's low in fat to begin with, you're better off yet. (For details, see our list of various beef cuts and their percentage of calories from fat in the table, Rating the Beef, on page 535.)

But what about saturated fat? Isn't beef higher in this kind of fat—believed to push cholesterol levels up—than chicken or fish? Generally, yes. But remember, generalizations can be deceiving. Choose the really lean cuts, like round, and ounce for ounce you've got a lot less saturated fat than we get from such common foods as stewed chicken, peanuts, cheese or even sunflower seeds.

A Good Source of Vitamins and Minerals

On the plus side, beef is an extremely good source of protein, B vitamins, iron and zinc. The latter two minerals are believed to be deficient in many diets, particularly those of women who are watching their weight.

Meat boosts iron absorption.

And even a small amount of beef can greatly increase the amount of iron our bodies can absorb from grains, potatoes and vegetables. (Enter beef stew, stage right.)

However you cut it—or cook it—beef does have more fat than vegetables or fruits. But this is true of most protein-rich foods, including dairy products, nuts and seeds. The trick is to balance these foods with others that are extremely low in fat—fruits, vegetables, corn, rice, wheat and other grains, beans of all kinds, potatoes and pasta. Go easy on the butter, and you wind up with a daily diet that includes meat but excludes excess fat.

Putting Meat in Perspective

Many health authorities recommend a diet that derives no more than 30 percent of its total calories from fat. To see how that works in practice, let's begin with a well-trimmed porterhouse steak—not an especially lean piece of meat. About 45 percent of its calories come from fat. But if you include a four-ounce baked potato, one slice of whole wheat bread, four ounces of broccoli, one pat of butter and eight ounces of skim milk with your broiled steak (a four-ounce serving), you've reduced the ratio of calories from fat to 27 percent. The total calories from this typical dinner is a quite moderate 596.

A low-fat meal with porterhouse steak.

Perhaps some comparisons with meatless dishes will help put beef's benefits in perspective.

A macaroni-and-cheese dish, made with 1½ cups of ricotta, fontina and cheddar cheeses, eight ounces of macaroni and 1 cup of milk, has about 45 percent of its calories tied up in fat. A sirloin steak, on the other hand, has only 33 percent of its calories in fat. In fact, many cuts of beef contain significantly less fat than comparable amounts of many cheeses (Brie, Gouda, cheddar, ricotta, Swiss and Romano among them).

Macaroni and cheese has more fat than sirloin steak.

A quiche made with two cups of cheddar, spinach, rice, three eggs and one cup of light cream has a staggering 74 percent of its calories coming from fat. No wonder real men don't touch the stuff.

Decoding Meat-Packing Labels

But short of taking a course in butcher-shop basics, what can a health-conscious consumer do to negotiate the meat morass? A good start would be to familiarize yourself with the meat industry's grading system. Its top rating is "prime," which means that, according to the U.S. Department of Agriculture (USDA), the meat is "the most tender, juicy and fla-

Prime is high in fat.

vorful." What makes a prime cut flavorful and juicy is fat, not only the trimmable fat but also the marbling, the flecks of fat within the lean that are impossible to eliminate. If you purchase a prime cut, it's best to cut away the trimmable fat before cooking.

The meat industry's "choice" rating goes to cuts that don't have quite enough marbling to warrant the prime label. Still, these cuts are high in fat content and so should be carefully trimmed.

The healthiest cuts of meat are neither "prime" nor "choice."

Ironically, as one moves down the meat industry's rating chart, one makes a healthful ascent. The "good" and "standard" ratings are given to cuts "which lack the juiciness and flavor of the higher grades," according to the USDA. The reason? There's less fat, so you have less waste, fewer calories and less cholesterol. Perhaps best of all, the healthier cuts cost less. Fortunately, the meat industry has been offering more of the leaner cuts in the market recently.

How to choose meat that's lean and tender.

So your choices are many. Beef's gamut runs from the cuts of the loin portion, which should be consumed in moderation and in careful balance with other foods, to the cuts of the round portion of the steer, which fall close to the government's 30 percent of calories from fat recommendation.

Identifying Meats on the Menu

When you eat out, however, another problem arises: identifying the cuts. While most supermarkets use standard names for the cuts of beef, restaurants use many aliases. And since there is no beef eater's thesaurus, you need a guide. Here are a few of the more common designations.

A guide to popular restaurant cuts.

Chateaubriand. This is a large tenderloin, sometimes called filet mignon. This is always at least a choice cut, and it might be prime. It costs the restaurant more to get, and it will cost you more.

Surf 'n' turf. You can ask the waiter wishfully if this is haddock and round steak, but typically this is a shellfish (usually lobster) and a tenderloin cut of beef that by itself would be filet mignon.

London broil. This is a flank steak and a highly recommended cut at home or out. It will cost you less in a market or a restaurant, and from a nutritional standpoint, it is one of the best cuts of beef.

Whether you're buying meat at the supermarket or ordering it at a restaurant, be assertive. Don't feel that you're inconveniencing the meat cutter by asking him to trim fat for you. And make it clear to the waiter that the size of the tip depends on whether or not you get the beef exactly the way you want it. This allows you to enjoy beef not only without reservation but also with the knowledge that you're doing something good for yourself.

How to get the beef you want.

Chapter 71

Happy Marriages: Foods That Go Together

Enjoying tasty, healthy food duos.

Spicing up popular combos.

Romeo and Juliet, Anthony and Cleopatra, Macaroni and Cheese....

Although it's true that Shakespeare never got around to immortalizing that last famous couple, it seems clear that certain foods are made for each other just the way people sometimes are. Liver and onions, spaghetti and meatballs, chicken and biscuits—the chemistry is just right.

And that's not all that's right. As luck would have it, many traditional food duos are compatible nutritionally as well as gastronomically. Corn tortillas and beans get together to form a more efficient form of protein. Cheese or meat adds protein to a pasta dinner, and the pasta helps stretch a modest amount of either. Fish and chips need only a green vegetable or salad to round out the dish. The same goes for chicken and biscuits.

Like many couples that have been together for a long time, however, some food partners can occasionally benefit from having their lives, well, spiced up a bit. Chili peppers added to liver and onions keep boredom at bay. So do herbs in biscuits and yogurt in chicken sauce. And who says macaroni and cheese can't have a little mustard added, and that you can't use three cheeses instead of just one? Or that fish and chips always have to be deep-fried and greasy? No one. So enjoy these variations on favorite old themes.

LIVER AND ONIONS

Overcooking is what usually gives liver that old-shoe texture. You can avoid that by cooking these liver strips a mere 2 minutes.

1   pound calves' liver
3   tablespoons lemon juice
1   canned green chili pepper, seeded and
        minced
2   cloves garlic, minced
1   teaspoon dried oregano
¼   teaspoon dried rosemary, crushed
4   large baking potatoes
3   medium-size onions, thinly sliced
¼   cup beef stock
2   teaspoons vegetable oil

Cut liver into strips about ½ inch wide and place in a shallow bowl. In a small bowl, mix lemon juice, chili pepper, garlic, oregano and rosemary. Pour over liver and toss to coat. Let stand for at least 2 hours.

About 1 hour before serving time, preheat oven to 425°F. Scrub potatoes and pat dry, then pierce each with a fork and bake for 1 hour.

In a large nonstick skillet, cook onions in stock over medium-low heat, stirring occasionally, for 15 to 20 minutes, or until stock evaporates and onions are tender and lightly browned. Remove onions to a plate.

Increase heat to medium-high. Heat oil in skillet for a few seconds, then add liver, reserving any marinade that remains in the bowl. Cook, stirring frequently, for about 2 minutes. Return onions to skillet, pour in reserved marinade, and toss to reheat onions. Serve over baked potatoes.

Yield: 4 servings

FISH AND CHIPS

Baked instead of fried, this rendition of the British favorite is much lower in calories. Although almost any kind of potato will work well for the chips, the small red type is exceptionally good for these crunchy morsels.

CHIPS
10 to 12 small red potatoes
1 teaspoon vegetable oil

FISH
1 pound flounder fillets
¼ cup whole wheat flour
pinch of ground red pepper
1 tablespoon vegetable oil
1 tablespoon margarine or butter
¼ cup lemon juice
paprika

To make the chips: Scrub potatoes, then dry thoroughly. Leaving skins on, cut them into strips roughly 2 inches long by ½ inch thick and wide. Pat dry again.

Preheat oven to 450°F.

Spread oil evenly over the bottom of a jelly-roll pan and distribute potatoes in a single layer in the pan. Bake for 30 minutes, turning frequently.

To make the fish: Pat fish dry. Place flour and ground red pepper in a plastic bag and add fish, one piece at a time. Shake well to coat lightly with flour. After coating each fillet, fold it in half or roll lengthwise. Set aside.

Heat a large cast-iron skillet or other heavy, ovenproof pan over medium-high heat until quite hot. Add oil and margarine or butter, then add fillets to pan in a single layer. Immediately tilt the pan so you can spoon some oil mixture over fish.

Place pan in the oven with chips. Bake for 10 to 15 minutes (depending on thickness of fillets), until fish is opaque and cooked through.

Remove chips and place on serving dish. Remove fish to a serving platter, then add lemon juice to the pan. Stir to loosen any browned bits from the bottom, then pour liquid over fish and sprinkle with paprika. Serve with chips.

Yield: 4 servings

TORTILLAS AND BEANS

Take your choice of beans. Serve with a salad of mixed greens or with marinated vegetables.

- 12 corn tortillas (6-inch diameter)
- ⅔ cup plain yogurt
- ⅓ cup sour cream
- 3 scallions, thinly sliced
- 2 cloves garlic, minced
- 1 tablespoon chili powder, or to taste
- ½ teaspoon ground cumin
- 4 cups coarsely chopped tomatoes
- 1½ cups cooked pinto, kidney or black beans, lightly mashed
- ¾ cup shredded cheddar or Monterey Jack cheese

Coat a deep-dish, 9-inch pie plate with vegetable spray. Use 4 tortillas to cover the bottom of the plate, overlapping them in the center.

Preheat oven to 375°F.

In a small bowl, mix yogurt, sour cream, scallions, garlic, chili powder and cumin. Spread a third of the mixture over tortillas. Top with 1⅓ cups tomatoes and ½ cup beans.

Repeat layering twice to use all tortillas, yogurt mixture, tomatoes and beans. Top with cheese.

Bake for 20 to 30 minutes, or until cheese has melted and ingredients are bubbly.

Yield: 4 servings

SPAGHETTI AND MEATBALLS

Serve up these favorites for a filling but not fatty supper entrée.

¾   pound lean ground beef
¼   cup bran
1   onion, minced
2   cloves garlic, minced
1   teaspoon dried thyme
½   teaspoon dried rosemary, crushed
1   egg
1   can (35 ounces) Italian plum tomatoes
¼   cup tomato paste
½   teaspoon dried oregano
½   teaspoon dried basil
⅛   teaspoon crushed red pepper flakes
1   bay leaf
8   ounces spaghetti

In a large bowl, mix beef, bran, onions, garlic, thyme, rosemary and egg until thoroughly combined. Using your hands or two soup spoons, shape meat into balls roughly the size of golf balls. Set aside.

In a 3-quart saucepan, combine tomatoes, tomato paste, oregano, basil, red pepper flakes and bay leaf. Bring to a boil, then reduce heat and simmer for 15 minutes. Add meatballs to pan and cook for 45 minutes. Stir occasionally. Before serving, remove bay leaf.

In a large pot, cook spaghetti in boiling water until just tender. Drain and place in a large serving bowl, then cover with meatballs and sauce.

Yield: 4 servings

MACARONI AND THREE CHEESES

This variation on the traditional dish is nice served with steamed peas and spinach salad.

- ½ pound macaroni
- 2 tablespoons whole wheat flour
- 1½ cups skim milk
- 1½ cups low-fat cottage cheese
- ½ cup grated Parmesan cheese
- ½ cup shredded cheddar cheese
- 1 teaspoon dry mustard
- ⅓ cup seasoned bread crumbs

In a large pot, cook macaroni in boiling water until just tender. Do not overcook. Drain and set aside.

Coat an 8 × 8-inch baking dish with vegetable spray.

In a 3-quart saucepan, whisk flour with about 2 tablespoons milk until blended to a smooth paste. Gradually whisk in remaining milk. Cook over medium heat, stirring constantly, until thickened. Remove from heat.

Preheat oven to 375°F.

Add macaroni, cheeses and mustard to the pan. Stir to mix. Pour into baking dish and sprinkle with bread crumbs. Bake for 30 minutes.

Yield: 4 servings

CHICKEN 'N' BISCUITS

This all-American combo gets added zip from chili powder. Start preparing the chicken. While it simmers, you can make the biscuits.

CHICKEN
6   whole chicken legs, with skin and all visible
        fat removed
3   tablespoons whole wheat flour
1½ teaspoons chili powder
1   tablespoon vegetable oil
1½ cups chicken stock
1   cup plain yogurt

BISCUITS
2   cups whole wheat flour
2¼ teaspoons baking powder
¼   teaspoon baking soda
3   tablespoons margarine or butter
½   cup plain yogurt
¼   cup skim milk
⅓   cup minced fresh parsley or chives

To make the chicken: With a sharp knife, cut each leg at the joint to make 2 pieces. Rinse pieces and pat dry. Place flour and 1 teaspoon chili powder in a plastic bag. Add chicken, 1 piece at a time, and shake to coat lightly with flour.

Heat oil in a large, heavy, well-seasoned skillet over medium heat for 30 seconds. Add chicken pieces, being careful not to crowd them. (If necessary, do chicken in several batches.) Cook over medium heat, turning pieces occasionally until lightly browned.

Pour 1 cup stock into skillet. Cover and simmer for 30 to 40 minutes, or until chicken is tender and juices run clear when you pierce a thigh with a fork.

To make the biscuits: In a large bowl, combine flour, baking powder and baking soda. With two knives or a pastry blender, cut in margarine or butter until mixture is crumbly and resembles coarse meal. Make a well in the center and add yogurt, milk and parsley or chives. Stir with a fork until all flour is moistened. Do not overmix.

Preheat oven to 450°F. Coat a baking sheet with vegetable spray.

Turn dough out onto a floured surface and gently knead for about 30 seconds. Pat or roll dough into a rectangle about ¾ inch thick. Cut into about 12 rounds with a floured 2½-inch biscuit cutter. Arrange on baking sheet and bake for 12 to 15 minutes, or until lightly browned.

To assemble: Remove chicken to a serving platter and keep warm. Add remaining stock and chili powder to skillet. Cook over medium heat for 3 minutes, stirring with a wooden spoon to scrape up browned bits. Turn off heat and whisk in yogurt. Pour sauce over chicken and serve immediately with warm biscuits.

Yield: 6 servings

Chapter 72

High-Calcium Cookery

Low-fat dairy products are the best.

W hat are the best food sources of calcium? Dairy products are particularly good, but you have to be selective. Full-fat products like whole milk, whole-milk yogurt, ice cream and many types of cheeses are too high in fat to be smart choices. Opt instead for skim milk, low-fat yogurt, buttermilk and low-fat or part-skim cheeses. Other good sources are salmon and sardines (bones included), broccoli, dried beans, blackstrap molasses, tofu, raisins, dried figs, oysters and green leafy vegetables.

You can beef up the calcium in foods by making a few adjustments as you cook.

A tip for increasing calcium in stock.

When cooking stock, soups or stews that contain bones, add a little vinegar or lemon juice or some chopped tomatoes to the pot. The acid in these ingredients will help leach the calcium from the bones. Stock made this way may have as much as 125 milligrams of calcium in each cup. That's as much as you'll find in ⅔ cup of cottage cheese.

Add skim milk to your finished soups just before serving to increase calcium even further.

Make good use of instant nonfat dry milk. With 52 milligrams of calcium (and only 15 calories) per tablespoon, it's an excellent calcium booster. Add it to fluid milk, yogurt, sauces, desserts, blender beverages, dips, soups, salad dressings and hot cereal.

Bone-Builder Recipes

The following recipes can help you get started on high-calcium cookery.

PIZZA NICOISE

DOUGH
½ cup plus 2 tablespoons unbleached flour
½ cup plus 2 tablespoons whole wheat pastry
    flour
½ teaspoon dry yeast
½ cup skim milk
1 teaspoon olive oil
½ teaspoon honey

TOPPING
⅔ cup thick tomato sauce
½ cup red onion slices
1 teaspoon dried basil
1 clove garlic, minced
1 can (3¾ ounces) low-sodium water-packed
    sardines
1 cup shredded part-skim mozzarella cheese

To make the dough: In a medium-size bowl, combine flours, yeast, milk, oil and honey. Knead for 5 minutes. Cover and let rest for about 10 minutes.

Preheat oven to 500°F.

Coat a pizza pan or baking sheet with vegetable spray. Press dough in pan to form a 12-inch round with raised edges. Bake for 5 minutes, or until light brown.

To make the topping: In a medium-size bowl, combine tomato sauce, onions, basil and garlic. Spread on baked pizza shell. Arrange sardines over sauce, then sprinkle with mozzarella. Bake for 5 minutes, or until cheese is golden and bubbly.

Yield: 4 servings

CORN CREPES WITH BEAN PÂTÉ

Masa harina, used in these crepes, is a fine corn flour popular throughout Mexico and Latin America. Soaked in lime water, masa harina gives tortillas their characteristic nutty-sweet flavor. Purchase the cornmeal in Mexican or Spanish grocery stores or in gourmet departments.

CREPES
¼ cup masa harina
¼ cup unbleached flour
¼ teaspoon turmeric
1 egg
½ cup skim milk
½ cup pureed corn kernels
2 teaspoons oil
1 tablespoon snipped chives

PÂTÉ
½ cup cooked white beans
½ cup cooked pinto beans
¼ cup minced fresh parsley
1 clove garlic, chopped
1 tablespoon lemon juice
1 teaspoon French-style mustard

ASSEMBLY
10 thin stalks broccoli, steamed
¼ cup shredded Monterey Jack cheese
½ cup chopped tomatoes

To make the crepes: In a large bowl, mix masa harina, flour, turmeric, egg, milk, corn, oil and chives. Let stand for 10 minutes. The batter should be the consistency of heavy cream. If it isn't, thin with additional milk.

Heat a nonstick crepe pan over medium heat and brush very lightly with oil. Add 2 tablespoons batter to pan, swirl to cover the bottom completely, then cook until top is dry and underside is lightly brown. Flip and cook other side briefly. Cool on a wire rack. Repeat with remaining batter, lightly brushing pan with oil, when necessary.

To make the pâté: In a blender or food processor, puree beans, parsley, garlic, lemon juice and mustard until smooth.

To assemble: Place a portion of pâté along edge of each crepe. Lay a broccoli stalk on top, then roll crepes to enclose filling. Arrange, seam-side down, on an ovenproof serving platter. Sprinkle with cheese. Broil for several minutes to warm crepes and melt cheese. Sprinkle with tomatoes.

Yield: 10 crepes

PESTO CHEESE

Serve as a spread for raw vegetables or whole grain crackers or as a topping for baked potatoes.

    4 cups plain yogurt
    ⅓ cup tightly packed basil leaves
    2 tablespoons sunflower seeds
    1 teaspoon olive oil
    1 teaspoon French-style mustard
    1 clove garlic

Spoon yogurt into a sieve lined with cheesecloth and allow to drain overnight. Transfer to a medium-size bowl.

Place basil, sunflower seeds, oil, mustard and garlic in a food processor or blender and process for 10 to 15 seconds, or until a paste forms. Add to yogurt, mixing with a spoon or wire whisk. Store in a covered container in the refrigerator.

Yield: about 1¼ cups

SMILING TOFU

This marinated tofu makes a face when you stuff it with savory shrimp filling.

MARINADE
⅓ cup chicken stock
1 tablespoon low-sodium soy sauce
1 tablespoon rice vinegar
1 teaspoon sesame oil
2 slices gingerroot, minced
1 clove garlic, minced

FILLING
3 ounces shelled, deveined shrimp (7 or 8 medium)
3 scallions, chopped
2 slices gingerroot, chopped
¼ cup sliced water chestnuts
1 clove garlic, chopped
1½ teaspoons cornstarch
1 tablespoon reserved marinade (above)
½ teaspoon sesame oil

ASSEMBLY
1 block (16 ounces) smooth, firm tofu
⅔ cup chicken stock
2 scallions, chopped

To make the marinade: In a shallow dish, combine stock, soy sauce, vinegar, sesame oil, ginger and garlic.

To make the filling: In a food processor or blender, combine shrimp, scallions, ginger, water chestnuts, garlic, cornstarch, marinade and sesame oil, and process until well mixed. Set aside.

To assemble: Cut tofu into 4 equal triangles by slicing an "X" through block. Cut each triangle in half horizontally to make 8 equal triangles. Make a pocket in each triangle by slicing each piece as you would a hamburger roll, starting at point and stopping ½ inch from wide end. Place tofu in marinade. Soak for 10 minutes, then turn and soak for 10 minutes more.

Divide filling into 8 portions. Gently stuff triangles, smoothing filled edges with your finger. (See the tofu smile?)

Coat a nonstick skillet with vegetable spray. Place 4 triangles in the pan, standing them on their filled edges. (The filling will not come out.) Cook for 1 minute on each edge. Then cook for 1 minute on each flat side. Add ⅓ cup stock and simmer for 3 minutes. Flip triangles and simmer for 3 minutes more. Remove to a serving platter. Repeat with remaining triangles and stock.

Add marinade to pan and reduce by half. Pour marinade over tofu and sprinkle with scallions.

Yield: 4 servings

ORANGE-ALMOND CHEESE

Serve this as a breakfast cheese with warm muffins or toast, or mixed into hot cereal. Or enjoy it as a dessert with sliced apples or fruit kabobs.

   4 cups plain yogurt
   2 tablespoons raisins, minced
   1 tablespoon slivered almonds, toasted and
         chopped
  1½ teaspoons honey
  1½ teaspoons frozen orange juice concentrate
         pinch of ground cinnamon

Spoon yogurt into a sieve lined with cheesecloth and allow to drain overnight. Transfer to a medium-size bowl. Mix in raisins, almonds, honey, orange juice concentrate and cinnamon. Store in a covered container in the refrigerator.

Yield: about 1¼ cups

ANTIPASTO WITH BAKED OYSTERS

OYSTERS

8 oysters on the half shell
½ teaspoon French-style mustard
¼ teaspoon fennel seeds, crushed
¼ cup minced tomato, well drained
1½ tablespoons minced scallions

SAUCE

¼ cup plain yogurt
1 tablespoon instant nonfat dry milk
¼ teaspoon French-style mustard
¼ teaspoon fennel seeds, crushed

ANTIPASTO

15 leaves kale (purple and green)
1 cup broccoli, steamed
1 can (6 ounces) salmon, drained and
   chunked
8 dried figs
½ cup ricotta cheese

To prepare the oysters: Preheat oven to 450°F. In a 9-inch pie plate, arrange oysters in their shells. In a small bowl, combine mustard and fennel. Spoon over oysters. Bake for 10 minutes, or until oysters change color from gray to whitish. Sprinkle with tomatoes and scallions.

To make the sauce: In a small bowl, combine yogurt, dry milk, mustard and fennel.

To make the antipasto: Line a serving platter with kale. Arrange broccoli, salmon and oysters on kale.

Slit the fat part of each fig with a sharp knife. Using a small spoon or a pastry bag fitted with a small tube, fill each fig with ricotta. Add to platter. Serve with yogurt sauce. Use kale leaves to scoop up other ingredients.

Yield: 4 to 6 servings

The Health Scoop
on Ice Cream

Americans are notorious trend followers, especially when it comes to edibles. One year crepes are in; the next year it's quiche, followed by pasta and kiwi dishes. But through all these years and fickle food fads, one thing has remained constant—our unflagging passion for ice cream.

Through thick (so to speak) and thin, feast or famine, recession, depression, rainy days and holidays, Americans have consistently taken their licks and come back for more. Even now, when it seems slightly out of character for a nation whose health consciousness has recently been raised, ice cream continues to be our major frozen asset.

Even health-conscious people can't resist ice cream.

According to the International Ice Cream Association (IICA) in Washington, D.C., almost 924 million gallons of ice cream were sold in 1986—that's up more than 4 percent from 1983 and almost 20 percent from 1973, with the greatest growth in the newer high-fat, super-premium ice creams.

Is Ice Cream More Nutritious than Other Snacks?

While ice cream's popularity has almost everything to do with taste, there persists the belief that it's somehow a step above other snack foods on the nutritional ladder. And that may indeed account for its appeal among both the health-conscious and the health-unconscious.

Whichever you are, we think it's time you were exposed to the cold facts about ice cream's nutritional status and how it stacks up against other common snack foods.

First of all, you have to know what goes into ice cream—and we're talking about commercial varieties, not homemade—before you can level any judgment against it. Basically, ice cream is made up of cream and milk combined with sugar (table sugar, corn syrup or honey), flavorings and fruits and nuts, in various proportions. To be called ice cream, federal standards require that vanilla contain at least 10 percent butterfat and chocolate 8 percent. Most supermarket store brands fall into this "economy" category. The more butterfat in the mix, the fancier the name, so there are the upscale, premium and superpremium (or gourmet) ice creams, with butterfat levels reaching 18 to 20 percent in certain cases.

Fancier brands are higher in fat.

The amount of sugar in ice cream, on the other hand, doesn't vary. Since ice cream is formulated to contain 15 to 16 percent sugar, sweetness is sometimes the most prominent taste. "Ice cream has to be extra sweet," says Gabe Mirkin, M.D., author of *Getting Thin*, "because cold numbs the taste buds for sweetness. Just let ice cream melt and see how much sweeter it tastes than when it was frozen," he says.

Why cold confections are so sweet.

Cold, Creamy, Sweet— and Not All Bad

On a more positive note, ice cream is, after all, a dairy product and contains many of the same good things that other dairy products do. It can boast reasonable amounts of protein, bone-strengthening calcium (though this should never be a main dietary source) and vitamin A—from 272 international units for a typical ½-cup (one large scoop) serving of the lower-fat ice cream to 449 international units for

Ice cream contains some protein, calcium and vitamin A.

higher-fat ones. And it's moderately low in cholesterol and sodium.

If you read the labels, you'll also notice that some manufacturers add stabilizers—such as guar gum, carrageenan, locust bean gum (which all come from plants) and gelatin—to protect the ice cream from the temperature fluctuations known as "heat shock." These additives help prevent large ice crystals, which tend to form when ice cream is partially melted and then refrozen. Emulsifiers (such as monoglycerides and diglycerides) help ensure easy scooping.

According to Michael Jacobson, Ph.D., executive director of the Center for Science in the Public Interest in Washington, D.C., "these additives never killed anybody like eating too much fat will."

Now for the Bad News....

Naturally, fat is about the worst thing (calorie-wise and health-wise) going for ice cream, and wouldn't you know, it's the main ingredient that separates ordinary ice cream from gourmet.

If you're going to eat ice cream, you should choose the one that's the lowest in fat and also get the one that's lowest in calories, right? Yes, but there's a hitch, and it has to do with the amount of air that's pumped into the ice cream (called "overrun"). The lower-fat (economy) ones are usually the fluffiest, so that a ½-cup serving may not be satisfying, and you might be inclined to eat more.

"Fluffier" ice creams are lower in fat.

The denser or heavier (gourmet) ice creams have very little added air, and because they are so concentrated, you may be satisfied with less.

Is ice cream really a superior snack? That depends on what you're comparing it with. Put against apples, oranges or just about any other fruit or vegetable, no. What about other snacks? Let's add up the calories of some common snacks and see how they

How ice cream compares with other snacks.

compare to a dish of economy and gourmet ice creams. The table, Nutritional Value of Ice Cream and Other Snack Foods, on pages 560–61, lists typical servings of popular snack foods, but if you're not typical, you could be getting less or more than the amounts listed.

For the sake of comparison, we'll use the lowest-calorie ice cream (159 calories per serving) and the highest (275 calories) and assume you'll be able to hold it to the average ½-cup serving.

Let's start with pretzels and beer. A typical serving of both adds up to 263 calories. By adding just one more beer, you've managed to tally up 409 calories.

Cookies and milk add up to a quick 300 calories, and that's if you can stop at two cookies.

If you decide on a serving of soda and chips, that's 312 calories. You can see that in calories alone a serving of the lower-fat ice cream is a clear winner. Besides, with the exception of milk, the snack foods we've mentioned don't have the nutrients that ice cream does, while they do contain some baddies, such as excessive salt, fat and/or sugar.

Calcium in Your Snacks

Not as calorie-rich as cheese and crackers.

"What about a snack of crackers and cheese?" you may ask. "That's not as bad as other snacks, is it?" As usual, there are pluses and minuses. How much cheese do you eat? For the purposes of compiling the table, two slices of American cheese sounded reasonable. If you cut them into quarters, you'd lay them on top of eight crackers, right? Want to wash it down with anything? A soda, maybe? Okay, you've just eaten 406 calories. That's too much for one snack, you say? Then let's cut it back to one slice of cheese and four crackers, plus the soda. Now the total is 278, still more than the lower-fat ice cream.

We can't forget to mention, however, that cheese is a good source of calcium and protein. Unfortunately, it's also high in sodium and fat.

Or, say you've decided to be very responsible about snacking, so you've switched to strawberry yogurt. And you're right—mostly. Yogurt is an excellent source of protein, calcium and some vitamins. Best of all, it's *very* low in fat. But even strawberry yogurt has a major drawback—sugar. And because of that, the calories mount up to 260 for an eight-ounce serving.

But what's lowest in calories may fail the percent-of-fat test. In fact, that's ice cream's greatest downfall. Look at the fat and calorie table again. You'll see that ice cream rates as high as or higher than candy bars, cheese, cookies, milk, and potato chips, and tortilla chips rate as high or higher than ice cream in percentage of calories from fat. The only positive note here is that while the fat levels are unfortunately high, the amount of cholesterol is on the low side—about 30 milligrams for the lower-fat varieties and 44 milligrams for the higher-fat ones. (Many doctors recommend that cholesterol be kept to a maximum of 300 milligrams per day.)

Ice cream's biggest drawback.

Like any snack food, ice cream has its negatives and positives. But there are more positives for ice cream than for many other snacks. So we're not about to tell you to never, ever put a spoon in your mouth again.

Instead, take a close look at your own diet and lifestyle. Are you overweight? Do your meals consist of lots of fast-food burgers and french fries? Do you routinely eat sausage, bacon and other fatty meats? Is the only exercise you get drawing your chair to the table? Then adding ice cream to your diet could help push both your calorie and fat consumption into the danger zone.

But if fresh vegetables, fruits, whole grains, chicken and fish are your mainstays and exercise is as routine as brushing your teeth, then go ahead and enjoy your just desserts—*once in a while.* Only consider softening the blow a little by choosing an ice cream that's lower in fat. Then put less in your dish and smother it with fresh fruit, like peaches or berries.

When ice cream is the right choice.

Nutritional Value of Ice Cream and Other Snack Foods

Product	Portion	Calcium (mg.)
Vanilla ice cream*		
Giant's Wellesley Farms, 10.2% fat	½ cup	55
Acme's Econo Buy, 10.2% fat	½ cup	64
Haagen-Dazs, 16.6% fat	½ cup	103
Frusen Gladje, 17.5% fat	½ cup	82
Apple †	1	10
Beer †	1 can (12 oz.)	18
Brownies, prepared from mix ‡	1 piece (2″ sq.)	Less than 0.02
Candy bar †	1 (2 oz.)	130
Cheese, processed American †	2 slices (¾ oz. ea.)	261
Chocolate chip cookies, prepared from mix ‡	2	Less than 0.02
Milk, whole, 3.3% fat †	1 cup	291
Milk shake, vanilla, fast-food §	10 oz.	344
Orange †	1	52
Potato chips †	1 oz. (14)	11
Pretzels †	1 oz. (5)	6.5
Saltines †	8	4
Soda, cola flavor †	1 can (12 oz.)	9
Strawberry yogurt ‡	8 oz.	280
Tortilla chips ‡	1 oz. (15)	30

NOTE: Where a dash appears, no data are available; food may or may not contain this element.

* Ice creams were analyzed by private laboratory.
† Nutritional information from USDA Handbooks No. 8–1, 8–14.
‡ Nutritional information calculated directly from package.
§ Nutritional information supplied by McDonald's.

Total Calories	Calories from Fat (%)	Protein (% of RDA for Adult Male)	Sodium (mg.)
159	47	4.6	—
181	46	5.5	—
272	59	8.8	—
275	61	8.2	—
81	5	0.5	1
146	0	1.6	19
130	35	1.8	95
302	60	9.3	46
159	75	16.8	609
150	48	1.8	95
150	48	14.3	120
211	35	17.5	232
62	2	2.2	0
161	63	2.7	As high as 284
117	10	5.3	1,008
96	23	3.6	123
151	0	0	14
260	10	17.9	—
145	50	3.6	183

Chapter 74

Selecting and Storing Vegetables for Maximum Nutrition

Vegetables are generally good sources of potassium, fiber and vitamins A and C. Some are good sources of B complex vitamins, calcium, magnesium and iron. Most are low in calories and fat. To maximize those nutrients, keep the following points in mind.

- The longer vegetables are exposed to air, heat, and water, the more nutrients they lose.
- Vegetables consumed raw immediately after harvesting have the most nutrients and best taste.
- Freshly picked produce from a nearby farmers' market or roadside stand is generally superior to vegetables that have been stored and then shipped in from faraway places.
- When shopping, look for healthy-colored, crisp vegetables with no signs of wilting or spoilage.

Overexposure to air, heat and water destroys nutrients.

Here is a listing of some specific vegetables and how to choose them.

Artichokes. Look for compact scales of a deep green color. If artichokes are fresh, they will squeak when rubbed against each other. If the leaves have started to spread, they are past their prime. Store in plastic bags or closed containers in the refrigerator for up to five days.

Giving artichokes the "rub" test.

Asparagus. Look for straight stalks with closed tips. Wrap in moist paper towels, enclose in a plastic bag, and store in the refrigerator for up to five days. An alternate storage method: Cut a thin piece off the bottom of each stalk, then stand the stalk upright in a tall container that has about an inch of water in the bottom. Slip a plastic bag over the top to hold in moisture.

Avocados. Also known as alligator pears, avocados are really fruit, but they're mostly used as a vegetable. Look for avocados that are fairly heavy, solid and free of bruises or black spots. Allow hard avocados to ripen at room temperature in a paper bag. When ready to eat, they'll feel soft if pressed gently between the palms. Ripe uncut avocados can keep in the refrigerator for four to seven days.

Ripen them in a paper bag.

Broccoli. Stalks should be tender and firm, not woody or limp. Flower buds should be tightly closed and dark green. If flowers are yellow or starting to open, the broccoli is past its prime. Plan to use soon after purchase. Store broccoli in a plastic bag in the refrigerator.

Garlic. Select firm, filled-out bulbs with clean skins. Store in a cool, dry place in a ventilated garlic jar or net bag. A hanging braid lasts a long time if properly cared for. If you must store garlic in the refrigerator, keep it in a closed container to prevent odor exchange with other foods.

How to store garlic.

Eggplant. Look for heavy, shiny eggplants that have almost black, patent-leather-like skins and bright green stem caps. The skin should feel firm when you press it with your thumb. Large eggplants contain more seeds and have tougher skins than small ones. Store in the refrigerator in a covered container or wrapped in plastic to minimize moisture loss. Use as soon as possible.

Mushrooms. Look for firm mushrooms with closed caps. Clean them with a damp paper towel or a mushroom brush. Store in the refrigerator, either on a shallow tray covered loosely with a damp paper towel or in a paper bag. Use within a few days.

How to keep mushrooms fresh longer.

Onions. Choose only firm bulbs with papery skins. Avoid onions that have begun to sprout. Store in a cool, dark, dry spot, preferably in a net sack for good circulation. Don't store near potatoes, which give off moisture and can cause onions to sprout or to rot.

A Harvest of Delights to Lighten Your Blood Pressure

You might want to go out today and hug a farmer. The prescription to keep your blood pressure down may be growing in his fields and orchards or grazing in his pastures right now.

Potassium, abundant in fresh fruits and vegetables, and calcium, found largely in dairy products, may be science's latest dietary one-two punch in the fight against hypertension.

During the last few years, studies have uncovered what may be an important link between dietary calcium and potassium and blood pressure. Researchers have found that people whose diets are potassium-rich—vegetarians, for example—have a low incidence of hypertension even if they're genetically disposed to the condition and don't control their salt intake.

Large-population surveys revealed the calcium connection: People with high blood pressure don't seem to get much calcium in the form of dairy products (and it's hard to get much without them). In one test, people who were mildly hypertensive and had lower levels of serum calcium experienced a moderate but consistent drop in blood pressure when they were given oral calcium supplements. The biggest improvement was seen in those people who had the lowest levels of calcium to start with. Studies like that are leading doctors to believe that there's much, much more to controlling blood pressure than cutting back on salt.

Battling high blood pressure with calcium and potassium.

Foods to Lower
Your Blood Pressure

The exact mechanisms by which the two essential nutrients regulate blood pressure continue to evade researchers. But both appear to help the body slough off excess sodium and are involved in important functions that control the workings of the vascular system.

Of course, the studies are relatively recent, and the evidence is far from voluminous. The calcium theory, in particular, is still so novel it falls into the hot-controversy category. But even some of the most cautious find it convincing, such as the nutritionist Patricia Hausman, author of *The Calcium Bible.* "It's a new idea," says Hausman. "There aren't a lot of studies, as there are on sodium. I'd call it preliminary but promising. The data there are impressive. I'm leaning toward thinking there's some effect here."

The calcium/hypertension link: "preliminary but promising."

For people who are used to the no-no diets for hypertension, the studies are promising in another way. "The thing that's nice about potassium and calcium is that they're positive nutrients, things people should eat more of," says Arlene Caggiula, Ph.D., associate professor of nutrition at the University of Pittsburgh Graduate School of Public Health. Dr. Caggiula's research focuses on dietary approaches to hypertension, and she has designed well-balanced diets for people with high blood pressure and education programs to help them stick to them. "With sodium you're saying to people, 'You can't eat it.' With potassium and calcium you're saying, 'You can and you should.' "

A Summer Harvest
of "Good Medicine"

The other nice thing about potassium and calcium is that they're easy to swallow, especially in the form of fruits and vegetables. Not only is it easy to work these two pressure-lowering nutrients into your menu, you can get them—deliciously—in the same dish. In fact, you can virtually build a diet around the foods they're in. All it takes is a little knowledge and a lot of ingenuity.

Tasty calcium-potassium dishes.

Getting potassium isn't tough. "It's in almost everything," says Hausman. It's abundant in foods that are wonderful for you: fruits, vegetables, beans, fish, poultry and lean cuts of meat.

Getting calcium is not quite as easy. Unfortunately, the foods that contain the most calcium tend to contain a fair amount of fat and sodium, too, which can spell trouble for hypertensives on fat- and salt-controlled diets. Difficult does not mean impossible, however. There are plenty of low-fat, low-sodium dairy alternatives—and some calcium-rich foods that haven't even been near the barnyard.

If you aren't hypertensive, by all means don't scratch milk and milk products off your shopping list. "For people to avoid milk because of sodium—unless you have hypertension—is not a good idea," says Leonard Braitman, Ph.D., a statistical consultant who worked on early calcium and hypertension studies. "For some people, like the lactose intolerant, it's not a good food. For other people, it's hard to beat. It's hard to make up your calcium intake with other foods. People should be aware that for people who have hypertension, sodium is a problem. But for others it's probably not."

The number one food source of calcium.

Creative Cookery in Ten Easy Steps

Ready to start a diet that may last—and lengthen—a lifetime? The first rule of all good menu planning is to make a list. Refer to the tables, Best Food Sources of Calcium, on pages 568–69, and Best Food Sources of Potassium, on pages 570–71, to help

Designing your own antihypertension diet.

Best Food Sources of Calcium

Food	Portion	Calcium (mg.)
Swiss cheese (LS)	2 oz.	544
Provolone cheese	2 oz.	428
Monterey Jack cheese	2 oz.	424
Yogurt, low-fat* (LS)	1 cup	415
Cheddar cheese	2 oz.	408
Muenster cheese	2 oz.	406
Colby cheese	2 oz.	388
Brick cheese	2 oz.	382
Sardines, Atlantic, drained solids*	3 oz.	372
American cheese	2 oz.	348
Ricotta cheese, part-skim	½ cup	337
Milk, skim* (LF, LS)	1 cup	302
Mozzarella cheese	2 oz.	294
Buttermilk*	1 cup	285
Limburger cheese	2 oz.	282
Ice milk, soft-serve* (LF, LS)	1 cup	274
Salmon, sockeye, drained solids* (LS)	3 oz.	271

SOURCES: Adapted from

Composition of Foods, Agriculture Handbook No. 8, by Bernice K. Watt and Annabel L. Merrill (Washington, D.C: Agricultural Research Service, U.S. Department of Agriculture, 1975).

Composition of Foods: Dairy and Egg Products, Agriculture Handbook No. 8–1, by Consumer and Food Economics Institute (Washington, D.C.: Agricultural Research Service, U.S. Department of Agriculture, 1976).

Nutritive Value of American Foods in Common Units, Agriculture Handbook No. 456, by Catherine F. Adams (Washington, D.C.: Agricultural Research Service, U.S. Department of Agriculture, 1975).

you design your own hypertension diet. We've marked the high-calcium foods that are low in fat and salt and high in potassium to help you make healthy choices. And here are a few tips to get you started.

1. Exercise your ingenuity. When you take a look at that list, envision new combinations of familiar foods: yogurt and bananas, salmon fillet with potatoes and broccoli, raisins and nuts. Imagine half a canta-

Food	Portion	Calcium (mg.)
Ice cream*	1 cup	176
Ice milk* (LF, LS)	1 cup	176
Tofu (LF, LS)	3 oz.	174
Pizza, cheese	⅛ of 14″ pie	144
Blackstrap molasses (LF)	1 tbsp.	137
Soy flour, defatted	½ cup	120
Almonds* (LS)	¼ cup	100
Broccoli, cooked* (LF, LS)	½ cup	89
Soybeans, cooked* (LS)	½ cup	88
Parmesan cheese	1 tbsp.	86
Collards, cooked (LF, LS)	½ cup	74
Dandelion greens, cooked	½ cup	74
Mustard greens, cooked (LF, LS)	½ cup	52
Kale, cooked (LF, LS)	½ cup	47
Broccoli, raw* (LF, LS)	1 cup	42
Chick-peas, cooked (LS)	½ cup	40

Nutrient Data Research Branch, U.S. Department of Agriculture, Washington, D.C.

NOTES:

If LF follows a food name, it indicates a low-fat food.
If LS follows a food name, it indicates a low-sodium food.

*Food is also high in potassium.

loupe filled with a scoop of ice milk or ricotta cheese. Think about a summer cooler made in the blender from orange juice, bananas and nonfat dry milk. Before you crack open a cookbook, experiment with your own combinations.

2. Browse through your cookbooks. Every home cookbook library is chock-full of recipes that are bypassed in lieu of family favorites. To rediscover

Best Food Sources of Potassium

Food	Portion	Potassium (mg.)
Potato, baked	1 medium	844
Avocado	½	602
Raisins	½ cup	545
Sardines, Atlantic, drained solids*	3 oz.	501
Flounder, baked	3 oz.	498
Orange juice	1 cup	496
Banana	1	471
Apricots, dried	¼ cup	448
Squash, winter, cooked	½ cup	445
Cantaloupe	¼ medium	413
Skim milk*	1 cup	406
Sweet potato, baked	1 medium	397
Salmon fillet, cooked*	3 oz.	378
Buttermilk*	1 cup	371
Whole milk*	1 cup	370
Round steak, trimmed of fat, broiled	3 oz.	352

SOURCES: Adapted from

Composition of Foods, Agriculture Handbook No. 8, by Bernice K. Watt and Annabel L. Merrill (Washington, D.C.: Agricultural Research Service, U.S. Department of Agriculture, 1975).

Composition of Foods: Dairy and Egg Products, Agriculture Handbook No. 8–1, by Consumer and Food Economics Institute (Washington, D.C.: Agricultural Research Service, U.S. Department of Agriculture, 1976).

Composition of Foods: Legumes and Legume Products, Agriculture Handbook No. 8–16, by Nutrition Monitoring Division (Washington, D.C.: Human Nutrition Information Service, U.S. Department of Agriculture, 1986).

Composition of Foods: Nut and Seed Products, Agriculture Handbook No. 8–12, by Nutrition Monitoring Division (Washington, D.C.: Human Nutrition Information Service, U.S. Department of Agriculture, 1984).

Scanning recipes that are high in potassium and calcium.

combos that will help lower your blood pressure, start by consulting the indexes of your old standbys for the ingredients featured in the two tables. Then zero in on dishes that are low in calories, fat and sodium. (Many recipes will still work even if you cut back on salt and fat.) You may discover new combinations of potassium- and calcium-rich foods that have been right under your nose for years. (If you reach a dead end,

Food	Portion	Potassium (mg.)
Cod, baked	3 oz.	345
Great Northern beans, cooked	½ cup	344
Sirloin, trimmed of fat, broiled	3 oz.	342
Apricots, fresh	3	313
Beef liver, pan-fried	3 oz.	309
Haddock, fried	3 oz.	297
Pork, trimmed of fat, cooked	3 oz.	283
Tomato, raw	1	279
Leg of lamb, trimmed of fat, cooked	3 oz.	274
Turkey, light meat, roasted	3 oz.	259
Perch, fried	3 oz.	243
Tuna, drained solids	3 oz.	225
Chicken, light meat, roasted	3 oz.	210
Broccoli, cooked*	½ cup	127

Composition of Foods: Vegetables and Vegetable Products, Agriculture Handbook No. 8–11, by Nutrition Monitoring Division (Washington, D.C.: Human Nutrition Information Service, U.S. Department of Agriculture, 1984).

Nutritive Value of American Foods in Common Units, Agriculture Handbook No. 456, by Catherine F. Adams (Washington, D.C.: Agricultural Research Service, U.S. Department of Agriculture, 1975).

The Calcium Bible, by Patricia Hausman (New York: Rawson Associates, 1985).

Nutrient Data Research Branch, U.S. Department of Agriculture, Washington, D.C.

*Food is also high in calcium.

your local library probably has shelves of cookbooks to give you ideas, and many may feature recipes low in calories, fat and sodium.)

3. Feature foods with high amounts of potassium and calcium. Not only can you get potassium and calcium in the same dish, you can get them in the same food. A few of the foods that are high in both nutrients are: sardines, scallops, skim milk, broccoli, salmon, buttermilk, whole milk, soybeans, blackstrap molasses, navy beans, almonds, ice milk and yogurt. If you're exercising your ingenuity, you can probably see a whole meal literally from soup to nuts, using just a few of these double-duty foods.

4. Stock up on low-fat yogurt. "It's a real bonanza food," says Dr. Caggiula. Not only is it low in fat and relatively low in sodium, it's high in calcium and potassium and can be used for everything from salad dressing to dessert. "Plain low-fat yogurt alone has 350 milligrams of potassium, and flavored low-fat yogurt has an average value of 450 milligrams," says Dr. Caggiula. "The best thing is that the low fat is even higher in potassium than regular yogurt." For high amounts of calcium, look for low-fat yogurt to which the manufacturer has added nonfat milk solids, suggests Patricia Hausman. It adds considerably more calcium and no more fat. She also suggests "dressing up" plain yogurt with potassium-rich foods such as frozen orange juice concentrate, raisins, sliced fresh fruit or shredded raw vegetables. If you're not a yogurt fan, you can get all its benefits by hiding it in blender shakes with fresh fruit and a sweetener such as honey or aspartame or in cold fruit soups.

5. Treat yourself to a Banana Smoothie. You can add high potassium and calcium nonfat milk solids to dishes simply by adding nonfat dry milk. Two tablespoons of nonfat dry milk added to half a glass of skim milk boosts the calcium from 150 to 255 milligrams. Add a banana, as Hausman does in her Banana Smoothie, and you've got a supercharged potassium/calcium breakfast.

To make a Banana Smoothie, combine ¾ cup skim milk, ¼ cup nonfat dry milk, ½ tablespoon peanut butter, a very ripe banana, one to two packets aspartame or 1 tablespoon honey and two ice cubes in a blender and process until smooth. One caveat: Though low in fat and sodium, this delicious drink is high in calories—282 per serving. If you're dieting, it's not the best snack or thirst quencher but a great and nutritious breakfast or lunch.

A nearly perfect antihypertension food.

A supercharged potassium/calcium breakfast.

When adding nonfat dry milk to milk products, use these proportions: 2 tablespoons milk powder to ½ cup milk, ¼ cup milk powder to 1 cup milk; 6 tablespoons milk powder to 1½ cups milk and ½ cup milk powder to 2 cups milk.

6. Reach for ricotta. While cottage cheese and fruit may be a favorite summer lunch, you can substantially increase the amount of calcium in the meal by substituting ricotta. Though it also has more fat and calories than cottage cheese, ricotta has about 260 milligrams of calcium in ½ cup compared to only about 80 milligrams in cottage cheese. You can cut out some fat by using part-skim ricotta or by mixing it with low-fat cottage cheese. It's great served with high-potassium vegetables, too.

A high-calcium cheese.

7. Toss together a stir-fry pizza. Make your own pizza dough—or buy it ready-made—but don't use the usual toppings. Vegetables like carrots, onions, peppers and broccoli (which is also high in calcium), either stir-fried in a bit of oil or steamed, take the place of tomato sauce. Top with part-skim mozzarella cheese and bake as usual.

Special toppings for pizza.

8. Improvise with canned pink salmon. Salmon is high in potassium and calcium—because of the tiny bones you can eat—and mixes well with cheese and vegetables. Served hot with vegetables or as the star of a cold vegetable-pasta salad, salmon can become a staple of your blood pressure diet.

9. Use soy foods for a calcium payoff. If you have to restrict your dairy intake, soy foods such as tofu and some cooked beans can provide a modest amount of calcium. Tofu, in particular, can be used in place of cheese in many dishes. It has about 150 milligrams of calcium per four-ounce serving. And it now comes packaged and tastes just like that summer treat, ice cream.

A good alternative to milk products.

10. Enjoy shrimp, the special occasion star. Though high in cholesterol, shrimp is a fair source of calcium and a delicious ingredient of a vegetable stir-fry high in potassium.

Chapter 76

A Healthy
Sandwich Sampler

A lot of folks think there's nothing new under the bun. "Sandwiches are just sandwiches," they say. "Big deal."

But sandwiches—with plenty of nutritious goodies tucked between two slices of whole grain bread—can be both handy and healthy.

Try no-salt condiments.

There's really no trick to it—you just have to be willing to experiment. You can stuff your sandwiches with vegetables, fish, fruit, nuts or eggs in any combination that pleases your taste buds. For toppers, you can use dressings made with tasty herbs and low-fat yogurt instead of salt and mayonnaise. And give the new no-salt mustards, ketchups and pickles a try.

Experiment with breads.

But that's not all. You can vary the *outside* as well as the inside of your sandwiches. Of course, whole wheat bread is always welcome, but rye, pumpernickel or pita may be just the thing to make your sandwiches sing.

Whether you like them hot or cold, plain or fancy, open-faced or closed, you can make sandwiches that stack up against the best. Just think of the possibilities.

Choice Sandwiches,
Fast and Easy

We've done a little of the thinking for you, and here are some of our best sandwich ideas.

PETITE PÂTÉ SANDWICHES

       1   pound chicken livers
       1   small onion, chopped
       1   tablespoon butter or margarine
           pinch of ground sage
           pinch of dried thyme
           pinch of dried rosemary
       1   teaspoon prepared mustard
           dash of hot pepper sauce
 4 to 6   crescent rolls
 ½ to ¾   cup coarsely chopped pimientos
 ½ to ¾   cup parsley sprigs

       In a medium-size skillet, sauté chicken livers
and onions in butter or margarine for 1 to 2 minutes.
Add sage, thyme, rosemary, mustard and hot pepper
sauce and sauté until livers are cooked. Place mixture
in a food processor and puree, then chill.
       Slice rolls in half horizontally. Spread bottoms
with pâté. Top with pimientos and parsley and replace
tops of rolls.

       Yield: 4 to 6 servings

GUACO TACOS

       2   avocados, chopped
 ⅓ to ½   cup thinly sliced scallions
       2   tablespoons lemon juice
 ¼ to ½   teaspoon hot pepper sauce
       8   taco shells
       1   cup shredded cheddar cheese
       1   cup shredded lettuce
       1   cup chopped tomatoes

       In a large bowl, combine avocados, scallions,
lemon juice and hot pepper sauce. Spoon into taco
shells. Top with cheese, lettuce and tomatoes.

       Yield: 4 servings

SIMPLE SALMON SANDWICHES

1 tablespoon mayonnaise
¼ cup plain yogurt
2 tablespoons chopped fresh dill
1 can (15½ ounces) salmon, drained and
    flaked
8 slices whole wheat bread, toasted
8 scallions
8 thin slices Swiss cheese

In a small bowl, combine mayonnaise, yogurt and dill. In a medium-size bowl, mix salmon with half of the dressing.

Spread salmon salad on four slices of toast. Place two scallions on top of each sandwich. Roll up slices of Swiss cheese and place two on each sandwich. Spread remaining slices of bread with remaining dressing and place on top.

Yield: 4 servings

MED CLUB

2 tablespoons olive oil or other vegetable oil
1 large eggplant, cut into ½-inch cubes
1 sweet red pepper, minced
1 onion, minced
3 cloves garlic, minced
¾ cup tomato sauce
2 tablespoons chopped fresh parsley
6 whole wheat pitas
½ pound thinly sliced cooked turkey breast
4 hard-cooked eggs, thinly sliced
½ pound thinly sliced provolone cheese

In a large, heavy skillet, heat 1 tablespoon oil and sauté eggplant over medium-high heat, stirring often, for 5 minutes, or until almost cooked through. Add remaining oil, peppers, onions and garlic. Sauté for 1 to 2 minutes. Add tomato sauce, reduce heat to medium and continue cooking until thick, about 5 minutes. Stir in parsley.

Cut pitas in half horizontally to make 12 slices. Roll up turkey slices and place on four of the pita bottoms, then top with sliced egg. Place a pita slice on each sandwich as the middle layer. Spoon on eggplant mixture. Roll up provolone slices and place on top of eggplant. Place remaining pita slices on top and cut sandwiches into quarters.

Yield: 4 servings

ZESTY PESTO HERO

Pesto, the Genoese sauce based on basil, cheese, garlic and oil, is not just for pasta or potatoes. As a sandwich spread, it blends beautifully with any salad vegetable from arugula to zucchini, stacked as high as you please!

    2   cloves garlic
 1½   cups loosely packed fresh basil
    ½   cup pine nuts
    ¾   cup grated Parmesan cheese
3 to 5   tablespoons olive oil or other vegetable oil
    2   loaves whole wheat French bread
    2   tomatoes, thinly sliced
    1   red onion, thinly sliced
   12   mushrooms, thinly sliced

In a food processor, mince garlic. Add basil and pine nuts and process until well minced. Add cheese and process until well blended. With the motor running, slowly pour in oil, adding only enough to make a thick spread. Continue processing until well blended.

Cut loaves of bread in half crosswise, then slice each piece in half horizontally. Spread cut side of each piece with pesto. On four bottom pieces, place a layer of tomatoes, then onions, then mushrooms. Place remaining pieces on top.

Yield: 4 servings

CURRIED CHICKEN AND FRUIT SANDWICHES

  3   cups cubed cooked chicken
  ⅓   cup chopped walnuts
  ⅓   cup halved grapes
  2   scallions, sliced
  3   tablespoons chopped fresh parsley
  2   tablespoons mayonnaise
  ¼   cup yogurt
1½   teaspoons curry powder
12   slices pumpernickel bread
  2   nectarines, peaches, apples or pears, thinly sliced

In a large bowl, combine chicken, walnuts, grapes, scallions and parsley. In a small bowl, combine mayonnaise, yogurt and curry powder.

Mix dressing into chicken mixture, then spoon salad onto six slices of bread. Top with fruit slices and remaining slices of bread.

Yield: 6 servings

ELEGANT MUSHROOM-CHEESE SANDWICHES

  2   tablespoons butter or margarine
  1   cup minced mushrooms
  1   tablespoon whole wheat pastry flour
  1   cup milk
  2   tablespoons minced fresh basil or
       1 tablespoon dried basil
16   asparagus spears
  4   slices whole wheat toast
  1   cup shredded cheddar cheese

In a medium-size saucepan, melt butter or margarine. Add mushrooms and sauté for 3 to 5 minutes. Stir in flour, reduce heat to low and cook for 1 to 2 minutes. Stir in milk gradually, blending well. Add basil and continue cooking over low heat, stirring frequently, until thick.

While sauce cooks, cut bottoms of asparagus, leaving 4- to 5-inch spears. Steam asparagus. Lay four asparagus spears on each slice of toast, then top each with one-quarter of the cheese. Place sandwiches on broiler pan and broil until cheese is bubbly. Place on serving plates and top with sauce.

Yield: 2 to 4 servings

SALAD-BAR SANDWICHES WITH SIX-HERB DRESSING

    ¼ cup plain yogurt
    1 tablespoon mayonnaise
    1 tablespoon ketchup
    1 teaspoon minced fresh parsley
    1 teaspoon minced chives
    ¼ teaspoon dillweed
    ¼ teaspoon dried basil
       pinch of dried tarragon
       pinch of dried thyme
    1 cup shredded or chopped cabbage
    1 cup shredded carrots
    ½ cup alfalfa sprouts
    ½ cup chopped tomatoes
    ½ cup chopped cucumbers
    ½ cup shredded cheddar cheese
    4 whole wheat pitas

In a medium-size bowl, combine yogurt, mayonnaise, ketchup, parsley, chives, dillweed, basil, tarragon and thyme and mix well.

In a large bowl, toss together cabbage, carrots, sprouts, tomatoes, cucumbers and cheese. Cut off an edge of each pita to form pockets. Spread inside of each pita with dressing, then stuff with the vegetable mixture.

Yield: 4 servings

WOK 'N' ROLL

    4 whole wheat sandwich rolls, cut in half
        horizontally
    ½ cup beef stock
    1½ teaspoons cornstarch
    2 teaspoons low-sodium soy sauce
    ½ pound beef round or sirloin, cut into thin
        strips
    1 tablespoon peanut oil
    1 green or sweet red pepper, cut into thin
        strips
    1 carrot, shredded
    1 onion, cut in half crosswise and sliced
    3 cloves garlic, minced
    ½ pound mushrooms, sliced
        pinch of ground red pepper

Hollow out each roll slightly by carefully removing some of the bread from the inside. Place rolls hollow-side up on serving plates.

In a medium-size bowl, combine stock, cornstarch and soy sauce and set aside.

In a wok or large skillet, stir-fry beef in oil just until browned. Add peppers, carrots and onions and stir-fry for about 30 seconds. Add garlic and stir-fry for another 30 seconds. Add mushrooms and continue stir-frying for 1 minute.

Add ground red pepper, pour in stock mixture and cook just until sauce thickens slightly, stirring occasionally. Spoon mixture onto rolls and serve immediately.

Yield: 4 servings

Low Sodium
from Soup to Nuts

G reat news! The food accent of the 1980s is on zingy flavor without salt.

Around the country, chefs are being trained to season their dishes so that when salt is removed, flavor isn't. The nation's food companies are developing lines of low-salt and no-salt products, and supermarkets are stocking them. Restaurants are offering no-salt gourmet dinners. Airlines and cruise lines are happy to serve low-sodium dishes.

The new era of low-sodium eating.

Yes, it's now possible to travel, entertain or go out on the town and enjoy foods that dance in your mouth but have hardly a grain of salt.

Of course, that makes not only your taste buds happy but your heart as well. Innumerable scientific studies have shown that there's a link between high-sodium intake and high blood pressure and that cutting back on sodium may help normalize blood pressure.

So be good to yourself and get in on the low-sodium boom. How? Do a little preliminary sodium sleuthing before you venture forth. Are you dining out, for instance? Check the restaurant to ascertain how they are using the saltshaker back in the kitchen. That's what we did, and here's what we discovered.

Dining out the low-salt way.

How the Pros Cut the Salt

We present here, of course, only a sampling of the use—or nonuse—of the saltshaker in the nation's restaurants. We suggest you do your own research in your hometown. Most chefs, we have found, are aware of the public's desire for less salt and are both creative and cooperative in their efforts to prepare healthy food without sacrificing good taste.

At the elegant Four Seasons in New York City, where chef Seppi Renggli has developed some innovative techniques for enhancing flavor without salt, you will find many items on the menu that are skillfully prepared without a grain of the stuff. For example, the whole wheat linguine with breast of quail is seasoned with garlic, shallots and cilantro. The bass and eggplant dish is flavored with a sweet red pepper pureé, spiked with a bit of hot red pepper. These salt-free menu items, dubbed Spa Cuisine, are proving to be very popular, manager Alex vonBidder told us.

Special seasonings replace salt.

If, however, you would prefer another item on the menu not included in the Spa Cuisine, you can request that no salt be added to the dish of your choice. In dishes that are made entirely from scratch, on the spot, that's rarely a problem. Soups and sauces may be exceptions. And the chef will compensate for the lack of salt with a judicious use of herbs and spices that will enhance the flavors of your particular dish.

Ask the chef to skip the salt.

In Hanover, New Hampshire, at the Hanover Inn, chef Michael Gray told us that very little salt is used behind the scenes. Since everything is made to order, that little bit can be eliminated and flavors enhanced with herbs, spices, fruit juices or vegetables. "Almost any dish, because it's cooked to order, can be prepared with little or no salt. And, when food is cooked fresh with local seasonal ingredients, flavors need little or no enhancement."

At the Blue Willow, also in New York City, they use nary a grain of salt in their cooking and make their own salt-free tomato sauce and salt-free spaghetti sauce, says chef Seth Lowenstein. They also provide commercial salt-free dill pickles and no-salt mustard, chutney and ketchup. Dishes that contain substances

A salt-free tomato sauce.

containing salt, such as cheese and bacon, are noted on the menu. Hamburgers and cheeseburgers have no added salt but are served in rolls that contain some salt. You may request low-sodium whole wheat Italian bread to replace the bun.

At La Normande and Le Bistro in Pittsburgh, where all dishes are made to order, chef Cathy

How Difficult Is It to Shake the Habit?

As with yogurt and brussels sprouts, acquiring a taste for low-sodium fare takes time—about two months.

That's what a group of volunteers found out when they attempted to gradually reduce their salt consumption for an experiment conducted by scientists at the University of Pennsylvania. For the first two months, they were allowed to eat anything they wanted, giving no thought to the amount of salt they were eating. They were then instructed to start reducing their sodium intake and were given a list of foods to avoid. Within two months, they discovered they were getting by quite happily on half the amount of salt they used to prefer (*American Journal of Clinical Nutrition*).

Their taste preference was tested by using Campbell's low-sodium soup and having salt added until the soup reached a level they considered tasty.

"Before they started restricting sodium, the level of salt they desired equaled about the same as in a regular can of soup," says Gary K. Beauchamp, Ph.D. "After two to three months, their preference was reduced by two-thirds to half the amount of salt."

Using salt-free stocks.

Armburger uses very little salt in food preparation. Upon request, she will eliminate salt entirely. "I prepare my own salt-free stocks using the process of reduction to intensify flavors," says Armburger.

Travel Meals Can Be Low in Sodium

To cut sodium intake while you travel, plan ahead. If you are planning a trip by air, you have only to call the airline and request low-salt or salt-free meals at least 24 hours before takeoff.

Taking a low-salt cruise.

"If you are planning a short cruise, say one or two weeks, just inform your travel agent when you book. If you neglect to do that, inform the cruise line at least one week before departure," says Tom Mittl of the Mittl Travel Agency in Allentown, Pennsylvania. "On the Carnivale line, it is suggested that you explain your dietary needs to the maître d' on the day of embarking. You may then see the menus for the week and choose the items you desire. That way there will be no waiting at mealtime.

"If you're taking a longer cruise—on an ocean liner, for instance—you should notify your travel agent or the cruise line as far in advance as possible— at least one month before departure. There are as many as seven meals a day served on these luxury cruises, and if your cruise is for 14 to 30 days, that's a lot of food to shop for."

"No Salt" at the Supermarket

Not too long ago, it was impossible to find prepared foods without added salt. But now you have a variety to choose from, and the number is growing.

Too busy to cook soup for dinner? Campbell's offers several varieties, all nicely flavored without added salt, including the ever-popular Chicken with Noodles, Chunky Vegetable Beef, Tomato, Split Pea, Chunky Chicken Vegetable, Chunky Beef and Mushroom. And as a boon to your quick, creative endeav-

Less salt in canned soups.

ors, several soups can double as sauces: Cream of Mushroom, Chicken Broth and French Onion.

That great refresher, V-8 juice, is now available without added salt, and so is Prego spaghetti sauce. In response to consumer interest, Campbell's has also reduced the sodium in its regular line.

And that's only the beginning. You can now enjoy all your favorite tomato foods from pasta to pizza the low-sodium way with Hunt's no-salt-added products: tomato sauce, tomato paste, tomato juice, whole tomatoes, stewed tomatoes, ketchup and spaghetti sauce.

Low-salt tomato products

Even canned vegetables have split with salt. Del Monte no-salt-added green beans, corn, peas, beets and tomato products are now on the grocer's shelf.

A pioneer in the field, Libby's offers a Natural Pack line of mushrooms and several varieties of vegetables that are free of added salt and sugar. "We pick that produce at its peak," says a company spokesperson, "in order to get the best flavor nature provides."

As a change from butter on your morning toast, for sandwiches and as a lift for your uncooked confections and baked goods, try the Westbrae line of sodium-free nut butters: almond, peanut, cashew and sesame tahini. To make your snack low-sodium all the way, spread any one of these butters on no-salt brown rice wafers.

Salt-free peanut butter.

LaChoy Food Products has introduced three no-salt-added oriental vegetables: bean sprouts, chop suey vegetables and fancy mixed Chinese vegetables.

A welcome addition to the no-salt menu are the Beatrice Foods' Eckrich delicatessen and luncheon meats, a category of foods that are usually highly salted. The no-salt versions will certainly enhance the low-sodium picnic basket.

Luncheon meats, minus the salt.

Kikkoman Lite Soy Sauce, now generally available in supermarkets all over the country, provides that rich soy flavor with 40 percent less sodium than the standard sauce.

Lawry's Season Salt-Free, available nationally, provides the same pungent herb blend as the original

An herb blend with potassium instead of salt.

Lawry's—with an important difference. "Potassium replaces the sodium," says Robin Saylor, head of Lawry's test kitchen. Other Lawry products that provide flavor without added salt are Season Pepper, Minced Onion with Green Onion Flakes and course-ground Garlic Powder with Parsley.

Chico-San's very popular rice cakes provide an excellent low-sodium alternative to bread. All four varieties are available with either no sodium or low sodium. You'll find them in supermarkets and in health food stores all over the country.

A delightful new breed: pickles without salt.

If you have been passing up the pickles because of their traditionally high-sodium content, rejoice! Under the Country Cuisine label, Salt Free Gourmet combines a blend of spices that delivers to your tongue a delightful taste sensation that makes the lack of salt go unnoticed. To perk up your picnic, try Country Cuisine Kosher dill slices in your tuna, egg, potato and macaroni salads. Country Cuisine no-salt-added spaghetti sauce is available at gourmet shops and many supermarkets. Soon you'll find Country Cuisine Dijon-style mustard and a salt-free ketchup.

Some cereals with no added salt.

"Quaker's Mother's Brand of cereals has no added salt and is available now in health food stores and supermarket nutrition centers across the country," says product manager Barbara Hinkes. "They include Oat Bran, Whole Wheat Rolled Flakes, Rolled Oats that make a thick porridge, Instant Oatmeal (a finer flake that needs no stove-top cooking) and Quick-Cooking Barley that is great for soups and vegetable pilafs." Quaker Rolled Oats in the familiar blue and red tube, both quick and old-fashioned, have no salt added and are available in most supermarkets.

Reduced-Salt Snacks and Condiments

Would you believe that Angostura bitters has been around since 1824? That's right—for over 160 years, and from the very beginning, according to a company spokesperson, it has been a no-salt-added flavor enhancer made from exotic herbs and spices. And it's all natural! It's a great condiment to pep up your no-sodium soups, casseroles, pilafs and beverages. Try it in tomato juice or ask for it with Perrier and a twist of lime or lemon so you can socialize at the bar *and* drive home! Because it is so versatile, you may find it in the condiment, gourmet, sodium-free or cocktail-mix section of your supermarket.

A 160-year-old flavor enhancer.

Diamond Crystal Specialty Foods has a great line of no-salt products that they've been providing to hospitals for five years and are now making available to the public by direct mail. They are offering five different types of low-sodium, sprinkle-on seasonings, seven sauce mixes, four soup mixes and two bouillon mixes—great for making low-sodium stock. Their lemon crystals are a convenient flavor enhancer for vegetables, salads and soups. Their meat loaf mix is popular because it acts as a binder, retaining flavorful juices. They also offer three flavors of low-calorie, no-salt-added salad dressings, which are dry mixes to be blended with yogurt, mayonnaise or buttermilk. To get their catalog, write to Diamond Crystal Specialty Foods, Inc., 10 Burlington Avenue, Wilmington, MA 01887.

No-salt salad dressings.

Interestingly, the Contadina Company's tomato paste not only has no salt added now but it never did! The same goes for their tomato puree. Furthermore, Contadina has successfully reduced the salt in their new tomato sauces by 25 percent.

The Hain Pure Foods Company makes many healthful, no-salt products, among them canned and dry soups, crackers, salad dressings, nut butters and condiments.

As if that weren't enough, you can now fill your snack dish with unsalted, dry-roasted or whole natural almonds, which are produced by Blue Diamond and literally go from low-sodium soup to nuts!

More Tasty, Low-Salt Foods for You and Your Guests

Low-salt entertaining.

One thing you don't want to give visiting friends and relatives is a big dose of sodium when they eat at your house. Not too long ago, hosting low-sodium dinners and parties was a bit of a problem. To control the amount of salt, you had to make nearly everything from scratch. Today, you can get a healthy hand from the scores of no-salt and reduced-sodium products available in stores. Here's how to make every milligram count when setting the buffet table.

Great low-sodium mixers.

• Make lavish use of club soda and sparkling water. Most contain less than 50 milligrams of sodium in an eight-ounce glass. The best have less than 10 milligrams. Read labels and choose brands that say they're low sodium or unsalted.

• Choose low-sodium vegetable-juice cocktails. A typical six-ounce serving has only 60 milligrams, compared with more than 500 milligrams for the salted kind.

• In the same vein, look for no-salt-added and reduced-sodium tomato juices.

• Zip up tomato-based drinks with a bit of horseradish, a pinch of ground red pepper, a few drops of hot-pepper sauce, a dash of bitters or a generous squeeze of lemon or lime juice.

Swiss cheese: naturally lower in sodium.

• Many low-sodium cheeses are making their way into dairy cases. The sodium savings can be impressive. For instance, choosing a 50 percent reduced-sodium cheddar can help you drop 130 milligrams of sodium per 1½-ounce piece. A 75 percent reduced-sodium Swiss cheese can have as few as 26 milligrams per 1½-ounce slice. Even regular Swiss cheese is a good idea because Swiss is naturally lower in sodium than most other cheeses. Swiss cheese has about half the sodium of cheddar or brick, for example, and only about one-fifth as much as blue cheese. Among other cheeses available in low- or reduced-sodium form are Gouda, Monterey Jack, Muenster and colby.

• No-salt and low-sodium crackers abound. Choose from wheat wafers, cracked-wheat wafers, bran wafers, rye wafers, melba rounds, melba toast, whole grain flatbreads, matzo, sesame crackers, herbed wheat crackers, rice crackers, plain bread sticks and sesame bread sticks. Other no-salt snack foods include potato chips, pretzels, corn chips and tortilla chips.

• Popcorn is a perennial holiday favorite. Make your own in a hot-air popper (to cut calories), then sprinkle it with your favorite herbs, no-salt herb blends or cinnamon.

Popping a low-salt snack.

• Pick no-salt and reduced-salt pickles. Choose from kosher dills or spears, dill chips and bread-and-butter chips.

• Add variety and color to a relish dish with no-salt hot cherry peppers or pickled sweet peppers.

• If you use olives, be aware that black olives usually contain about one-third the sodium of green ones. But also be aware that neither is low sodium.

• Set out no-salt ketchup, mayonnaise, chili sauce, spicy chutney, green-peppercorn sauce and barbecue sauce. Use low-sodium soy sauce.

• Seek out no-sodium mustards. Salted mustards average 100 to 200 milligrams per tablespoon. Some types go as high as 445 milligrams. No-salt and low-sodium brands can slash that amount. Among the varieties available are hot, mild, sweet, sassy, coarse, smooth and lemon sesame.

• Season your homemade dips with no-salt herb blends. There are a million (almost) to choose from. Try lemon herb, hot and spicy, Italian, oriental, French, Mexican, and curry. Look for blends that are targeted especially for vegetables, fish, chicken and steak.

Herb blends make great dips.

• For fish dips, use no-salt tuna, salmon and sardines. If you've got salted varieties you'd like to use up, empty the cans into a colander, then rinse under cold water for a full minute. You'll wash away up to 90 percent of the sodium.

• When shopping, scan the shelves for salt-free vegetable dips, salsas, taco sauces, curry sauces, and sweet-and-sour sauces, often sold with dietetic foods.

Serve unsalted nuts.

• Serve unsalted roasted almonds, cashews, peanuts, sunflower seeds and mixed nuts. An ounce of unsalted cashews, for instance, can have less than 10 milligrams of sodium; salted cashews can weigh in at around 180 milligrams.

• Buy peanuts that were roasted in their shell. Roast chestnuts on an open fire (or in your oven). Be sure to cut an X-shaped steam vent in each chestnut before heating.

• Cook with unsalted margarine and butter. Or use oil, which is salt-free.

• Standard baking powders contain a lot of sodium. A typical brand has 405 milligrams in a teaspoon. A low-sodium version can contain as little as 2 milligrams.

Quick 'n' Tasty Low-Sodium Recipes

Cooking from scratch, of course, gives you even more control over sodium input. Here are seven recipes that offer good taste without superfluous salt.

CORNY MEAT LOAF

Serve at supper, then slice for "cold cuts."

2 pounds ground beef
½ cup rolled oats
⅓ cup wheat germ
½ cup minced onions
¼ cup chopped fresh parsley
1 can (17 ounces) no-salt corn, drained
2 tablespoons no-salt herb blend
1 tablespoon low-sodium soy sauce
2 eggs, beaten
¼ cup plain yogurt
½ cup no-salt tomato juice or tomato soup
no-salt ketchup (optional)

In a large bowl, combine beef, oats, wheat germ, onions, parsley, corn, herb blend and soy sauce. In a small bowl, mix eggs and yogurt, then add to meat mixture. Add tomato juice and mix well.

Coat a 9 × 5-inch loaf pan with vegetable spray. Place meat mixture in pan, packing firmly. Place in refrigerator and allow to rest for 10 minutes.

Preheat oven to 350°F.

Run a knife around edge of meat loaf to loosen, then carefully turn out onto a large, shallow baking pan. Coat loaf with ketchup, if desired. Place pan on middle rack of oven and bake for 1¼ hours. Remove from oven and allow to rest for 10 minutes before slicing.

Yield: 6 to 8 servings

STRING BEANS
IN TARRAGON MARINADE

Help yourself to these savory beans—you'll never miss the salt.

2 tablespoons olive oil
½ cup plain yogurt
⅓ cup tarragon vinegar
1 large clove garlic, minced or crushed
1 pound string beans, lightly steamed
1 large onion, thinly sliced
1 cup shredded low-sodium cheddar cheese

In a large bowl, combine oil, yogurt, vinegar and garlic. Add beans and toss, then marinate for 20 minutes at room temperature. Add onions, cover and refrigerate for several hours, then toss with cheese.

Yield: 4 to 6 servings

NUTTY PÂTÉ APPETIZER

A zippy make-ahead pâté to please the crowd.

2 tablespoons no-salt butter or margarine
2 cups sliced mushrooms
1 cup shredded zucchini or yellow squash
½ cup chopped onions
2 cloves garlic, crushed
¾ cup cooked brown rice
1 egg
1¾ cups ground no-salt or low-salt nuts
½ cup chopped fresh parsley
¼ cup wheat germ
4½ teaspoons Worcestershire sauce
1 tablespoon no-salt herb blend
pinch of ground red pepper (optional)

In a large skillet, melt butter or margarine over medium heat. Add mushrooms, squash and onions. Sauté until onions are translucent but not brown. Add garlic and cook for 2 minutes. In a food processor or blender, puree vegetables. Transfer mixture to a large bowl.

In a food processor or blender, puree rice and egg. Add rice mixture to vegetable mixture, then add nuts, parsley, wheat germ, Worcestershire sauce, herb blend and ground red pepper, if used. Mix well.

Preheat oven to 375°F.

Coat a 9 × 5-inch loaf pan with vegetable spray. Turn pâté mixture into pan, packing firmly. Bake for 30 minutes, or until edges are golden. Remove from oven and let stand for 30 minutes. Unmold pâté and allow to cool to room temperature. Wrap and refrigerate. Slice to serve.

Yield: 6 servings

TANGY RELISH SALAD

This soft-set relish makes a nice accompaniment to meats, chicken or fish.

   1 packet low-calorie lime gelatin dessert
   1 cup boiling water
1½ cups cold water
   2 tablespoons lime juice
1½ cups shredded cabbage
   ¼ cup chopped no-salt dill pickles
   2 tablespoons prepared horseradish
   1 tablespoon chopped pimientos
     pinch of ground red pepper (optional)

In a 2- or 3-quart saucepan, add gelatin to boiling water, then turn off heat and stir until gelatin is dissolved, about 2 minutes. Add cold water and lime juice. Chill until slightly thickened.

Stir in cabbage, pickles, horseradish, pimientos and ground red pepper. Pour into a serving bowl and chill until firm.

Yield: 6 to 8 servings

QUICK CHICKEN DIVAN

A good way to use leftovers.

> 1 tablespoon no-salt butter or margarine
> 1 small onion, minced
> 1 small green or sweet red pepper, minced
> 1 clove garlic, crushed
> 2 cups broccoli florets, lightly steamed
> 2 cups cubed cooked chicken
> 1 can (10½ ounces) low-sodium cream of mushroom soup
> 1 tablespoon no-salt herb blend
> 1 teaspoon low-sodium soy sauce
> ½ teaspoon cornstarch
> ½ cup shredded low-sodium cheddar or Swiss cheese

In a medium-size skillet, melt butter or margarine over medium heat. Add onions and peppers and sauté until onions are translucent but not brown. Add garlic and sauté for 2 minutes more. Set aside.

Arrange broccoli evenly in a 1½-quart baking dish, then arrange chicken over broccoli.

Preheat oven to 450°F.

In a medium-size bowl, combine sautéed peppers and onions, soup, herb blend, soy sauce and cornstarch. Pour over chicken and sprinkle with cheese. Bake for 15 minutes.

Yield: 4 servings

GARBURE

This is a traditional, thick soup of southwestern France.

       1 cup dried navy or pea beans, soaked
             overnight
       8 cups water
       2 potatoes, sliced
       2 onions, sliced
1 or 2 leeks, sliced
       2 medium-size turnips, sliced
       2 carrots, sliced
       ½ cup dried split peas
       1 bay leaf
       1 teaspoon thyme
       1 teaspoon marjoram
       ¼ cup minced fresh parsley
       3 cloves garlic, minced
       1 hot chili pepper
       ½ small head cabbage, shredded
 ½ to 1 pound roasted pork, chicken, goose, duck or
             other meat (optional)
       ½ cup finely shredded low-sodium cheddar or
             Swiss cheese

Drain beans and set aside.

In a large stock pot, bring water to a boil. Add beans, potatoes, onions, leeks, turnips, carrots, split peas, bay leaf, thyme, marjoram, parsley, garlic and chili pepper. Cover and bring quickly to a boil, then reduce heat and simmer for 1 hour.

Add cabbage and meat, if used. Cover and bring quickly to a boil, then reduce heat and simmer for 30 minutes.

Discard bay leaf and chili pepper. If meat was used, remove and slice it, then place a serving in each bowl. Add soup. Garnish with cheese.

Yield: 4 to 6 servings

CHUNKY SALSA

Use this crunchy southwestern sauce on tacos, tosadas, burritos—you name it!

1   medium carrot
½ small onion
1   can (14½ ounces) no-salt stewed tomatoes, drained
1   can (4 ounces) chopped green chili peppers
½ teaspoon ground cumin
½ teaspoon dried oregano
    hot pepper sauce, to taste

In a food processor, coarsely chop carrot and onion. Add tomatoes and chop coarsely. (If working by hand, chop carrot and onion, then chop tomatoes and blend them in a bowl.)

Transfer tomato mixture to a serving bowl. Stir in chilies, cumin, oregano and pepper sauce. Let stand for 1 hour to blend flavors. Then serve at room temperature.

Yield: 2½ cups

More Sneaky Maneuvers for Cutting Back on Salt

There are a lot of outrageous ways to cut back on your salt intake—like plugging up the holes in your saltshakers, declaring the anchovy an endangered species or sealing the golden gateway to fast-food land.

Then there are subtle ways.

Take a cup of no-salt-added tomato sauce, for instance. Add it to your stew in lieu of the salted variety, and you'll be eliminating over 1,400 milligrams of sodium from your meal!

Simple ways to cut sodium.

If life with green beans is just not bearable without salt, then try them with half the salt. Blend the unsalted variety (less than 10 milligrams of sodium per ½ cup) with the salted (442 milligrams). No loss of the flavor here, either.

A 50 percent reduction.

Sodium Cutbacks Are a Cinch

Getting the picture? With all of the brand-new no-salt-added products on the market today, there are literally hundreds of low-salt cuts you can make in your meals without surrendering a smack of flavor. And they aren't all limited to the can.

So you say you really like that salty taste you get when biting into a peanut butter cracker? Well, you can go halfway here, too. Regular peanut butter atop an unsalted cracker (or vice versa) can still have you yearning for more. The same is true of dip. Unsalted crackers can only enhance the flavor of the dip. The savings may be small, but they add up in the long run.

Unsalted crackers are a plus.

Low-sodium cheeses can be a boon to the cook who wants to cut back. Some people missed sodium when eating cheese out-of-hand, but the difference is not as pronounced when a mixture of low-sodium cheddar and Swiss is melted on a homemade pizza or casserole.

Enhancing Flavors and Seasoning with Less Salt

With some of the new flavor enhancers and some knowledge of how to use the right blends of herbs and spices, you really could plug up the holes in the saltshaker if you wanted to.

- Kikkoman makes "lite" soy sauce with 43 percent less salt—or 170 milligrams of sodium per teaspoon. That's something that can really add up to savings in the long run.

A no-salt tenderizer.

- Adolph's has a tenderizer that enables you to enhance the flavor of meat without any added salt.
- A dash of Angostura aromatic bitters can make up for that "missing something" when making gravies, sauces or salad dressings.

Three tasty herbs.

- A bay leaf, a generous sprinkling of oregano and a dash of garlic powder can spruce up a low-sodium spaghetti sauce if the taste doesn't suit you.
- Certain spices and fruits are natural for some foods. Curry, paprika, parsley, sage, tarragon, marjoram, orange, cherries and pineapple are well suited for chicken dishes. For fish, try bay leaf, marjoram, parsley, anise, dry mustard, green pepper and ginger. For pork, try applesauce (there's no salt added there), apples and sage.

Peppers are a good choice.

- Sweet peppers, paprika, chili peppers and ground chilies go well in soups and stews. Nutmeg can really highlight a vegetable dish. Don't be afraid to experiment with some bold flavors—coriander, cardamom, cumin, cloves, anise and ginger—but proceed cautiously.

• When a recipe calls for bread crumbs and you haven't any no-salt bread, substitute no-salt dry cereal reduced to crumbs in a food mill, food processor or electric blender.

• To pep up a meat loaf, use chopped onions, low-salt vegetable juice and celery, including the tops.

• Low-salt or no-salt vegetable juice makes an excellent stock for a vegetable beef soup.

• Allspice does wonders for low-salt cottage cheese and ricotta dishes.

• A few drops of lemon juice add zip to salt-free chicken, nut breads and vegetables. Chicken soup without salt, for example, gets a nice lift from a bay leaf and a little lemon juice.

A few drops of lemon juice.

Is Your Saltshaker Oversalting Your Food?

Trying to shake the salt habit? Start with your saltshaker, says a group of researchers from Australia. They found that the size and number of the holes in a shaker can have a dramatic effect on the amount of salt sprinkled on food at the table.

"Consumers have a poor perception of the amount of salt being delivered to the food and apply a similar manual action to all shakers, regardless of hole size," the researchers say. This results in higher amounts of salt being used from shakers with bigger holes.

Multiholed saltshakers are okay to use, they say, if the holes are small enough. But for best restriction, the Australians recommend a shaker with a single three-millimeter (about ⅛ inch) hole. That can reduce total salt shaken from a maximum of 1.2 grams to a mere 0.37 grams per meal (*Human Nutrition: Applied Nutrition*).

Chapter 79

A Guide to Healthful Cooking Techniques

There's more than one way to cook your goose—baking, frying, stewing, boiling, poaching, braising, roasting—you get the idea. But putting convenience aside, are there any *nutritional* advantages to some cooking techniques over others? Or is heat heat—and a fried potato just as healthful as a baked one?

The Nutritional Effects of Cooking Methods

Scientists have been playing Julia Child in their laboratories for quite some time, trying to figure out just exactly what cooking does to the nutritional value of our food. What follows is a brief summary of those findings.

Baking. If you do it to bread (or pastry or potatoes), it's called baking; if you do it to a piece of meat or fowl, it sometimes goes by the name of roasting. It's the same process, however—cooking with hot air as opposed to hot water or hot oil. And it does have its nutritional advantage: There is no water for nutrients to leach into.

Boiling. Is boiling healthful? It depends. If you use lots of water and boil for a long time, you're going to lose more nutrients than if you boil quickly and use relatively little water. (Even then, use the cooking

Boil quickly.

water for broths or soups to save nutrients that would otherwise be lost.)

Broiling. Broiling is healthful in the sense that it lets fats drip out and away from what's being cooked—hence cutting calories—but it can be unhealthful if these fats are allowed to ignite, forming smoke and the suspected carcinogen, benzo[a]pyrene. The solution? Broil from *above* (as opposed to charcoal-grilling, from below). Studies have shown that by broiling from above, you can keep the production of benzo[a]pyrene to a minimum.

Broil from above.

Charcoal-grilling. There are ways to minimize problems with this method of cooking: (1) Cook only lean meats (steak rather than spareribs, for instance) over charcoal because it's the fat dripping into the fire that forms the chemical; (2) don't keep the meat right next to the coals; and (3) place meats on foil to shield them from benzo[a]pyrene.

Three ways to grill.

Deep-frying. While baking, broiling and barbecuing uses hot air to cook food, deep-frying uses hot oil. What are the advantages? There are none. There are only disadvantages, as a matter of fact. Oil is an added expense, and it also adds a lot of calories. A piece of broiled fish, for example, might contain 100 calories; if it is breaded and deep-fried, it can contain twice that many.

Deep-frying adds calories and expense.

Pressure-cooking. Pressure-cooking is actually a better way of steaming. By shortening the amount of time foods need to be in contact with heat, pressure-cooking reduces the amount of vitamin and mineral loss.

Steaming. Steaming involves cooking *over* rather than *in* water and can be healthful (with vegetables, especially) because it doesn't allow water to come into actual contact with what's being cooked. A drawback, however, is that some vegetables may require longer steaming, thus offsetting the nutritional advantage gained by avoiding immersion. Steaming can also leave vegetables pale.

Minimizing nutrient losses.

How to remove fat from a stew.

Lock in nutrients with wok cookery.

Stewing. Stewing's blessings are mixed. Unless you brown meats first and pour off the fat, all that fat stays in either the meat or the broth. Stewing can, however, be healthful if you're including lots of vegetables with your meat, because any vitamins that leach out of the veggies leach into the broth. (A trick for removing some of the fat from a stew is to refrigerate it and then scoop off the hardened, white lard that rises to the surface.)

Stir-frying. Stir-frying is a relatively new technique to the Western world (although Orientals have been using it for centuries), and it's potentially very healthful if you use lean cuts of meat and low to moderate amounts of oil. Because it's fast, stir-frying sears the outside of what's being cooked, locking nutrients inside. This is an especially healthful way to cook vegetables. (One or two teaspoons of oil, incidentally, is plenty for cooking four or five servings of vegetables.)

Two Nutrient-Saving Reminders

So there you have it: a guide to healthful cooking. Is there a rule of thumb or two to be discerned from it all?

Yes. For vegetables, "cook them, don't kill them." And for meats, "you're better off cooking the fat out than in."

For the lowdown on microwave cooking, see chapter 81.

A Guide to
"Healthier"
Kitchenware

There was a time when all it took to be a good cook was a wooden club. As long as your main course wasn't kicking you in the face, it was pretty much as ready for the fire as it was ever going to be. Meat tenderizing was an act of self-defense.

Nowadays, though, we've got everything from waffle irons to popcorn poppers to help us prepare our food. This is great, but it's also a little confusing. With so much to choose from, where is a good cook to draw the line?

We posed that question to some experts in the field—people who either cook or write about cooking for a living—and here are the instruments they find most useful and the most healthful. A cotton-candy machine might be fun, but it's not worth its counter space as far as whipping up good nutrition is concerned.

We asked the experts.

A Roundup
of Nutrient-Saving Equipment

So here we go: healthful cooking's "Basic 11" kitchen gizmos.

1. Good pots and pans. Quality pays off in cookware, not only in terms of durability but also in terms of saving nutrients and energy. Good cookware has tight-fitting lids (reducing cooking time and hence

Why metals make a difference.

vitamin damage), and it tends to be made of energy-wise and nutrient-wise materials (such as enameled iron, heavy stainless steel and specially anodized aluminum) that distribute heat evenly and quickly.

2. Good knives and cutting boards. Again, the word *good* makes a difference. A sharp, well-balanced knife just might encourage you to do more trimming of unhealthful fats from your meats and more slicing of healthful fruits and vegetables as well. A good-sized acrylic cutting board is important, too: It acts as the proper "shock absorber" for top-notch cutlery and gives you plenty of "elbow room" for cutting up meat and veggies for vitamin- and mineral-packed stews, stir-fries and casseroles. (Always wash knives and cutting boards in hot, soapy water and rinse thoroughly after using them to cut or chop meat.)

Cooking gently saves nutrients.

3. A steamer. Perhaps no other kitchen device safeguards the nutritional value of food the way a steamer does. Anything it cooks, it cooks gently, but quickly. Nutrient losses are kept to a bare minimum, whether it's meat, vegetables or rice that you're subjecting to a steamer's care. Better yet, steamers come in all shapes and sizes, from fold-out basket types that work on top of your stove to the new electric models that can steam practically anywhere.

"If I could have only one pot or pan . . . ."

4. A wok. "If I could have only one pot or pan, I'd have a wok," says one gourmet cook. That's how adaptable the "oriental frying pan" is. You can stir-fry with a wok (using oil), but you can also boil an egg, cook cereal, simmer soup, steam vegetables—it's a very versatile and nutrition-oriented device. It's great for cooking foods fast enough so that a minimum of vitamins is lost, and it's inexpensive, too.

5. A colander. This simple, sturdy strainer is ideal for draining pastas, rinsing fruits and vegetables, making cottage cheese or yogurt cheese or draining tuna fish of its salt brine.

6. A blender. No, not made obsolete by the food processor, the blender still deserves its counter space. For pureeing vegetables, blending batters, emulsifying sauces, grinding seeds and spices and whipping up frothy fruit punches and "health cocktails," the good old blender, whether it's a 5-speed or a 15-speed, is still hard to beat.

An ever-useful standby: the blender.

7. A juicer. For getting down to the nectar of things, the juicer is tops. Whether it's the liquid essence of an orange, peach or carrot you're after, a juicer is the gadget for the job. Great for thirsty fitness buffs and kids who seem to be hooked on soda pop.

8. A mixer. Not just for blending cake batter, the electric mixer is proudest of all to put muscle into the wholesome art of baking bread. Kneading is a cinch for most of the new models, and attachments are available that will even allow you to grind your own grains.

9. A toaster oven. So who needs a toaster oven in addition to a regular oven? You do if you're energy-conscious and an aficionado of top-browned, open-faced sandwiches, of if you frequently bake or reheat quantities of food that look lost inside the oven of your stove. A toaster oven also can be just what the chef ordered for toasting homemade breads that are just too voluptuous (or crumbly) for your regular toaster.

Saving energy while toasting food.

10. A food processor. It's the Cadillac of kitchen gizmos, but a food processor performs many tasks *fast*. Slice or shred pounds of fruit or vegetables in minutes. Process meat or fish into a pâté without adding eggs or cream, or make cream soups without thickeners. Indeed, uses for the food processor are limited by imagination only.

11. A pressure cooker. A pressure cooker can save time (by cooking some foods four times as fast as an oven or ordinary pot), it can save money (via the energy savings from those shortened cooking times), and it can save nutrients (studies show that pressure-cooking is one of the kindest methods of all on nutrients). Pressure cookers work their magic by doing just as their name implies—cooking under pressure—and

The pressure cooker—a top-notch nutrient saver.

they can do this to nearly any type of food. Soups, stews, pot roasts, even casseroles and individually wrapped items such as fillets can feel right at home in a pressure cooker. Pressure cookers are available in both stove-top and electric models.

The Microwave:
Healthy Cooking
Is Its Forte

I f you're part of a two-career couple, you're probably already sold on the incredible convenience of
a microwave appliance. But what you may not realize
is that it's also a superb way to make healthful, low-fat
meals that taste great and look even better. That's
because microwaves work particularly well on fresh
foods with a high water content, such as vegetables,
fish and fruits.

A microwave will not brown, grill or roast meats
well; you may not be able to use it for pies or breads.
But when it comes to poaching fish, cooking vegetables or making stews, it's wonderful. For busy week-
nights, when it's impractical to conventionally cook
such vegetables as potatoes and squash, a microwave
can have them done in minutes. Instead of sautéing
fish in a lot of butter, you can microwave it tenderly
using lemon and herbs for flavoring. Best of all, because microwaves cook so quickly, fewer nutrients
are lost in the process.

Perfect potatoes in minutes.

Healthy Food Cooked in a Flash

Successful microwave cooking is a learned art.
Here are a few tips for busy cooks who like to eat well
but don't have the time for conventional ovens.

Tips for Perfect Vegetables

It's important that each piece you're cooking is
the same size to ensure even cooking. For vegetables

Arranging veggies for just-right cooking.

like broccoli and asparagus, which have tough, thick stalks, arrange the stalks in a circle, with the delicate buds facing toward the middle. This will ensure that the stalks get a more intense cooking.

If you like crisp skin on baked potatoes, don't depend on your microwave. It simply won't do it. Instead, when the potato is nearly cooked, heat it under a conventional broiler for a few minutes.

For very crisp vegetables, don't use any water. Just cover them with waxed paper or plastic wrap and cook. For fresh corn, leave the green outer leaves on to retain the corn's moisture.

Be sure to cover everything to help preserve flavors and keep moisture from escaping.

Moist, Tender Fish—in Four Minutes

The secret of tasty, evenly cooked fish.

The key to microwaving fish well is to be sure it's at room temperature before starting. If the fish is chilled, it creates a texture problem. Because it takes so long for the microwaves to warm the outside, you wind up overcooking.

The best fish for microwaving also happen to be the ones lowest in fat and highest in water: whitefish such as flounder and shellfish such as scallops. Smother the fish in chopped fresh tomatoes and basil and microwave it on full power for approximately four minutes.

How to Make Rich, Thick Sauces and Stews

Melding flavors.

A microwave can be a great convenience when making long-cooking sauces and stews. But there's one problem. One of the delights of a stew is the slow blending of flavors. Since a microwave cooks everything so quickly, herbs, spices and other flavorings don't have time to work their magic. The solution? Put the sauce together the night before, cook it quickly in the microwave, then leave it in your refrigerator overnight. By the time you arrive home at the end of a long day, the flavors will have melded and all you'll have to do is heat it up.

When preparing a stew, try to use vegetables that are similar in texture, such as all root vegetables. This will ensure that the stew ingredients cook evenly. If you want to add some delicate vegetable like mushrooms, do so at the last minute.

Chapter 82

Slices of Life: A Guide to Better Bread

A report card on regional breads.

Which bread is the most nutritious? Which is the least? Those are questions that a lot of people have wanted to know the answer to for a long time. The Kansas-based American Institute of Baking (AIB) has been curious, too. So it undertook a study of eight types of variety breads—pumpernickel, raisin, oatmeal, whole wheat, cracked wheat, mixed grain, Italian, French—and three other kinds—bagels, pita and tortillas. AIB researchers looked at these bread types as produced in four representative cities: New York, Atlanta, San Francisco and Kansas City.

Pumpernickel: a tale of two cities.

What they found was that there is nearly as much variation from city to city as there is from bread to bread. One man's nutrient-filled croissant, it seems, is another dough-schlepper's heap of empty calories. Or worse. AIB discovered, for example, that even though the level of sodium is especially high in pumpernickel bread in general, where you buy it can make a world of difference: In Atlanta, 100 grams (about 3½ ounces) of pumpernickel contained 849 milligrams of sodium, while the same amount of pumpernickel in San Francisco had only about half as much. That's a pretty wide gap for two items labeled "pumpernickel."

The same lack of standardization and uniformity was found in each of the 11 bread categories. It may, to some extent, reflect regional taste or texture preferences. Still, there are a few overall trends that can be discerned.

• Most whole wheat, French, Italian and pita breads and bagels were high in protein.

• Raisin and whole wheat breads were high in fat.

• Whole wheat, cracked wheat, and mixed-grain breads and tortillas were high in dietary fiber and magnesium.

For benchmark nutrient values for various types of bread, see Appendix B. Perhaps this information will help you to become the well-bread individual you always thought you were.

Why Whole Wheat Bread Stands above the Rest

Whole wheat bread is on the rise—in the kitchen and in popularity—and for very good reasons. White bread simply can't measure up in flavor and health-giving qualities.

That's because to become white flour, the wheat kernel undergoes a lot of processing that strips it of valuable vitamins, minerals and fiber. And the label "enriched" on many white breads only means that food manufacturers returned a few of those nutrients. Most are junked for good.

Nutrients that are never replaced.

Take fiber, for instance. Whole wheat bread contains three times more fiber than white bread—three times more health power to help lower your cholesterol, discourage diabetes and keep away hemorrhoids and varicose veins.

Whole wheat bread also contains three times more magnesium than white bread, a nutrient that some scientists say is a must to prevent heart attacks. And whole wheat is loaded with B vitamins. In fact, whole wheat has more of just about everything but calories. It has 15 fewer calories per slice than white bread.

Three times more magnesium—and loaded with B vitamins.

Whole Wheat Bread That's Easy to Bake

There's no whole wheat bread like homemade. The smell alone is enough to make you healthy. But when you think of actually baking that bread, you probably conjure up an image of your grandma kneading dough for half the afternoon. Baking bread seems like about as much fun as washing clothes in the river.

Well, our recipe is for life on the go. You won't have to knead it, it requires very little time, and it's easy. Even inexperienced bread bakers can whip it up like a pro.

WHOLE WHEAT BREAD

    ¼   cup plus ½ tablespoon honey
    ¼   cup warm water
    1   package dry yeast
6 to 7   cups whole wheat flour
    1   teaspoon salt (optional)
    2½   cups hot water
    ⅓   cup oil

Dissolve ½ tablespoon honey in warm water and sprinkle yeast on top. Do not stir. Set aside to proof.

In a large mixing bowl, combine 4 cups flour with salt, if used, hot water, remaining honey and oil. With an electric mixer, blend on low speed until thoroughly mixed. Add yeast mixture.

Add remaining flour 1 cup at a time, blending after each addition, until dough is consistency of cookie dough. Knead for 10 minutes on low speed.

Grease 2 large bread pans with solid shortening. Oil hands and mold dough into 2 loaves. (Lightly oil countertop so dough doesn't stick.) Place dough in pans, cover and let rise in a warm place until increased in bulk by one-third.

Preheat oven to 350°F.

Bake for 40 to 45 minutes, or until loaves sound hollow when tapped. Remove from pans and cool on wire racks.

Yield: 2 large loaves

Chapter 83

Using More Whole Grains

Whole grains are excellent sources of fiber, nutrients and complex carbohydrates. Use a variety of grains to provide low-cost, vitamin-rich eating pleasure and to add new interest to your meals. Replace some of the meat in your menu with grains to cut saturated fat and calories.

Wonderful Ways with Grains

To help you, here is a handy guide to the grains.

Barley. Available as pearl barley (which is white and translucent and has had its outer husk removed) and pot, or Scotch, barley (which has had only a single outer layer removed and must be soaked overnight before cooking). Either makes a delicious pilaf when cooked in broth with mushrooms and onions. Also used to flavor and thicken soups and stews. To prepare, cook one cup barley in three cups water for 55 minutes.

Two choices.

Buckwheat groats. This is not a true grain, but it is treated as such. It is used most often as flour in pancakes, biscuits and muffins. The groats make a fine breakfast cereal or pilaf. Kasha is the name given to toasted groats, which make a delicious substitute for potatoes. Cook one cup groats in two cups water for 15 minutes.

A great substitute for potatoes.

Bulgur. This is cracked wheat that has been hulled and parboiled, which conserves most of the nutrients by leaching them from the outer layer into the center of the grain. Use in casseroles, tabbouleh, vegetable dishes and as a rice substitute. Cook one cup bulgur in two cups water for 15 to 20 minutes.

Cornmeal. Available in white, yellow and blue varieties—the blue is favored in Tex-Mex and American Indian foods—cornmeal can be used to thicken sauces, gravies and soups. It can also be made into polenta and used in unleavened breads, pones, muffins, griddle cakes and tortillas. Cook one cup cornmeal in four cups water for 25 minutes.

Millet. Also known as proso and broomcorn, millet makes a delicious breakfast cereal when topped with fruit and maple syrup. Boil like rice for main dishes or use to thicken and flavor soups and stews. Cook one cup millet in three cups water for 45 minutes.

Oats. Steel-cut and rolled oats are available. Steel-cut oats are made by cutting the groats into pieces with steel rollers. Rolled oats, the more familiar form, are made by flaking the groats, which make the nutrients more available for digestion. Use to thicken and enrich soups or to extend meat dishes. Also great in stuffings, pilafs, breads, pancakes and granola. Cook one cup of steel-cut oats in three cups water for 30 to 40 minutes. Cook rolled oats in two cups water for 8 to 10 minutes, or until thick.

A grain that holds onto its nutrients.

Try it for breakfast.

The most versatile grain of all.

Chapter 84

Using More
Dried Beans

B eans in their infinite variety can bring new vitality to your menu. They're high in protein and a good source of iron, calcium, magnesium and fiber. They're low in fat, easy to store and inexpensive.

The ABCs of Beans

Here are some tips on how to make good use of beans.

How to store dried beans.

• Store dried beans in tightly covered jars in a cool, dry place. Add a couple of bay leaves to each jar to discourage insects.

• Most dried beans should be presoaked to restore water lost in drying and to shorten cooking time.

How to soak beans.

• When soaking beans, use a container large enough to permit expansion by 2½ times. Use six cups of water for one pound of beans. Let stand overnight in a cool place. (Split peas and lentils need no presoaking.)

• To have presoaked beans always on hand, soak some overnight and the next morning, pour off the soaking water, spread beans on a cookie sheet and freeze. When they're as hard as marbles, transfer to a plastic bag. They will not stick together and can be used directly from the freezer.

• If you forget to presoak your beans, place them in boiling water and boil for two minutes, then let stand for one hour, covered. Then cook them in the usual way.

• If you are one of those who get a lot of "back talk" from beans, try this cooking method: Discard the soaking water, cover beans with fresh water and cook for 30 minutes. Discard that water, too. Add more fresh water and resume cooking.

How to "de-gas" beans.

• If molasses or tomatoes is called for in a recipe, don't add it at the beginning of the cooking process because there is a substance in molasses and tomatoes that will toughen the outside covering of the beans. Add the molasses or tomatoes later, when the beans are tender.

A Nutritional "Supplement"

You can also use bean puree made in the blender or processor to boost the nutritional value and flavor of baked goods, casseroles, stuffings, soups and sandwich fillings. Use immediately, refrigerate for up to six days or freeze for up to six weeks.

Here are some other tips.

• Keep a jar of marinated beans in the refrigerator. Spoon some over salads or over mounds of cottage cheese, or serve in bowls with crackers or crisp raw vegetables.

• Add bean flour to baked goods as a nutritional booster. Grind any kind of dried beans very finely, but grind only as much as you need for immediate use— bean flour has a short shelf life.

Try bean flour.

• To use bean flour in baked goods, substitute two or three tablespoons for an equal amount of wheat flour. The protein in beans complements and enhances the protein of baked goods.

Chapter 85

Upgrading Leftovers

W hy build nutrition into your meals only to discard the leftovers? With a little ingenuity, you can make leftovers tasty and nutritious the second time around.

Stovetop Magic with Odds and Ends

Here are some suggestions on ways to incorporate orphaned foods into tasty new dishes.

- Leftover brown rice can add body to today's soup or ground meat. So can leftover oatmeal.
- For leftover liver sauté onions, mushrooms and peppers in a tablespoon of oil and a little chicken broth. Cut the liver into small cubes, then add to the vegetables, along with some cooked brown rice, if you have any. Bring to serving temperature. It's delicious and goes a long way. Or chop the liver with hard-cooked eggs, an onion, a few lettuce leaves for moisture and some soy nuts for nutrients and crunch. Add a bit of chicken fat for flavor, if you wish. Serve as a pâté with crisp raw vegetables and whole grain crackers.

A delicious way to re-work leftover liver.

- Leftover boiled or baked potatoes make a creamy, heartwarming soup. Sauté onions briefly, then puree with potatoes in a blender or processor.

Add milk or stock and a few herbs, such as parsley, dill, bay leaf or a bit of allspice.

Leftover spuds make great soup.

• The next time you make ratatouille, plan to have some of this great eggplant, pepper, zucchini and tomato dish left over. Then use it as the filling for a Spanish omelet. Or heat it slightly, add a tablespoon of nutritional yeast and place about ½ cup of the mixture in individual heatproof serving dishes. Drop an egg on each serving and heat in the oven until eggs are set.

You can also mix ratatouille with cooked brown rice, cover with a few slices of mozzarella cheese and heat until the cheese melts. Fantastic! Or use ratatouille as a filling for crepes.

• A cup of leftover sautéed sliced mushrooms, minced and combined with one tablespoon of minced onions, ½ cup of bread or cracker crumbs and a little melted butter or margarine makes a great crust for a quiche. You can freeze the crust until you're ready to make the quiche.

• Leftover corn can be cut off the cob and joined with sliced red peppers and onions in the sauté pan for delicious Mexican corn as a side dish. Or cover cooked vegetables with shredded cheese, broil until the cheese melts and serve as a main dish.

Corn—even better the second time around.

Chapter 86

Shaping Up Your Potato

Mashed, baked or steamed, the versatile potato can fill you up without filling you out. It's low in fat, high in fiber, packed with vitamins and minerals, and by itself has only a few more calories than an apple. So where did its fattening reputation come from? From the company it too often keeps: butter, sour cream and other diet stressors.

12 Ways to Perk Up Potatoes

Jettison those heavyweights and try these lighter alternatives.

1. Sprinkle with fresh or dried herbs (alone or in combination). For starters, try basil, caraway seeds, celery seeds, dill, chives, oregano or thyme.

2. Top your baked potato with low-fat yogurt and chopped chives or dill. For a "richer" topping, drain the yogurt for an hour in a sieve lined with cheesecloth. The yogurt will thicken to the consistency of sour cream.

3. Another sour cream alternative: Blend low-fat cottage cheese until smooth in a blender or food processor. Add a tablespoon of lemon juice for tang. If needed, thin with a bit of skim milk.

4. Combine a cup of low-fat cottage cheese with ½ cup of low-fat yogurt and chopped herbs for a high-protein spud topper.

Baked potato topping without the fat.

5. For a gourmet presentation, lightly sauté mushrooms and onions. Blend about ½ cup of this mixture into your baked or mashed potatoes.

A gourmet spud.

6. For added flavor and unusual color, add a cup of mashed, cooked butternut squash to your mashed potatoes.

7. If you're in a hurry, mix a dollop of cream of mushroom soup with your mashed spuds.

8. Mix some cream of tomato soup with a dash of Worcestershire sauce, a bit of powdered mustard and a little shredded cheddar cheese. Use to top baked potatoes.

9. Stuck with a few leftovers but not enough for a full meal? Serve them over baked potatoes. Good choices include stir-fried vegetables, meat sauce, chicken Parmesan and tuna casserole.

Combine with leftovers.

10. For pizza lovers: Top baked potatoes with spaghetti sauce, a touch of oregano and some part-skim mozzarella. Broil to melt the cheese.

A potato pizza.

11. Enjoy home fries without frying. Cut potatoes into slabs ¼ inch thick. Brush lightly with oil on both sides. Bake on a cookie sheet for 20 minutes at 450°F; turn once during baking.

Try "oven fries."

12. Cut the calories in potato salad by using yogurt, flavored with mustard in place of mayonnaise.

Chapter 87

Who's Who in the New Health Milks

R emember when buying a carton of milk was easy? There was regular and skim. But now there's 1 percent fat, 2 percent fat, protein-fortified milk, cultured buttermilk, acidophilus milk, Lactaid (for the lactose intolerant) and now something called CalciMilk, which is beefed up with extra calcium.

It's enough to make you wonder what was wrong with milk-the-original.

Milk-the-original was, and still is, a little high in fat. The American Heart Association recommends that no more than 30 percent of our calories come from fat, but nearly 50 percent of the calories in whole milk comes from fat. Whole milk also can be a real pain for some people to digest, namely those who lack the enzymes necessary for breaking down the sugar (called lactose) in milk.

So the dairy industry has been busy, not just slimming milk down but also pumping it up—with added protein, enzymes (to make it more digestible) and now even calcium (to make it better still for the bones). Few foods have been as responsive to the health and fitness movement as milk.

Whole milk is high in fat.

Milk That's Fit to Drink

Be confused no longer by all those newcomers to your dairy case. What you're looking at are examples of a good food made even better.

Low-fat milk. Low-fat milks start with 2 percent milk fat by weight and go as low as 0.5 percent milk

Fat Content of Milk

Type	Calories from Fat (%)	Calories*	Cholesterol (mg.)
Whole milk (3.3% milk fat by weight)	48.0	150	33
2% fat milk	34.0	121	18
1% fat milk	22.0	102	10
Skim milk	4.5	86	4

NOTE: Figures are based on an 8-ounce serving.

* Figure may be slightly higher if milk is fortified with nonfat milk solids or protein.

fat. Any milk lower than 0.5 is called skim. These might not seem like significant reductions from whole milk's fat content of around 3.5 percent, but in terms of calories and percentage of calories from fat, these reductions are significant, as the table above shows.

Low-fat milks reduce the percentage of calories from fat.

Protein-fortified milk. This is usually low-fat milk to which protein, in the form of nonfat milk solids, has been added. Per eight-ounce serving, the increase comes to more than 1.5 grams, or 20 percent more protein than normal milk.

Buttermilk. Buttermilk can be made from whole milk, low-fat milk or skim milk. The process involves exposing the milk to bacteria similar to that which produces yogurt. In some cases, flakes of actual butter may be added, as may salt. Read the label.

Buttermilk may contain salt.

Acidophilus milk. Acidophilus refers to the friendly type of bacteria that give this milk its slightly sweet taste. The bacteria are friendly in that they are thought to improve the bacterial environment of the intestines, so they may do more than just aid in the digestion of milk. There is also preliminary evidence from an animal study that acidophilus milk, if consumed regularly, may help control cholesterol by reducing the amount the body absorbs.

A milk to control cholesterol.

Lactaid. Lactaid is a specially formulated milk for people who are unable to digest regular milk. It also is a low-fat milk, containing only 1 percent milk fat, but otherwise it is the same as regular milk in nutritional content.

CalciMilk. CalciMilk is a low-fat milk (containing only 100 calories and two grams of fat per serving) to which calcium has been added—enough, in fact, so that just two eight-ounce glasses a day satisfy 100 percent of an adult's Recommended Dietary Allowance for this important, bone-building mineral.

Two glasses will give you the RDA.

If Milk Doesn't Agree with You . . .

How do you know if you are lactose intolerant? If your tummy rumbles or feels crampy and bloated 15 to 30 minutes after you have drunk a glass of milk, you probably have lactose intolerance. And if you experience gas or diarrhea an hour or two later, you almost certainly have the problem.

The symptoms of lactose intolerance.

If you do, you're not alone. Seventy percent of the people of the world cannot digest milk. And that is especially true of adults of certain ethnic groups like Orientals, Jews and blacks. What's more, many people don't become aware of their intolerance until after they've suffered from intestinal flu (which breaks down lactose activity) or increased their milk consumption, such as during pregnancy.

Orientals, Jews and blacks have the highest incidence.

That reaction is only natural, says Theodore Bayless, M.D., who is associated with the National Digestive Diseases Education and Information Clearinghouse in Baltimore. What happens as we grow older is that we develop a decline in the amount of lactose, the enzyme that is responsible for digesting lactose, or milk sugar. Our intestines, which produce the enzyme in the first place, fail to make enough, so the milk sugar passes directly into the colon. There it eventually breaks down, leaving behind gas, bloated bellies, cramps and even diarrhea.

A problem of aging.

If you suspect or discover that you have lactose intolerance, you need not be deprived of milk's nutrients or taste, says Dr. Bayless. (See the table below for a list of food alternatives.) Besides drinking Lactaid, you can get calcium from almonds, leafy green vegetables and fish such as sardines, which have edible bones, as well as from calcium supplements. Just remember to avoid those labeled "calcium lactate." You might also try eating smaller amounts of milk products or having them with your meals, a trick that may delay the release of lactose in the intestines.

Sources of calcium for nondrinkers.

Reading labels can lead you to satisfying milk-free alternatives. Some watchwords to look for are "pareve" and "parve," found in bread and baked goods, which mean that they conform to kosher food laws and are made without milk. Beware, however, of words like "caseinate," "lactose" and "whey," which are all milk additives. If you like to cook without milk, you can try substituting water, eggs, oil or fruit juice in recipes.

Ways to Tolerate Lactose Intolerance

"No" Foods	"Yes" Foods
Milk	Buttermilk; milk and milk products treated with Lactaid (a lactase enzyme that comes in powdered, liquid and tablet forms) or acidophilus (bacteria that break down lactose)
Ice cream	Frozen yogurt; Tofutti; Ice Bean and other soybean desserts
Butter	Nut butters; soy margarine
Soft cheese	Firm cheeses like brick, Swiss, Edam, cheddar, provolone; cottage cheese

Chapter 88

Bottled Water
Fit to Drink

There's a whole new group of beverage connoisseurs emerging from the ranks of thirsty consumers. They're skipping the soft drinks, dumping the diet colas and reaching for . . . water?

That's right. Today, water is the number one beverage of choice for health-conscious people. It helps regularity and provides important minerals like calcium and potassium. For the weight-conscious, it's lower than low-cal—it's no-cal. For the athlete, it helps replenish lost fluids. For the no-sugar-alcohol-caffeine-or-additives buffs, it's simply a pure and pleasant way to quench their thirst.

Tips for the Sodium-Conscious

The "real" question, though, is just what kind of water is best? Water running from the tap has its problems. It may be softened to make it suitable for sudsing, and that means that good minerals like calcium (and the taste) have often been sacrificed for bad minerals like sodium. Then there is the matter of substances either left in or added to tap water, such as bacteria or chlorine or toxic minerals like lead and mercury.

But bottled water can be contaminated, too, and there's often no way of knowing whether it is. Brands sold exclusively in the state where they're bottled are not subject to federal purity regulations. Furthermore, no standards are set for the amount of sodium al-

Hard facts about the content of water.

lowed in bottled water. Sodium levels can vary and may be quite high (see the table below). The U.S. Food and Drug Administration requires that only bottlers who make low-salt or no-salt claims must list sodium content. Now, granted, there is still a lot less sodium in water than in most diet drinks, but the sodium content may be as changeable as the seasons. And that's something people on salt-restricted diets should know.

One thing that is crystal clear, however, is that as the grocery aisles become flooded with bottled waters, our decisions get more difficult. Here are some pointers to help you make a naturally good selection.

Sorting out your choices.

• Look for labels that say natural spring water (that means the water naturally rises to the earth's surface without pumping or processing). If the word *natural* is left off the label, minerals have been artificially added.

Sodium Content of Some Bottled Waters

Brand	Sodium* (mg.)
Still Waters	
Poland Spring	0.32
Deer Park	0.39
Mountain Valley	0.65
Evian	1.18
Sparkling Waters	
Perrier	3.04
San Pellegrino	10.02
Canada Dry Club Soda	44.00
Vichy (Celestins)	277.40

NOTE: Figures are based on an 8-ounce serving.

* The recommended safe sodium levels are from 1,100 to 3,300 mg. a day.

The more minerals, the more taste.

• Keep in mind that minerals give water its taste—the more there are, the stronger the flavor. Some sparkling waters, like the imported Vichy, are so mineral rich that they may take on an alkaline, soapy or even bicarbonate taste. Still waters (those without bubbles) may refresh more because they have little aftertaste.

• Remember that while most waters contain important minerals like calcium, phosphorus and magnesium, they are no substitute for mineral-rich foods.

• If you are avoiding your tap water because you are unsure of its quality or taste, don't forget to make your ice cubes from bottled water, too.

Finding a healthful club soda.

• Seltzer and unflavored soda beverages are simply tap water that has been filtered and carbonated with bubbles. Club soda has had minerals and mineral salts added, so look for the ones labeled low-sodium or no-salt. Note also that club soda may contain small amounts of alcohol or caffeine.

Answers to Your Questions about Food and Health

I n some respects, the cornucopia of new and exciting foods on the market makes choosing a nutritious diet easier than ever. In other respects, though, the choices are harder: Unfamiliar choices raise intelligent questions among nutrition-conscious consumers. Here are answers to questions commonly posed by curious and concerned shoppers.

Blackberries, Bancha Tea and "Milk" Shakes

Q. I believe I read that blackberries are high in vitamin C. Is that right? What about blackberry jam?

A. Blackberries are a fairly good source of vitamin C. One cup has 30.2 milligrams. By comparison, a cup of blueberries has 18.9 milligrams, a cup of raspberries, 30.8 milligrams and a cup of strawberries, 84.5 milligrams. By the way, that classic source of vitamin C, the orange, holds 95.8 milligrams per cup of segments.

Unfortunately, when you make jam out of blackberries—or any fruit, for that matter—only a trace of vitamin C remains, for two reasons. First, heating the fruit destroys at least one-third to one-half of the vitamin. Second, the actual fruit is diluted in the jam by the addition of other ingredients such as honey, sugar and pectin.

Jam is low in vitamin C.

Q. A friend told me that a kind of tea called bancha has a lot of vitamin A and calcium in it. What exactly is bancha, and is it nutritious?

A. Bancha is a poor grade of green tea made from the leaves of the common tea plant. Samples tested in a laboratory showed that brewed bancha contains no vitamin A (or beta-carotene) and insignificant amounts of calcium and magnesium.

Bancha *does* contain caffeine, however; one cup has about 44 milligrams of caffeine. That compares to an average of 117 milligrams in a cup of brewed coffee and an average of 80 milligrams in a cup of brewed black tea.

Bancha tea has caffeine, but little nutritional value.

Q. A friend told me that "shakes" sold in fast-food restaurants actually contain no milk, which is why they aren't called milk shakes. Is that correct?

A. A drink's name can be an important clue to its ingredients. In most states, to be called a milk shake, a drink must include a milk product with a certain amount of butterfat in it. But in others, only a drink made with ice cream can be called a milk shake.

If a drink is just called a shake, you can't tell for sure whether it contains butterfat, vegetable fat substituted for the butterfat, or a combination of both.

One way you can be sure that your drink has real milk in it is to look for the "Real" seal of the American Dairy Association. For instance, a ten-ounce McDonald's shake—with whole milk or cream, sugar, butterfat and stabilizers—carries the "Real" seal and provides 324 milligrams of calcium, 9.4 grams of protein and about 331 calories. In a ten-ounce glass of milk, you would get 363 milligrams of calcium and 10 grams of protein, but only 186 calories.

"Real" milk shakes are usually labeled.

Nutritional Gold in Citrus, Potatoes, and Melons

Q. My neighbor told me that the white inner rind of oranges and grapefruits is full of nutrients and that I should eat some of the rind. Is my neighbor right?

A. Your neighbor is a smart cookie. If you eat the white inner rind of oranges or grapefruits, you'll be getting extra vitamin C, bioflavonoids, pectin and potassium.

Inner rinds are nutrient rich.

Q. I know that when you french-fry potatoes, you're adding fat and, of course, calories. But is there a nutritional difference between french-fried and, say, baked potatoes?

A. Yes, there is, and baked potatoes come out on top. In a study done at Cornell University, researchers compared the effect of deep-fat frying and baking on the protein and mineral content of several varieties of potatoes. The fried potatoes lost from 35 to 45 percent of their amino acids. The baked potatoes lost only 5 percent of their amino acids in the skin and the area directly under the skin (cortex), but the amino acid content in the center (pith) actually increased by 13 percent, apparently because protein migrates toward the middle during baking.

As for minerals, the loss was consistently greater for fried potatoes. For example, the fried potatoes lost an average of 24 percent of their pith calcium, 31 percent of their cortex calcium, 13 percent of their pith potassium and 40 percent of their cortex potassium. By contrast, the baked potatoes lost only 4 percent of their cortex calcium but gained 5 percent in their pith, and they lost 16 percent of their cortex potassium but gained 22 percent in their pith.

Why baked potatoes are better than fried.

So, for better nutrition, baked potatoes are your best bet.

Q. I know that cantaloupe is high in vitamin A. I assume that honeydew, because it isn't orange, doesn't have very much. Am I right?

A. Yes, but you can't always go by color alone. It's true that cantaloupe's orange color indicates it's a good source of beta-carotene—a food pigment the body converts to vitamin A. One cup of cubed cantaloupe holds the equivalent of 5,158 international units of vitamin A (a good day's supply), while honeydew has a mere 68 international units. Other orange or red fruits and vegetables—apricots, winter squash, red peppers and carrots, for instance—are likewise loaded with vitamin A.

But here's the tricky part. Some foods that have lots of beta-carotene pigment, explains Micheline Mathews Roth, M.D., a carotenoid expert from Harvard Medical School, also contain chlorophyll, a green pigment that hides the beta-carotene. A cup of raw spinach, for example, has 3,760 international units of vitamin A; a cup of raw broccoli, 1,356 international units; a cup of cooked asparagus, 1,492; and a cup of cooked kale, 9,620.

Some "green" foods are high in A.

Sushi: Proceed with Caution

Q. A few months ago, I read that eating sushi is unsafe because of possible parasites in raw fish. My wife and I have enjoyed sushi for years and never had a bad experience. Is sushi safe, or are we taking a risk?

A. A parasitologist at the Centers for Disease Control (CDC) in Atlanta says that eating sashimi, or raw fish (sushi is merely the most popular way to serve sashimi), is reasonably safe. There is always a chance that uncooked fresh fish harbors parasitic worms, but this rarely happens at a sushi bar. The researcher at the CDC says that eating sushi is safer than eating raw clams or oysters.

At the worst, you could pick up an anisakis worm from sushi. But in the past ten years, fewer than ten people in the United States have reported this happening.

Although anisakis can cause abdominal pain, bowel inflammation and possibly death, if untreated, a doctor who knows what's ailing you (and you should definitely mention that you've eaten raw fish) can easily treat you.

So far, public health officials have given sushi a tentative green light. The U.S. Food and Drug Administration (FDA) has been under mild pressure to regulate sushi's use by restaurants and the public, but without harder evidence of a hazard, the agency is hesitant to tarnish sushi's good reputation or to harm its popularity.

Where does that leave the sushi lover? If you want to enjoy sushi while minimizing the risk, you should do the following.

How to safeguard against bad sushi.

• Eat only fish that has light-colored flesh. Fish with dark-colored flesh is more likely to carry undetected parasites.

• Find out whether the fish has been frozen solid and defrosted before being served. Freezing may detract a bit from the texture, but it also kills any parasites.

• Dine at a restaurant where the chefs are Japanese or Japanese-trained. They're more likely to know good raw fish from bad.

• If possible, find out if your fish came from one of the fishing fleets that specializes in catching fish for sushi. Fish intended for sushi requires special handling as soon as it is caught.

Organ Meats, Imitation Crab and Hydrogenated Fats

Q. Are organ meats like sweetbreads, liver and kidneys good or bad for you?

A. Sweetbreads, which are the thymus glands of very young animals, give you plenty of protein but not too many other nutrients. Other organ meats, however, provide not only protein but high levels of vitamin C and iron. Also, livers, kidneys, hearts and brains are all relatively low in fat when compared with red meats.

Most organ meats are iron rich.

Some people think that certain animal organs aren't safe to eat because they collect and concentrate the toxins in an animal's body. But the U.S. Department of Agriculture carefully monitors the levels of organ toxins to ensure they don't reach concentrations that would be dangerous.

So if you enjoy organ meats, use them in moderation. They're all relatively high in cholesterol. Compare 3½ ounces of beef, containing 70 milligrams of cholesterol, with equal portions of organ meats. You'll find 150 milligrams of cholesterol in hearts, 250 milligrams in sweetbreads, 300 milligrams in liver, 375 milligrams in kidneys and 2,000 milligrams in brains.

Q. My store recently began carrying what they say is imitation crabmeat. What is this stuff? Is it good for you?

A. The product you're referring to is called surimi (*sur-EE-mee*).

Surimi: It's inexpensive, but content varies.

Technically, surimi is a "structured fish product." That means it contains a relatively inexpensive and available fish, such as pollack or turbot, mixed with some crabmeat or just crab flavoring and processed with egg whites, wheat starch, sugar and sometimes salt. Some brands may also contain monosodium glutamate (MSG) and Red Dye No. 3. At least one brand, called Wakefield Gems, is said to have no MSG and to be comparable to canned crabmeat for protein, fat and calories.

Q. I know that hydrogenated fats aren't good for me, so I try to avoid products that have hydrogenated fats listed on the ingredients label. But now I'm wondering: If the label doesn't list hydrogenated fats, does that mean all fats in the product are unhydrogenated?

Labels must list hydrogenated fat.

A. Yes. According to the FDA, if a label doesn't list hydrogenated fats and the label complies with FDA regulations, then there are no hydrogenated fats in the product. Conversely, if a fat has been completely or partially hydrogenated, then this must be stated on the label.

Notes on Frozen Pizza, Chocolate and Parsnips

Q. I like to eat frozen pizzas, but I hear they contain a lot of sodium. Is that true? And what about the sodium content of other frozen entrees?

A. Yes. In a study of the sodium content of frozen pizzas, researchers discovered that a six-ounce serving of baked frozen cheese pizza provides about 1,100 milligrams of sodium. That's quite a hefty amount: You could get along quite nicely on a daily *total* of only 200 to 300 milligrams.

Some frozen pizzas may be high in sodium.

And the National Academy of Sciences recommends people without high blood pressure consume no more than 1,100 to 3,300 milligrams of sodium per day. Frozen pizzas with bacon or pepperoni toppings have even more than 1,100 milligrams per six ounces.

But frozen pizza is certainly not unique in having lots of sodium. For example, a 5.5-ounce portion of a certain commercial frozen fried chicken breast has 1,362 milligrams of sodium; an 8-ounce frozen chicken pie has 999 milligrams; 6.5 ounces of frozen beef-and-bean burritos, 910 milligrams; and a 5-ounce portion of frozen veal Parmesan has 1,014 milligrams. (Some frozen entrées have slightly less sodium than those mentioned above.)

Q. I've heard that chocolate has a lot of caffeine in it. Does it?

A. Not really. A typical chocolate bar has anywhere from 4 to 10 milligrams of caffeine per ounce, and a cup of cocoa has between 0.5 and 5 milligrams. By comparison, a cup of regular percolated coffee has from 64 to 124 milligrams; a cup of regular instant coffee, 40 to 108 milligrams; and a cup of decaffeinated coffee, 2 to 8 milligrams.

Chocolate not high in caffeine.

Q. Recently I was served whipped parsnips in a fancy restaurant. I was surprised that they tasted sweet. The waiter claimed no sugar had been added to them. Are parsnips quite naturally sweet?

A. Yes, they are. On the average, 3.4 percent of a parsnip is composed of the sugars glucose, fructose and sucrose. But other vegetables have even more sugars. Carrots, for instance, are 5.94 percent sugar, and beets are 6.45 percent. In contrast, vegetables that are low in sugar include broccoli (1.82 percent), celery (1.23 percent) and escarole (0.58 percent).

Some vegetables are naturally sweet.

Understanding Vinegar and Nuts

Q. A while ago, I found a strange-looking "clot" in my vinegar bottle. I threw it all out, but then someone told me this was the "mother" and was not harmful. What's going on?

A. A "clot" is an unsightly addition to your vinegar bottle, but that vinegar you threw out wasn't harmful. Vinegar is made from fruit juice that first undergoes an alcoholic fermentation by yeast, then an oxidative fermentation by bacteria. The oxidizing bacteria are called the "mother of vinegar." They convert the alcohol into acetic acid, the stuff that gives vinegar its sour flavor. The "mother" is normally skimmed off or filtered out of the finished product. Your "mother" obviously slipped through this step. It would have been perfectly safe to strain out the mother and use the vinegar.

Q. I've always been told that some foods, like nuts, are more difficult to digest than others. Is that true?

A. Not exactly. It would be accurate to say that some foods take *longer* to digest than others.

How quickly you digest a food depends on how much carbohydrate, protein and fat it contains. You can digest carbohydrate the fastest, followed by protein and then fat.

Since nuts are high in fat, they may take a little longer to digest. Also, remember to chew nuts thoroughly to ensure complete digestion of their valuable nutrients—unchewed pieces may pass through the digestive tract undigested.

Don't let vinegar clots alarm you.

Nuts take longer to digest. Chew them well.

A Reader's Guide to Recommended Dietary Allowances

These charts show the Recommended Dietary Allowances (RDAs) of essential nutrients for men, women and children—the recognized yardstick for measuring nutritional needs. The nutrient intakes listed are based on available scientific evidence and are considered adequate for practically all healthy persons. The Food and Nutrition Board of the National Research Council of the National Academy of Sciences established these values. The U.S. Recommended Daily Allowances (USRDAs), referred to from time to time throughout this book, are simplified versions of the RDAs. They were proposed by the U.S. Food and Drug Administration to be used primarily in food labeling.

Recommended Dietary Allowances

Vitamins

Age (yr.)	Weight (lb.)	Height	Protein (g.)	Vitamin A (I.U.)	Thiamine (B$_1$) (mg.)	Riboflavin (B$_2$) (mg.)
■ Men						
11–14	99	5'2"	45	5,000	1.4	1.6
15–18	145	5'9"	56	5,000	1.4	1.7
19–22	154	5'10"	56	5,000	1.5	1.7
23–50	154	5'10"	56	5,000	1.4	1.6
51+	154	5'10"	56	5,000	1.2	1.4
■ Women						
11–14	101	5'2"	46	4,000	1.1	1.3
15–18	120	5'4"	46	4,000	1.1	1.3
19–22	120	5'4"	44	4,000	1.1	1.3
23–50	120	5'4"	44	4,000	1.0	1.2
51+	120	5'4"	44	4,000	1.0	1.2
■ Pregnant						
—	—	—	+30	+1,000	+0.4	+0.3
■ Lactating						
—	—	—	+20	+2,000	+0.5	+0.5
■ Infants						
0–0.5	13	2'0"	13	2,100	0.3	0.4
0.5–1	20	2'4"	18	2,000	0.5	0.6
■ Children						
1–3	29	2'11"	23	2,000	0.7	0.8
4–6	44	3'8"	30	2,500	0.9	1.0
7–10	62	4'4"	34	3,500	1.2	1.4

Niacin (mg.)	Vitamin B$_6$ (mg.)	Vitamin B$_{12}$ (mcg.)	Folate (mcg.)	Vitamin C (mg.)	Vitamin D (I.U.)	Vitamin E (I.U.)
18	1.8	3.0	400	50	400	12
18	2.0	3.0	400	60	400	15
19	2.2	3.0	400	60	300	15
18	2.2	3.0	400	60	200	15
16	2.2	3.0	400	60	200	15
15	1.8	3.0	400	50	400	12
14	2.0	3.0	400	60	400	12
14	2.0	3.0	400	60	300	12
13	2.0	3.0	400	60	200	12
13	2.0	3.0	400	60	200	12
+2	+0.6	+1.0	+400	+20	+200	+3.0
+5	+0.5	+1.0	+100	+40	+200	+4.5
6	0.3	0.5	30	35	400	4.5
8	0.6	1.5	45	35	400	6
9	0.9	2.0	100	45	400	9
11	1.3	2.5	200	45	400	9
16	1.6	3.0	300	45	400	10.5

(continued)

Minerals

Age (yr.)	Weight (lb.)	Height	Calcium (mg.)	Iodine (mcg.)
■ Men				
11–14	99	5'2"	1,200	150
15–18	145	5'9"	1,200	150
19–22	154	5'10"	800	150
23–50	154	5'10"	800	150
51+	154	5'10"	800	150
■ Women				
11–14	101	5'2"	1,200	150
15–18	120	5'4"	1,200	150
19–22	120	5'4"	800	150
23–50	120	5'4"	800	150
51+	120	5'4"	800	150
■ Pregnant				
—	—	—	+400	+25
■ Lactating				
—	—	—	+400	+50
■ Infants				
0–0.5	13	2'0"	360	40
0.5–1	20	2'4"	540	50
■ Children				
1–3	29	2'11"	800	70
4–6	44	3'8"	800	90
7–10	62	4'4"	800	120

Iron (mg.)	Magnesium (mg.)	Phosphorus (mg.)	Zinc (mg.)
18	350	1,200	15
18	400	1,200	15
10	350	800	15
10	350	800	15
10	350	800	15
18	300	1,200	15
18	300	1,200	15
18	300	800	15
10	300	800	15
10	300	800	15
30–60	+150	+400	+5
30–60	+150	+400	+10
10	50	240	3
15	70	360	5
15	150	800	10
10	200	800	10
10	250	800	10

(continued)

Estimated Safe and Adequate Daily Intakes for Other Minerals and Trace Elements

Age (yr.)	Chloride (mg.)	Chromium (mcg.)	Copper (mg.)	Fluoride (mg.)
■ Men				
All	1,700–5,100	50–200	2.0–3.0	1.5–4.0
■ Women				
All	1,700–5,100	50–200	2.0–3.0	1.5–4.0
■ Infants				
0–0.5	275–700	10–40	0.5–0.7	0.1–0.5
0.5–1	400–1,200	20–60	0.7–1.0	0.2–1.0
■ Children				
1–3	500–1,500	20–80	1.0–1.5	0.5–1.5
4–6	700–2,100	30–120	1.5–2.0	1.0–2.5
7–10	925–2,775	50–200	2.0–2.5	1.5–2.5
11+	1,400–4,200	50–200	2.0–3.0	1.5–2.5

SOURCE: *Recommended Dietary Allowances*, 9th ed. (Washington, D.C.: National Academy of Sciences, 1980).

Manganese (mg.)	Molybdenum (mg.)	Potassium (mg.)	Selenium (mcg.)	Sodium (mg.)
2.5–5.0	0.15–0.50	1,875–5,625	50–200	1,100–3,300
2.5–5.0	0.15–0.50	1,875–5,625	50–200	1,100–3,300
0.5–0.7	0.03–0.06	350–925	10–40	115–350
0.7–1.0	0.04–0.08	425–1,275	20–60	250–750
1.0–1.5	0.05–0.10	550–1,650	20–80	325–975
1.5–2.0	0.06–0.15	775–2,325	30–120	450–1,350
2.0–3.0	0.10–0.30	1,000–3,000	50–200	600–1,800
2.5–5.0	0.15–0.50	1,525–4,575	50–200	900–2,700

A Reader's Guide to
the Nutrient Content
of Foods

The following is a nutritional analysis of over 500 foods, listing the precise amount of selected vitamins and minerals contained in each one. Consult this data bank when you're trying to incorporate more of a specific nutrient into your diet, when you're planning meals and menus for your family or when you want to assess your daily nutrient intake.

Nutrient Content of Foods

Food	Portion	Vitamin A (I.U.)*	Thiamine (mg.)	Riboflavin (mg.)	Niacin (mg.)	Vitamin B$_6$ (mg.)	Vitamin B$_{12}$ (mcg.)	Folate (mcg.)
■ **Beverages** (*See also* Dairy Products; Fruits and Fruit Juices)								
Alcoholic								
Beer, regular	12 fl. oz.	0.000	0.021	0.093	1.613	0.178	0.060	21.400
Cordial/liqueur, coffee,								
53 proof	1½ fl. oz.	0.000	0.002	0.006	0.075	——	——	0.000
Whiskey, gin, rum,								
vodka, 80, 86, 90								
proof	1½ fl. oz.	0.000	0.003	0.002	0.005	0.000	0.000	0.000
Wine, dessert	2 fl. oz.	——	0.011	0.011	0.126	0.000	0.000	0.200
Wine, red, table	3½ fl. oz.	0.000	0.005	0.029	0.083	0.035	0.010	2.100
Wine, white, table	3½ fl. oz.	0.000	0.004	0.005	0.069	0.014	0.000	0.200
Carbonated								
Club soda	12 fl. oz.	0.000	0.000	0.000	0.000	0.000	0.000	0.000
Cola, aspartame-								
sweetened	12 fl. oz.	0.000	0.018	0.082	0.000	0.000	0.000	0.000
Cola, Dr. Pepper-type	12 fl. oz.	0.000	0.000	0.000	0.000	0.000	0.000	0.000
Cola, regular	12 fl. oz.	0.000	0.000	0.000	0.000	0.000	0.000	0.000
Cream soda	12 fl. oz.	0.000	0.000	0.000	0.000	0.000	0.000	0.000
Ginger ale	12 fl. oz.	0.000	0.000	0.000	0.000	0.000	0.000	0.000
Grape soda	12 fl. oz.	0.000	0.000	0.000	——	0.000	0.000	0.000
Root beer	12 fl. oz.	0.000	0.000	0.000	0.000	0.000	0.000	0.000
Chocolate								
Cocoa, home recipe,								
w/milk	1 cup	318.000	0.102	0.435	0.365	0.107	0.870	12.000
Drink powder, no milk	1 serving	5.080	0.010	0.030	0.100	0.004	0.000	——
Malted milk, fortified								
mix, w/milk	1 cup	3058.000	0.734	1.259	10.902	1.020	0.870	31.800
Milk, mix, w/milk	1 cup	312.000	0.101	0.428	0.317	0.104	0.870	12.200
Coffee								
Brewed	6 fl. oz.	——	0.000	0.000	0.393	0.000	0.000	0.300
Instant, prepared	6 fl. oz.	0.000	0.000	0.002	0.507	0.000	0.000	0.000
Substitute, prepared	6 fl. oz.	——	——	0.002	0.389	——	0.000	——
Fruit punch drink, canned	6 fl. oz.	26.000	0.041	0.043	0.039	0.000	0.000	2.300

Vitamin C (mg.)	Vitamin D (I.U.)	Vitamin E (I.U.)	Calcium (mg.)	Copper (mcg.)	Iron (mg.)	Magnesium (mg.)	Potassium (mg.)	Sodium (mg.)	Zinc (mg.)
0.000	—	—	18.000	32.000	0.110	23.000	89.000	19.000	0.060
0.000	—	—	1.000	45.000	0.030	1.000	15.000	4.000	0.010
0.000	—	—	0.000	9.000	0.020	0.000	1.000	0.000	0.020
0.000	—	—	5.000	27.000	0.140	5.000	54.000	5.000	0.040
0.000	—	—	8.000	21.000	0.440	13.000	115.000	6.000	0.100
0.000	—	—	9.000	22.000	0.330	11.000	82.000	5.000	0.070
0.000	—	—	17.000	—	—	4.000	6.000	75.000	0.360
0.000	—	—	12.000	—	0.110	4.000	—	21.000	0.280
0.000	—	—	12.000	22.000	0.140	1.000	2.000	38.000	0.150
0.000	—	—	9.000	41.000	0.130	3.000	4.000	14.000	0.050
0.000	—	—	19.000	30.000	0.190	3.000	4.000	43.000	0.240
0.000	—	—	12.000	66.000	0.660	3.000	5.000	25.000	0.180
0.000	—	—	12.000	82.000	0.310	4.000	3.000	57.000	0.260
0.000	—	—	19.000	26.000	0.180	4.000	3.000	49.000	0.260
2.400	100.000	—	298.000	—	0.780	56.000	480.000	123.000	1.220
0.000	—	0.083	10.400	197.000	0.600	22.900	142.000	75.000	0.343
33.800	278.000	—	384.000	156.000	3.770	53.000	620.000	244.000	1.150
2.500	100.000	—	300.000	176.000	0.800	54.000	498.000	165.000	1.260
0.000	—	—	3.00	12.000	0.720	10.000	96.000	4.000	0.030
0.000	—	—	6.00	13.000	0.090	8.000	64.000	6.000	0.050
—	—	—	5.00	16.000	0.120	7.000	43.000	7.000	0.060
55.100	—	—	14.000	95.000	0.380	4.000	47.000	41.000	0.230

(continued)

Food	Portion	Vitamin A (I.U.)*	Thiamine (mg.)	Riboflavin (mg.)	Niacin (mg.)	Vitamin B₆ (mg.)	Vitamin B₁₂ (mcg.)	Folate (mcg.)
Beverages—continued								
Mineral water, Perrier	1 cup	0.000	0.000	0.000	0.000	0.000	0.000	0.000
Tea								
Brewed	6 fl. oz.	0.000	0.000	0.025	0.000	0.000	0.000	9.200
Instant, lemon flavor	1 cup	0.000	0.000	0.019	0.090	——	0.000	——
Instant, sugar and lemon flavor	1 cup	0.000	0.000	0.047	0.093	——	0.000	9.600
■ Breads								
Bagels								
Egg	1	17.600	0.209	0.160	1.940	0.024	0.052	13.200
Water	1	0.000	0.209	0.160	1.940	0.024	0.000	13.200
Biscuit, home recipe	1	0.000	0.080	0.080	0.700	——	——	——
Bread								
Cornbread, home recipe	1 slice	61.700	0.081	0.081	0.675	0.032	0.077	4.500
Cracked wheat	1 slice	0.000	0.095	0.095	0.840	0.023	0.000	——
French, enriched	1 slice	0.000	0.161	0.123	1.400	0.019	0.000	13.000
Italian, enriched	1 slice	0.000	0.120	0.070	1.000	0.016	0.000	10.500
Mixed grain	1 slice	0.000	0.098	0.095	1.040	0.026	0.000	16.300
Mixed grain, toasted	1 slice	0.000	0.079	0.097	1.060	0.026	0.000	16.500
Pita	1 pocket	0.000	0.171	0.076	1.400	——	——	——
Pumpernickel	1 slice	0.000	0.109	0.166	1.060	0.049	0.000	——
Raisin, enriched	1 slice	0.000	0.083	0.155	1.020	0.009	0.000	8.750
Rye, American, light	1 slice	0.000	0.103	0.080	0.828	0.023	0.000	9.750
Vienna, enriched	1 slice	0.000	0.115	0.088	1.000	0.013	0.000	9.250
Wheat, home recipe, toasted	1 slice	11.000	0.055	0.040	0.812	0.051	0.028	12.500
White, firm	1 slice	0.000	0.108	0.071	0.863	0.008	0.000	8.050
Whole wheat, home recipe	1 slice	10.800	0.068	0.038	0.798	0.050	0.027	12.300
Bread stick, Vienna-type	1	0.000	0.020	0.030	0.300	——	——	——
English muffin, plain, toasted	1	0.000	0.239	0.207	2.430	0.026	0.000	20.700
French toast, home recipe	1 slice	111.000	0.124	0.163	1.010	0.038	0.291	17.600
Muffins								
Blueberry, home recipe	1	90.000	0.090	0.100	0.700	——	——	——

Vitamin C (mg.)	Vitamin D (I.U.)	Vitamin E (I.U.)	Calcium (mg.)	Copper (mcg.)	Iron (mg.)	Magnesium (mg.)	Potassium (mg.)	Sodium (mg.)	Zinc (mg.)
0.000	—	—	32.000	0.000	0.000	1.000	0.000	3.000	0.000
0.000	—	—	0.000	18.000	0.040	5.000	66.000	14.250	0.040
0.000	—	—	5.00	19.000	0.020	4.000	49.000	14.000	0.080
0.000	—	—	6.000	210.000	0.050	5.000	50.000	—	0.080
0.000	—	—	23.100	46.000	1.460	11.000	40.700	198.000	0.286
0.000	—	—	23.100	46.000	1.460	11.000	40.700	198.000	0.286
0.000	—	—	34.000	—	0.400	6.160	33.000	175.000	—
0.000	7.000	—	48.600	18.000	0.671	8.100	42.300	126.000	0.212
0.000	—	0.037	16.300	—	0.665	8.750	33.300	108.000	—
0.000	—	0.063	38.500	51.000	1.080	7.000	30.100	193.000	0.221
0.000	—	0.054	5.000	—	0.700	—	22.000	152.000	—
0.000	—	0.037	26.000	71.000	0.815	12.300	54.500	103.000	0.300
0.000	—	0.037	26.600	72.000	0.832	12.500	55.700	105.000	0.306
0.000	—	—	30.800	—	0.916	—	44.800	215.000	—
0.000	—	—	22.700	—	0.877	21.800	139.000	173.000	0.365
0.000	—	—	25.500	34.000	0.775	6.250	60.000	94.000	0.155
0.000	—	—	20.000	25.000	0.680	6.000	51.000	174.000	0.318
0.000	—	0.045	27.500	36.000	0.770	5.000	21.500	138.000	0.158
0.000	—	0.037	20.000	65.000	0.682	23.500	86.500	90.600	0.572
0.000	—	0.042	29.000	50.000	0.653	4.830	25.800	118.000	0.143
0.000	—	0.037	19.800	64.000	0.670	23.300	85.000	89.000	0.562
0.000	—	—	16.000	—	0.300	—	33.000	548.000	—
0.000	—	—	105.000	201.000	1.830	12.200	364.000	414.000	0.466
0.000	10.000	—	72.200	59.000	1.340	11.700	85.800	257.000	0.553
0.000	—	—	34.000	32.000	0.600	10.000	46.000	252.000	—

(continued)

Food	Portion	Vitamin A (I.U.)*	Thiamine (mg.)	Riboflavin (mg.)	Niacin (mg.)	Vitamin B$_6$ (mg.)	Vitamin B$_{12}$ (mcg.)	Folate (mcg.)
Breads—continued								
Muffins—continued								
Bran, home recipe	1	206.000	0.100	0.112	1.260	0.111	0.092	16.800
Corn, mix, w/egg and								
milk	1	100.000	0.080	0.090	0.700	——	——	——
Rolls								
Hamburger/hot dog	1	0.000	0.196	0.132	1.580	0.014	——	14.800
Hard, enriched	1	0.000	0.200	0.120	1.700	0.018	0.000	29.500
Submarine/hoagie,								
enriched	1	0.000	0.540	0.320	4.500	0.047	——	——
Stuffing, mix, prepared	1 cup	910.000	0.130	0.170	2.100	——	——	——
■ Cereals								
All Bran	1 oz.	1250.000	0.369	0.426	4.991	0.509	——	100.200
Bran Buds	1 oz.	1250.000	0.369	0.426	4.991	0.509	——	100.200
Bran flakes, Kellogg	1 oz.	1250.000	0.363	0.436	5.016	0.509	1.527	100.300
Cheerios	1 oz.	1250.000	0.368	0.426	4.996	0.511	1.499	6.232
Cornflakes, Kellogg	1 oz.	1250.000	0.368	0.426	4.996	0.511	——	100.000
Corn grits, enriched	1 cup	——	0.240	0.150	1.960	0.058	——	1.000
Cream of wheat, regular	1 cup	——	0.200	0.100	1.500	——	——	9.000
Grape-Nuts	1 oz.	1250.000	0.368	0.425	4.999	0.510	1.502	99.970
Millet, cooked	1 cup	92.000	0.180	0.060	2.280	0.280	——	0.000
Oatmeal								
Cooked	1 cup	38.000	0.260	0.050	0.300	0.047	——	9.000
Instant	1 packet	1514.000	0.530	0.290	5.490	0.742	——	150.000
Oats, rolled, regular, dry	1 cup	——	0.480	0.110	0.800	——	——	0.000
100% Bran	1 cup	0.000	0.687	0.773	8.978	0.902	2.706	0.000
Raisin bran, Ralston	1.33 oz.	1247.000	0.404	0.404	4.983	0.471	1.481	99.650
Rice Chex	1 oz.	16.990	0.369	——	4.995	0.511	1.507	100.100
Total	1 oz.	5000.000	1.460	1.718	20.020	1.976	6.014	400.300
Wheat germ, toasted	1 oz.	47.170	0.474	0.233	1.583	0.278	——	99.850
Wheaties	1 oz.	1250.000	0.391	0.391	4.986	0.489	1.466	8.798
■ Combination Dishes								
Beans and frankfurters,								
canned	1 cup	330.000	0.180	0.150	3.300	——	——	——
Beans w/pork and tomato								
sauce, canned	1 cup	330.000	0.200	0.080	1.500	——	——	——

Vitamin C (mg.)	Vitamin D (I.U.)	Vitamin E (I.U.)	Calcium (mg.)	Copper (mcg.)	Iron (mg.)	Magnesium (mg.)	Potassium (mg.)	Sodium (mg.)	Zinc (mg.)
2.480	—	—	53.600	85.000	1.260	35.200	98.800	168.000	1.080
0.000	—	—	96.000	—	0.600	—	44.000	191.000	—
0.000	—	0.024	53.600	66.000	1.190	7.600	36.800	241.000	0.248
0.000	—	0.030	24.000	50.000	1.200	11.500	49.000	312.000	0.300
0.000	—	0.080	58.000	—	3.000	—	122.000	761.000	—
0.000	—	—	92.000	—	2.200	—	126.000	1254.000	—
15.040	—	0.630	22.960	324.000	4.492	105.800	349.700	319.800	3.727
15.040	—	0.447	19.000	300.000	4.492	90.170	474.200	174.000	3.727
—	101.000	0.177	13.810	210.000	8.142	51.610	180.300	263.900	3.707
14.990	—	—	48.460	144.000	4.509	39.090	101.200	307.200	0.786
14.990	50.580	0.043	0.851	19.000	1.786	3.397	26.100	350.900	0.080
—	—	0.432	1.000	29.000	1.560	11.000	54.000	0.000	0.170
—	—	—	51.000	75.000	10.300	10.000	43.000	2.000	0.330
—	49.990	—	10.770	94.000	1.231	18.970	94.750	197.000	0.624
0.200	—	—	4.000	—	2.300	48.000	76.000	8.000	1.820
—	—	5.260	20.000	129.000	1.590	56.000	132.000	1.000	1.150
—	—	1.579	163.000	98.000	6.320	—	100.000	286.000	—
—	—	—	42.000	—	3.600	—	282.000	2.000	—
27.060	—	—	19.760	447.000	3.488	134.000	353.900	196.300	2.466
1.347	98.980	—	18.180	205.000	4.511	56.560	193.200	327.200	1.124
15.080	—	0.016	3.971	75.000	1.789	7.087	32.850	237.400	0.392
60.140	—	—	48.110	122.000	18.040	31.790	105.700	351.400	0.670
1.756	8.505	5.944	12.540	176.000	2.584	90.820	268.400	1.004	4.717
14.660	0.000	0.177	43.010	131.000	4.497	31.280	105.600	354.900	0.635
0.000	—	0.836	94.000	—	4.800	—	668.000	1392.000	—
5.000	—	0.836	138.000	—	4.600	—	536.000	1180.000	—

(continued)

Food	Portion	Vitamin A (I.U.)*	Thiamine (mg.)	Riboflavin (mg.)	Niacin (mg.)	Vitamin B$_6$ (mg.)	Vitamin B$_{12}$ (mcg.)	Folate (mcg.)
Combination Dishes—continued								
Beef and vegetable stew	1 cup	2400.000	0.150	0.170	4.700	——	0.002	——
Beef potpie, home recipe	1 serving	1720.000	0.300	0.300	5.500	——	——	——
Chili con carne w/ beans,								
canned	1 cup	150.000	0.080	0.180	3.300	0.263	——	——
Enchilada	1	0.000	0.184	0.253	——	0.253	2.070	——
Macaroni and cheese								
Canned, enriched	1 cup	260.000	0.120	0.240	1.000	——	——	——
Home recipe, enriched	1 cup	860.00	0.200	0.400	1.800	——	——	——
Pizza								
Cheese, baked	1 slice	750.000	0.336	0.288	4.210	0.120	0.480	55.200
Pepperoni, baked	1 slice	532.000	0.324	0.288	5.150	0.096	0.360	78.000
Soufflés								
Cheese, home recipe	1 cup	760.000	0.050	0.230	0.200	——	——	——
Spinach	1 cup	3461.000	0.091	0.305	0.477	0.120	0.680	61.900
Spaghetti								
Tomato and cheese,								
home recipe	1 cup	1080.000	0.250	0.180	2.300	——	——	——
Tomato and meat,								
home recipe	1 cup	1590.000	0.250	0.300	4.000	——	——	——
Taco	1	420.000	0.089	0.065	1.410	0.122	0.405	11.300
■ Dairy Products								
Cheese								
American, processed	1 oz.	347.300	0.008	0.101	0.020	0.020	0.199	2.025
Blue	1 oz.	206.600	0.008	0.109	0.292	0.048	0.349	10.130
Brick	1 oz.	310.800	0.004	0.101	0.033	0.018	0.360	6.075
Brie	1 oz.	191.400	0.020	0.149	0.109	0.068	0.474	18.230
Cheddar, cut pieces	1 oz.	303.800	0.008	0.107	0.023	0.021	0.237	5.063
Cheddar, shredded	¼ cup	299.300	0.008	0.106	0.023	0.021	0.234	5.250
Cottage, 1% fat	1 cup	84.000	0.047	0.373	0.289	0.154	1.430	28.000
Cottage, 2% fat	1 cup	158.000	0.054	0.418	0.325	0.172	1.610	30.000
Cottage, large-curd,								
4% fat	1 cup	367.000	0.047	0.367	0.284	0.151	1.400	27.000
Cream	1 oz.	410.100	0.005	0.057	0.029	0.013	0.122	4.050
Edam	1 oz.	263.300	0.010	0.111	0.023	0.022	0.440	5.063
Feta	1 oz.	——	——	——	——	——	——	——
Gouda	1 oz.	185.300	0.009	0.096	0.018	0.023	——	6.075
Gruyère	1 oz.	350.300	0.017	0.080	0.030	0.023	0.460	3.038

Vitamin C (mg.)	Vitamin D (I.U.)	Vitamin E (I.U.)	Calcium (mg.)	Copper (mcg.)	Iron (mg.)	Magnesium (mg.)	Potassium (mg.)	Sodium (mg.)	Zinc (mg.)
17.000	0.000	0.767	29.000	183.000	2.900	——	613.000	1006.000	——
6.000	——	1.758	29.000	——	3.800	——	334.000	596.000	——
——	0.000	——	82.000	——	4.300	——	594.000	1354.000	——
——	——	0.411	96.600	299.000	3.290	75.900	653.000	1332.000	1.290
0.000	——	0.572	199.000	——	1.000	——	139.000	729.000	——
0.000	——	0.477	362.000	——	1.800	52.000	240.000	1086.000	——
2.400	——	——	220.000	144.000	1.610	31.200	230.000	698.000	1.670
2.400	——	——	196.000	——	2.520	——	216.000	817.000	——
0.000	——	——	191.000	——	1.000	——	115.000	346.000	——
2.900	——	——	230.000	120.000	1.340	37.000	202.000	763.000	1.290
13.000	——	——	80.000	——	2.300	——	408.000	955.000	——
22.000	5.000	0.000	124.000	——	3.700	——	665.000	1009.000	——
0.810	5.860	——	109.000	105.000	1.150	36.500	263.000	456.000	1.560
0.000	——	0.270	176.200	17.000	0.111	6.075	46.580	411.100	0.861
0.000	——	0.270	151.900	11.000	0.091	7.088	73.910	401.000	0.759
0.000	——	0.270	193.400	7.000	0.122	7.088	38.480	161.000	0.749
0.000	——	0.270	52.650	——	0.142	0.000	43.540	180.200	——
0.000	——	0.270	206.600	31.000	0.192	8.100	28.350	178.200	0.891
0.000	——	0.270	203.800	31.000	0.193	7.750	27.750	175.300	0.878
0.000	5.000	2.161	138.000	——	0.320	12.000	193.000	918.000	0.860
0.000	5.000	2.161	155.000	——	0.360	14.000	217.000	918.000	0.950
0.000	5.000	2.146	135.000	43.000	0.315	11.300	189.000	911.000	0.833
0.000	——	0.270	23.290	11.000	0.344	2.025	34.430	85.050	0.152
0.000	23.790	0.270	209.600	8.000	0.122	8.100	53.660	277.400	1.073
0.000	——	0.270	141.800	——	0.182	5.063	18.230	320.000	0.830
0.000	——	0.270	200.500	——	0.071	8.100	34.430	234.900	1.124
0.000	——	0.270	290.600	——	——	——	23.290	96.190	——

(continued)

Food	Portion	Vitamin A (I.U.)*	Thiamine (mg.)	Riboflavin (mg.)	Niacin (mg.)	Vitamin B_6 (mg.)	Vitamin B_{12} (mcg.)	Folate (mcg.)
Dairy Products—continued								
Cheese—continued								
Limburger	1 oz.	367.500	0.023	0.145	0.046	0.024	0.299	16.200
Monterey Jack	1 oz.	272.400	——	0.112	0.000	——	——	——
Mozzarella, skim-milk	1 oz.	168.100	0.005	0.087	0.030	0.020	0.235	2.025
Mozzarella, whole-milk	1 oz.	227.800	0.004	0.070	0.024	0.016	0.187	2.025
Muenster	1 oz.	322.000	0.004	0.092	0.029	0.016	0.423	3.038
Neufchâtel	1 oz.	325.000	0.004	0.056	0.036	0.012	0.076	3.038
Parmesan, grated	1 tbsp.	43.810	0.003	0.024	0.020	0.007	——	0.500
Provolone	1 oz.	233.900	0.005	0.092	0.045	0.021	0.420	3.038
Ricotta, skim-milk	1 cup	1063.00	0.052	0.455	0.192	0.049	0.716	——
Ricotta, whole-milk	1 cup	1205.000	0.032	0.480	0.256	0.106	0.831	——
Romano	1 oz.	164.000	——	0.106	0.022	——	——	2.025
Roquefort	1 oz.	300.700	0.011	0.168	0.211	0.035	0.184	14.180
Swiss	1 oz.	243.000	0.006	0.104	0.026	0.024	0.481	2.025
Cream								
Half-and-half	1 tbsp.	65.630	0.005	0.023	0.012	0.006	0.050	0.375
Light	1 tbsp.	108.000	0.005	0.022	0.009	0.005	0.033	0.375
Sour, cultured	1 tbsp.	113.600	0.005	0.021	0.010	0.002	0.043	1.563
Whipped, imitation, frozen	1 tbsp.	40.380	0.000	0.000	0.000	0.000	0.000	0.000
Whipped, pressurized can	1 tbsp.	34.250	0.001	0.002	0.003	0.002	0.011	——
Eggnog, commercial	1 cup	894.000	0.086	0.483	0.267	0.127	1.140	2.000
Milk								
Chocolate, whole	1 cup	302.000	0.092	0.405	0.313	0.100	0.835	12.000
Evaporated, skim, canned	1 fl. oz.	125.000	0.014	0.099	0.056	0.018	0.076	2.875
Nonfat, fluid	1 cup	500.000	0.088	0.343	0.216	0.098	0.926	13.000
1% fat	1 cup	500.000	0.095	0.407	0.212	0.105	0.898	12.000
2% fat	1 cup	500.000	0.095	0.403	0.210	0.105	0.888	12.000
Whole, 3.3% fat	1 cup	307.000	0.093	0.395	0.205	0.102	0.871	12.000
Milk shakes								
Chocolate, thick	10 fl. oz.	258.000	0.141	0.666	0.372	0.075	0.945	15.000
Vanilla, thick	10 fl. oz.	357.000	0.094	0.610	0.457	0.131	1.630	21.000
Yogurt								
Fruit flavor, low-fat	1 cup	104.000	0.084	0.404	0.216	0.091	1.060	21.000
Plain, low-fat	1 cup	150.000	0.100	0.486	0.259	0.111	1.280	25.000
Plain, nonfat	1 cup	16.000	0.109	0.531	0.281	0.120	1.390	28.000
Plain, whole-milk	1 cup	279.000	0.066	0.322	0.170	0.073	0.844	17.000

Vitamin C (mg.)	Vitamin D (I.U.)	Vitamin E (I.U.)	Calcium (mg.)	Copper (mcg.)	Iron (mg.)	Magnesium (mg.)	Potassium (mg.)	Sodium (mg.)	Zinc (mg.)
0.000	——	0.270	142.800	——	0.041	6.075	36.450	229.800	0.608
0.000	——	0.270	214.700	9.000	0.203	8.100	23.290	153.900	0.861
0.000	——	0.270	185.300	8.000	0.061	7.088	24.300	133.700	0.790
0.000	——	0.270	148.800	——	0.051	5.063	19.240	107.300	0.638
0.000	——	0.270	205.500	9.000	0.122	8.100	38.480	180.200	0.810
0.000	——	0.270	21.260	——	0.081	2.025	32.400	114.400	0.152
0.000	——	0.060	86.000	23.000	0.059	3.188	6.688	116.400	0.199
0.000	——	0.270	216.700	7.000	0.152	8.100	39.490	251.100	0.932
0.000	——	2.339	669.000	——	1.080	36.000	308.000	307.000	3.300
0.000	——	2.339	509.000	85.000	0.940	28.000	257.000	207.000	2.850
0.000	——	0.270	305.800	——	——	——	——	344.300	——
0.000	——	0.270	190.400	10.000	0.162	8.100	26.330	519.400	0.597
0.000	28.350	0.270	275.400	36.000	0.051	10.230	31.390	74.930	1.124
0.130	——	——	15.880	——	0.011	1.563	19.630	6.125	0.077
0.114	——	——	14.440	33.000	0.006	1.313	18.250	5.938	0.041
0.124	1.200	——	16.750	——	0.009	1.625	20.690	7.688	0.039
0.000	——	——	0.313	——	0.006	0.063	0.875	1.188	0.001
0.000	——	——	3.813	——	0.002	0.375	5.500	4.875	0.014
3.810	57.000	——	330.000	18.000	0.510	47.000	420.000	138.000	1.170
2.280	103.000	0.335	280.000	——	0.600	33.000	417.000	149.000	1.020
0.395	28.000	——	92.500	——	0.093	8.613	105.900	36.630	0.287
2.400	103.000	0.219	302.000	100.000	0.100	28.000	406.000	126.000	0.980
2.370	102.000	0.218	300.000	——	0.120	34.000	381.000	123.000	0.950
2.320	102.000	0.218	297.000	——	0.120	33.000	377.000	122.000	0.950
2.290	102.000	0.218	291.000	500.000	0.120	33.000	370.000	120.000	0.930
0.000	39.000	——	396.000	——	0.930	48.000	672.000	333.000	1.440
0.000	42.200	——	457.000	——	0.310	37.000	572.000	299.000	1.220
1.500	——	——	345.000	——	0.160	33.000	442.000	133.000	1.680
1.820	——	——	415.000	——	0.180	40.000	531.000	159.000	2.020
1.980	——	——	452.000	——	0.200	43.000	579.000	174.000	2.200
1.200	——	——	274.000	——	0.110	26.000	351.000	105.000	1.340

(continued)

Food	Portion	Vitamin A (I.U.)*	Thiamine (mg.)	Riboflavin (mg.)	Niacin (mg.)	Vitamin B$_6$ (mg.)	Vitamin B$_{12}$ (mcg.)	Folate (mcg.)
■ Desserts								
Brownie, home recipe, w/nuts	1	40.000	0.040	0.030	0.200	——	——	——
Cake								
Angel food, mix, prepared	1 slice	0.000	0.064	0.122	0.594	0.007	0.015	4.770
Coffee, mix, prepared	1 slice	120.000	0.140	0.150	1.300	——	——	——
Devil's food, mix, w/icing, prepared	1 slice	100.000	0.070	0.100	0.600	——	——	4.140
Pineapple upside-down, home recipe	1 slice	272.000	0.112	0.077	0.742	0.044	0.059	8.400
Pound, home recipe	1 slice	80.000	0.050	0.060	0.400	——	——	1.980
Sponge, home recipe	1 slice	125.000	0.092	0.132	0.726	0.037	0.332	14.500
White, w/chocolate icing, home recipe	1 slice	21.300	0.071	0.107	0.675	0.017	0.058	3.550
Cheesecake, commercial	1 slice	216.000	0.026	0.111	0.391	0.054	0.421	15.300
Cookies								
Chocolate chip, home recipe	1	4.300	0.015	0.015	0.146	0.002	0.010	0.900
Chocolate chip, mix	1	6.090	0.014	0.022	0.195	0.002	——	0.945
Fig bar	1	15.700	0.020	0.018	0.182	0.015	0.000	0.840
Gingersnap, home recipe	1	2.520	0.014	0.012	0.122	0.004	0.006	0.560
Cupcake, w/chocolate icing	1	60.000	0.050	0.060	0.400	——	——	——
Custard, baked	½ cup	465.000	0.055	0.250	0.150	——	——	——
Danish pastry, plain	1	69.600	0.156	0.150	1.470	——	——	——
Doughnut, cake, plain	1	14.300	0.060	0.050	0.428	0.009	——	2.000
Éclair, custard, w/chocolate icing	1	340.000	0.040	0.160	0.100	——	——	——
Fruitcake, dark, home recipe	1 slice	20.000	0.020	0.020	0.200	——	——	——
Granola bar	1	——	0.067	0.026	——	——	0.000	——
Ice cream								
Sundae, hot fudge	1	231.000	0.066	0.314	1.120	0.132	0.660	9.900
Vanilla, hard, 10% fat	1 cup	543.000	0.052	0.329	0.134	0.061	0.625	3.000
Ice Milk								
Vanilla, hard, 4.3% fat	1 cup	214.000	0.076	0.347	0.118	0.085	0.875	3.000
Vanilla, soft, 2.6% fat	1 cup	175.000	0.117	0.541	0.184	0.133	1.370	5.000

Vitamin C (mg.)	Vitamin D (I.U.)	Vitamin E (I.U.)	Calcium (mg.)	Copper (mcg.)	Iron (mg.)	Magnesium (mg.)	Potassium (mg.)	Sodium (mg.)	Zinc (mg.)
0.000	—	0.766	8.000	—	0.400	3.000	38.000	50.000	0.000
0.000	—	2.131	50.000	20.000	0.451	5.830	51.900	142.000	0.106
0.000	—	2.891	44.000	—	1.200	—	78.000	310.000	—
0.000	—	2.771	41.000	—	1.000	—	90.000	180.000	—
3.500	—	0.887	50.400	84.000	1.110	11.900	119.000	167.000	0.378
0.000	—	1.323	6.000	—	0.500	20.000	58.000	—	
0.000	—	2.652	25.100	33.000	1.110	7.260	59.400	164.000	0.799
0.000	—	2.846	70.000	78.000	0.682	13.500	76.700	200.000	0.263
4.250	18.200	—	47.600	51.000	0.408	8.500	83.300	189.000	0.357
0.000	—	0.398	3.300	32.000	0.249	3.500	20.500	20.600	0.044
0.000	—	0.417	2.940	12.000	0.228	2.520	13.500	37.800	0.053
0.000	—	0.557	10.100	41.000	0.339	3.640	40.600	44.900	0.090
0.000	—	0.279	2.590	9.000	0.161	1.330	13.700	19.700	0.031
0.000	—	0.075	47.000	—	0.400	—	42.000	120.000	—
0.500	—	0.000	148.500	—	0.550	—	193.500	104.500	—
0.000	—	0.000	68.900	—	1.200	9.750	60.500	249.000	0.546
0.000	—	0.268	11.000	33.000	0.365	5.750	27.300	139.000	0.128
0.000	—	0.000	80.000	—	0.700	—	122.000	82.000	—
0.000	—	—	11.000	—	0.400	—	74.000	23.000	—
—	—	0.000	14.400	—	0.763	—	78.200	66.700	0.000
3.300	16.000	0.148	216.000	132.000	0.611	34.700	413.000	177.000	0.990
0.700	—	0.119	176.000	200.000	0.120	18.000	257.000	116.000	1.410
0.760	—	0.118	176.000	—	0.180	19.000	265.000	105.000	0.550
1.170	—	0.000	274.000	—	0.280	29.000	412.000	163.000	0.860

(continued)

Food	Portion	Vitamin A (I.U.)*	Thiamine (mg.)	Riboflavin (mg.)	Niacin (mg.)	Vitamin B₆ (mg.)	Vitamin B₁₂ (mcg.)	Folate (mcg.)
Desserts—continued								
Pie								
Apple, home recipe	1 slice	25.700	0.149	0.108	1.240	0.035	0.000	6.750
Blueberry, home recipe	1 slice	40.000	0.150	0.110	1.400	—	0.000	—
Cherry, home recipe	1 slice	590.000	0.160	0.120	1.400	—	0.000	—
Chocolate cream, home recipe	1 slice	264.000	0.100	0.170	0.720	0.047	0.366	9.000
Lemon meringue, home recipe	1 slice	167.000	0.096	0.120	0.720	0.029	0.191	10.800
Pumpkin, home recipe	1 slice	3210.00	0.110	0.180	1.000	—	—	—
Pudding								
Chocolate, mix, cooked, w/milk	½ cup	170.000	0.025	0.195	0.150	—	—	—
Rice, w/raisins	½ cup	145.000	0.040	0.185	0.250	—	—	—
Tapioca cream, home recipe	½ cup	240.000	0.035	0.150	0.100	—	—	—
Sherbet, orange, 2% fat	1 cup	185.000	0.033	0.089	0.131	0.025	0.158	14.000
Turnover, apple	1	11.400	0.028	0.020	0.332	0.011	0.028	1.140
■ Eggs								
Large, fried w/butter	1	286.000	0.033	0.126	0.026	0.050	0.581	22.000
Large, hard-cooked, no shell	1	260.000	0.037	0.143	0.030	0.057	0.657	24.000
Substitute, liquid	¼ cup	1356.000	0.069	0.188	0.069	—	0.187	—
White only, large, raw	1	0.000	0.002	0.094	0.029	0.001	0.021	5.000
Whole, large, poached	1	259.000	0.035	0.127	0.026	0.051	0.616	24.000
Whole, large, raw	1	260.000	0.044	0.150	0.031	0.060	0.773	32.000
Yolk only, large, raw	1	313.000	0.043	0.074	0.012	0.053	0.647	26.000
■ Fats and Oils								
Butter, regular	1 tsp.	142.700	0.000	0.002	0.002	0.000	—	0.140
Margarine								
Corn oil, regular, hard	1 tsp.	155.000	0.000	0.002	0.001	0.000	0.004	0.060
Corn oil, regular, soft	1 tsp.	155.000	0.000	0.002	0.001	0.000	0.004	0.050
Safflower oil, soft	1 tsp.	155.000	0.000	0.002	0.001	0.000	0.004	0.050
Mayonnaise								
Imitation, soy	1 tbsp.	—	—	—	—	—	—	—
Soy, commercial	1 tbsp.	39.000	0.000	0.000	0.000	—	—	—

Vitamin C (mg.)	Vitamin D (I.U.)	Vitamin E (I.U.)	Calcium (mg.)	Copper (mcg.)	Iron (mg.)	Magnesium (mg.)	Potassium (mg.)	Sodium (mg.)	Zinc (mg.)
2.000	——	3.204	12.200	72.000	1.220	10.800	115.000	207.000	0.230
4.000	——	3.204	15.000	——	1.400	9.450	88.000	361.000	——
0.000	——	3.204	19.000	——	0.900	9.450	142.000	410.000	——
0.000	——	2.369	84.000	119.000	1.080	25.000	142.000	273.000	0.660
3.660	——	2.846	15.600	28.000	0.900	7.200	52.800	223.000	0.336
0.000	——	3.084	66.000	——	1.000	16.900	208.000	278.000	——
1.000	——	0.000	132.500	——	0.400	——	177.000	167.500	——
0.000	——	0.000	130.000	——	0.550	0.000	234.500	94.000	——
1.000	——	0.000	86.500	33.000	0.350	——	111.500	128.500	——
3.860	——	0.000	103.000	——	0.310	15.000	198.000	88.000	1.330
0.284	——	0.673	3.980	14.000	0.312	2.560	13.900	109.000	0.054
0.000	24.800	——	26.000	92.000	0.920	5.000	58.000	144.000	0.640
0.000	24.000	0.574	28.000	100.000	1.040	6.000	65.000	69.000	0.720
0.000	34.750	——	33.250	——	1.318	——	207.000	111.000	0.815
0.000	0.000	——	4.000	25.000	0.010	3.000	45.000	50.000	0.010
0.000	28.000	0.574	28.000	100.000	1.040	6.000	65.000	146.000	0.720
0.000	28.000	0.522	28.000	100.000	1.040	6.000	65.000	69.000	0.720
0.000	27.000	0.520	26.000	45.000	0.950	3.000	15.000	8.000	0.580
0.000	1.400	0.110	1.120	1.000	0.007	0.093	1.213	38.670	0.002
0.008	15.000	0.903	1.410	——	——	0.120	1.990	44.300	——
0.007	15.000	0.745	1.250	——	0.000	0.110	1.770	50.700	——
0.007	15.000	0.820	1.250	——	——	0.110	1.770	50.700	——
——	——	4.634	——	——	——	——	——	74.600	0.020
——	5.600	4.321	2.000	34.000	0.100	0.000	5.000	78.400	0.020

(continued)

Food	Portion	Vitamin A (I.U.)*	Thiamine (mg.)	Riboflavin (mg.)	Niacin (mg.)	Vitamin B₆ (mg.)	Vitamin B₁₂ (mcg.)	Folate (mcg.)
Fats and Oils—continued								
Salad Dressing								
Blue Cheese	1 tbsp.	32.100	0.000	0.020	0.000	—	—	—
French	1 tbsp.	—	—	—	—	—	—	—
Italian	1 tbsp.	—	0.000	0.000	0.000	—	—	—
Russian	1 tbsp.	106.000	0.010	0.010	0.100	—	—	—
Thousand Island	1 tbsp.	50.000	0.000	0.000	0.000	—	—	—
Vegetable oil								
Corn	1 tbsp.	—	0.000	0.000	0.000	0.000	0.000	0.000
Olive	1 tbsp.	—	0.000	0.000	0.000	0.000	0.000	0.000
Soybean	1 tbsp.	—	0.000	0.000	0.000	0.000	0.000	0.000
■ Fish and Shellfish								
Bass, striped, broiled	3 oz.	98.660	0.128	0.119	2.466	—	—	—
Bluefish, raw	3½ oz.	398.000	0.058	0.080	5.950	0.402	5.390	1.590
Caviar, from sturgeon	1 tsp.	—	—	—	—	—	—	—
Clams, meat only, raw	3½ oz.	300.000	—	0.213	1.765	0.079	49.440	2.650
Cod, Atlantic, cooked, dry heat	3 oz.	39.200	0.075	0.067	2.140	0.241	0.890	—
Crab								
Blue, cooked, moist heat	½ cup	1680.00	0.125	0.060	2.150	—	5.690	—
Deviled	⅓ cup	—	0.063	0.086	1.188	—	—	—
Crabcake	3 oz.	249.000	0.061	0.091	1.519	—	5.040	—
Fish sticks and portions, frozen, reheated	3 oz.	89.900	0.108	0.151	1.809	0.051	1.530	15.490
Haddock, cooked, dry heat	3 oz.	53.900	0.034	0.038	3.940	0.294	1.180	—
Halibut, cooked, dry heat	3 oz.	150.000	0.081	0.077	6.050	0.337	1.160	—
Lobster, cooked, moist heat	3 oz.	74.000	0.006	0.056	0.909	0.065	2.640	9.450
Mackerel, Atlantic, cooked, dry heat	3 oz.	152.800	0.135	0.350	5.820	0.390	16.150	—
Perch, cooked, dry heat	3 oz.	—	—	—	—	—	—	—
Oysters								
Eastern, breaded, fried	3 oz.	—	—	0.170	1.400	0.050	13.280	11.550
Eastern, raw	⅓ cup	—	—	0.133	1.040	0.040	15.300	7.900

Vitamin C (mg.)	Vitamin D (I.U.)	Vitamin E (I.U.)	Calcium (mg.)	Copper (mcg.)	Iron (mg.)	Magnesium (mg.)	Potassium (mg.)	Sodium (mg.)	Zinc (mg.)
0.300	—	—	12.400	—	0.000	—	6.120	167.000	—
—	—	—	1.700	—	0.100	—	12.300	214.000	0.010
—	—	—	1.000	103.000	0.000	—	2.000	116.000	0.020
1.000	—	—	3.000	—	0.100	—	24.000	133.000	0.070
0.000	—	—	2.000	—	0.100	0.000	18.000	109.000	0.020
0.000	—	2.897	0.000	—	0.000	0.000	0.000	0.000	0.000
0.000	0.000	2.393	0.024	10.000	0.052	0.001	0.000	0.005	0.008
0.000	—	1.648	0.000	56.000	0.000	0.000	0.000	0.000	0.000
0.000	0.740	—	39.970	—	1.616	36.570	—	57.070	—
—	—	—	6.880	53.400	0.477	33.250	372.200	59.900	0.807
—	—	—	14.670	—	0.633	—	9.667	117.300	—
—	—	0.530	46.140	344.240	13.979	9.240	314.100	55.800	1.365
0.870	—	—	11.800	30.600	0.414	35.800	207.700	66.400	0.490
—	—	—	33.500	503.000	0.600	26.350	252.300	286.000	3.290
4.620	—	—	37.290	—	0.957	—	131.300	686.700	—
0.000	—	—	89.500	518.500	0.917	28.020	275.700	280.100	3.480
—	—	—	17.000	85.900	0.630	21.250	222.200	495.000	0.563
—	—	—	36.100	28.050	1.140	42.590	339.000	74.360	0.406
—	—	—	50.880	29.750	—	90.540	489.900	58.850	0.450
—	—	—	51.600	1649.000	0.330	29.660	299.200	323.000	2.480
0.349	—	—	13.000	79.900	1.330	82.560	340.500	70.900	0.800
—	—	—	86.960	163.200	0.980	32.700	292.800	67.300	1.210
—	—	—	52.620	3650.000	5.910	48.900	207.700	354.800	74.100
—	—	1.180	357.200	3569.00	5.400	43.520	183.200	89.400	72.760

(continued)

Food	Portion	Vitamin A (I.U.)*	Thiamine (mg.)	Riboflavin (mg.)	Niacin (mg.)	Vitamin B$_6$ (mg.)	Vitamin B$_{12}$ (mcg.)	Folate (mcg.)
Fish and Shellfish—continued								
Salmon								
Pink, solids w/bones and liquid, canned/ water	3 oz.	46.800	0.020	0.158	5.560	——	——	13.060
Smoked	3 oz.	74.970	0.020	0.086	4.010	0.240	2.770	1.650
Sockeye, cooked, dry heat	3 oz.	177.800	0.180	0.145	5.670	0.186	4.930	——
Sardines								
Atlantic, canned/oil, drained	3 oz.	190.100	0.680	0.193	4.460	0.140	7.600	10.030
Pacific, canned/tomato sauce, drained	3 oz.	310.300	0.040	0.198	3.570	0.105	7.650	20.700
Scallops, raw	3½ oz.	——	0.012	0.065	1.150	——	1.530	——
Shrimp								
Breaded, fried	3 oz.	——	0.110	0.120	2.610	0.080	1.590	6.900
Raw	3½ oz.	——	0.028	0.034	2.550	0.104	1.610	3.000
Swordfish, raw	3½ oz.	119.000	0.037	0.095	9.680	0.330	1.750	——
Tuna								
Canned/water	½ cup	——	——	——	——	0.302	——	3.760
Light, canned/oil	½ cup	62.500	0.030	——	——	0.088	——	4.200
Tuna salad	½ cup	99.400	0.032	——	——	0.083	——	7.460
■ Fruits and Fruit Juices								
Apple butter	1 tbsp.	0.000	——	——	——	——	——	——
Apples								
Canned, sweetened, heated	½ cup	56.500	0.009	0.010	0.083	0.045	0.000	0.150
Dried, uncooked	¼ cup	0.000	0.000	0.034	0.199	0.027	0.000	——
Juice, canned or bottled	1 cup	2.000	0.052	0.042	0.248	0.074	0.000	0.200
Raw, unpeeled	1	74.000	0.023	0.019	0.106	0.066	0.000	3.900
Applesauce, canned, unsweetened	½ cup	35.000	0.016	0.031	0.230	0.032	0.000	0.700
Apricots								
Canned/juice	½ cup	2098.000	0.023	0.024	0.427	——	0.000	0.000
Dried, uncooked	¼ cup	2353.000	0.003	0.049	0.975	0.051	0.000	3.350
Nectar, canned	1 cup	3304.000	0.023	0.035	0.653	——	0.000	3.300
Raw	3	2790.000	0.033	0.042	0.642	0.057	0.000	9.180

Vitamin C (mg.)	Vitamin D (I.U.)	Vitamin E (I.U.)	Calcium (mg.)	Copper (mcg.)	Iron (mg.)	Magnesium (mg.)	Potassium (mg.)	Sodium (mg.)	Zinc (mg.)
0.000	—	0.480	181.400	86.300	0.720	28.500	277.400	470.700	0.780
—	—	1.300	8.900	195.500	0.720	15.400	148.750	666.400	0.260
—	—	—	5.990	57.000	0.470	26.300	319.000	55.800	0.430
—	—	—	324.300	158.100	2.480	33.200	337.000	429.300	1.100
0.870	—	—	203.700	231.200	1.960	28.900	290.000	352.000	1.200
—	—	1.010	24.200	53.300	0.290	56.000	321.900	161.000	0.950
—	—	—	57.200	223.000	1.070	33.600	190.900	292.000	1.170
—	—	1.590	51.900	264.000	2.400	36.500	185.100	148.400	1.100
1.050	—	—	4.400	126.000	0.810	26.900	228.000	—	1.150
—	—	—	9.600	8.800	2.560	23.600	251.000	285.000	0.350
—	—	2.150	10.700	56.900	1.110	24.700	—	—	—
2.250	—	—	17.660	148.600	—	—	—	—	—
—	—	—	3.000	—	0.100	—	50.000	0.000	—
0.200	—	0.076	4.000	52.000	0.245	2.500	71.000	3.500	0.050
0.825	—	—	3.000	41.000	0.302	3.500	96.750	18.750	0.043
2.300	—	0.037	16.000	55.000	0.920	8.000	296.000	7.000	0.070
7.800	—	1.213	10.000	52.000	0.250	6.000	159.000	1.000	0.050
1.450	—	0.164	3.500	32.000	0.145	3.500	91.500	2.500	0.030
6.100	—	1.646	15.000	67.000	0.370	12.000	204.500	4.500	0.135
0.775	—	—	14.750	140.000	1.527	15.250	447.800	3.250	0.243
1.400	—	—	17.000	183.000	0.960	13.000	286.000	9.000	0.230
10.680	—	1.417	14.940	96.000	0.576	8.550	315.000	1.068	0.279

(continued)

Food	Portion	Vitamin A (I.U.)*	Thiamine (mg.)	Riboflavin (mg.)	Niacin (mg.)	Vitamin B$_6$ (mg.)	Vitamin B$_{12}$ (mcg.)	Folate (mcg.)
Fruits and Fruit Juices—continued								
Avocado, California,								
raw	1	1322.000	0.233	0.264	4.150	0.605	0.000	141.000
Banana, raw, peeled	1	96.400	0.054	0.119	0.643	0.688	0.000	22.700
Blackberries, raw	1 cup	237.000	0.043	0.058	0.576	0.084	0.000	18.000
Blueberries, raw	1 cup	145.000	0.070	0.073	0.521	0.052	0.000	9.300
Boysenberries, frozen,								
unsweetened	1 cup	89.000	0.070	0.049	1.010	0.074	0.000	83.600
Carambola, raw	1	626.000	0.036	0.034	0.522	——	0.000	——
Cherries								
Sour, frozen,								
unsweetened	1 cup	1349.000	0.068	0.053	0.212	0.104	0.000	7.000
Sweet, raw	10	146.000	0.030	0.040	0.270	0.020	0.000	2.860
Cranberries								
Juice, bottled	1 cup	0.000	0.013	0.040	0.127	——	0.000	0.506
Raw, chopped	1 cup	50.000	0.033	0.022	0.110	0.072	0.000	1.900
Sauce, canned,								
sweetened	½ cup	27.500	0.021	0.029	0.139	0.020	0.000	——
Currants, Zante, dried	¼ cup	26.000	0.058	0.051	0.582	0.107	0.000	3.675
Dates								
Natural, dried,								
chopped	¼ cup	22.250	0.040	0.045	0.980	0.086	0.000	5.600
Natural, dried, whole	5	21.000	0.040	0.040	0.915	0.080	0.000	5.200
Elderberries, raw	1 cup	870.000	0.102	0.087	0.725	0.334	0.000	24.700
Figs								
Dried, uncooked	¼ cup	66.000	0.035	0.044	0.345	0.112	0.000	3.750
Raw	1	71.000	0.030	0.025	0.200	0.057	0.000	5.000
Fruit cocktail								
Canned/juice	½ cup	378.500	0.015	0.020	0.500	——	0.000	0.000
Canned/syrup	½ cup	261.000	0.023	0.024	0.477	0.064	0.000	0.000
Fruit salad								
Canned/juice	½ cup	747.000	0.014	0.018	0.443	——	0.000	——
Canned/water	½ cup	538.500	0.019	0.026	0.458	0.039	0.000	——
Grapefruit								
Juice, canned, raw	1 cup	1082.000	0.099	0.049	0.494	——	0.000	51.200
Juice, canned,								
sweetened	1 cup	0.000	0.100	0.058	0.798	0.050	0.000	25.900
Juice, canned,								
unsweetened	1 cup	18.000	0.104	0.049	0.571	0.049	0.000	25.600

Vitamin C (mg.)	Vitamin D (I.U.)	Vitamin E (I.U.)	Calcium (mg.)	Copper (mcg.)	Iron (mg.)	Magnesium (mg.)	Potassium (mg.)	Sodium (mg.)	Zinc (mg.)
17.100	——	5.185	23.800	575.000	2.550	88.600	1369.000	25.900	0.907
10.800	——	0.478	7.140	124.000	0.369	34.500	471.000	1.190	0.190
30.200	——	7.510	46.000	202.000	0.830	29.000	282.000	0.000	0.390
18.900	——	——	9.000	88.000	0.240	7.000	129.000	9.000	0.160
4.100	——	——	36.000	106.000	1.120	21.000	183.000	2.000	0.290
26.900	——	——	6.000	152.000	0.330	12.000	207.000	2.000	0.140
2.600	——	——	20.000	140.000	0.820	13.000	192.000	1.000	0.160
4.800	——	0.134	10.000	70.000	0.260	8.000	152.000	0.000	0.040
108.000	——	——	8.000	33.000	0.400	8.000	61.000	10.000	0.050
14.800	——	——	8.000	——	0.220	6.000	78.000	1.000	0.140
2.750	——	——	5.000	28.000	0.305	4.000	35.500	40.000	0.070
1.675	——	——	31.000	169.000	1.173	14.750	321.300	2.750	0.235
0.000	——	——	14.500	128.000	0.512	15.750	290.300	1.250	0.130
0.000	——	——	13.500	120.000	0.480	14.500	270.500	0.100	0.120
52.200	——	——	55.00	——	2.320	——	406.000	9.000	——
0.425	——	——	71.500	156.000	1.112	29.500	354.500	5.500	0.250
1.000	——	——	18.000	35.000	0.180	8.000	116.000	1.000	0.070
3.400	——	——	10.000	77.000	0.265	8.500	117.500	4.500	0.105
2.450	——	——	8.000	88.000	0.365	7.000	112.000	7.500	0.105
4.150	——	——	14.000	63.000	0.310	10.500	144.000	6.500	0.180
2.350	——	——	8.500	82.000	0.365	6.500	95.500	4.500	0.090
93.900	——	0.146	22.000	82.000	0.490	30.000	400.000	2.000	0.130
67.300	——	0.149	20.000	120.000	0.890	24.000	405.000	4.000	0.150
72.000	——	0.148	18.000	94.000	0.500	24.000	378.000	3.000	0.210

(continued)

Fruits and Fruit Juices—continued

Food	Portion	Vitamin A (I.U.)*	Thiamine (mg.)	Riboflavin (mg.)	Niacin (mg.)	Vitamin B₆ (mg.)	Vitamin B₁₂ (mcg.)	Folate (mcg.)
Grapefruit—continued								
Pink and red, raw	½	318.500	0.049	0.025	0.246	0.052	0.000	11.550
White, raw	½	11.800	0.044	0.024	0.318	0.051	0.000	11.800
Grapes								
American type, raw	1 cup	92.000	0.085	0.052	0.276	0.101	0.000	3.600
Juice, canned and								
bottled	1 cup	20.000	09.066	0.094	0.663	0.164	0.000	6.580
Guava, common, raw	1	713.000	0.045	0.045	1.080	0.129	.000	0.000
Kiwi fruit, raw	1	133.000	0.015	0.038	0.380	——	0.000	0.000
Kumquats, raw	4	228.000	0.060	0.076	——	——	0.000	0.000
Lemons								
Juice, raw	1 tbsp.	3.063	0.005	0.002	0.015	0.007	0.000	0.000
Raw, peeled	1	21.500	0.030	0.015	0.074	0.059	0.000	7.840
Limes								
Juice, raw	1 cup	1082.000	0.099	0.049	0.494	——	0.000	51.200
Raw, peeled	1	21.500	0.030	0.015	0.074	0.059	0.000	7.840
Mango, raw	½	4030.000	0.060	0.059	0.605	0.139	0.000	0.000
Melons								
Cantaloupe, raw,								
cubed	1 cup	5158.000	0.058	0.034	0.918	0.184	0.000	27.300
Casaba, raw, cubed	1 cup	51.000	0.102	0.034	0.680	——	0.000	0.000
Honeydew, raw, cubed	1 cup	68.000	0.131	0.031	1.020	0.100	0.000	0.000
Watermelon, raw,								
cubed	1 cup	585.000	0.128	0.032	0.320	0.230	0.000	3.400
Mixed fruit, canned/syrup	½ cup	247.500	0.019	0.051	0.765	——	0.000	0.000
Mulberries, raw	1 cup	35.000	0.041	0.141	0.868	——	0.000	0.000
Nectarine, raw	1	1001.000	0.023	0.056	1.350	0.340	0.000	5.100
Oranges								
All varieties, raw	1	269.000	0.114	0.052	0.369	0.079	0.000	39.700
Juice, frozen, diluted	1 cup	194.000	0.197	0.045	0.503	0.110	0.000	109.000
Juice, raw	1 cup	496.000	0.223	0.074	0.992	0.099	0.000	136.000
Papayas								
Nectar, canned	1 cup	277.000	0.015	0.010	0.375	0.023	0.000	5.200
Raw, cubed	1 cup	2819.000	0.038	0.045	0.473	0.027	0.000	0.000
Passionfruit								
Juice, yellow	1 cup	5953.000	——	0.249	5.530	——	0.000	0.000
Purple, raw	4	504.000	——	0.092	1.080	——	0.000	0.000

Vitamin C (mg.)	Vitamin D (I.U.)	Vitamin E (I.U.)	Calcium (mg.)	Copper (mcg.)	Iron (mg.)	Magnesium (mg.)	Potassium (mg.)	Sodium (mg.)	Zinc (mg.)
45.500	——	0.459	18.450	54.000	0.148	9.850	156.000	0.000	0.086
39.300	——	0.440	14.150	59.000	0.071	10.600	174.500	0.000	0.083
3.700	——	0.960	13.000	37.000	0.270	5.000	176.000	2.000	0.040
0.200	——	——	22.000	71.000	0.600	24.000	334.000	7.000	0.130
165.000	——	——	18.000	93.000	0.280	9.000	256.000	2.000	0.210
74.500	——	——	20.000	——	0.310	23.000	252.000	4.000	——
28.400	——	——	32.000	80.000	0.280	8.000	148.000	4.000	0.080
4.506	——	——	1.375	5.000	0.005	0.875	16.750	0.125	0.009
39.200	——	——	19.200	27.000	0.444	——	102.000	1.480	0.044
93.900	——	0.146	22.000	82.000	0.490	30.000	400.000	2.000	0.130
39.200	——	——	19.200	27.000	0.444	——	102.000	1.480	0.044
28.650	——	1.728	10.500	114.000	0.130	9.000	161.000	2.000	0.035
67.500	——	0.334	17.000	67.000	0.340	17.000	494.000	14.000	0.250
27.200	——	0.355	9.000	——	0.680	14.000	357.000	20.000	——
42.100	——	0.355	10.000	70.000	0.120	12.000	461.000	17.000	——
15.400	——	——	13.000	51.000	0.280	17.000	186.000	3.000	0.110
88.000	——	——	1.500	74.000	0.460	6.500	107.000	5.000	0.090
51.000	——	——	55.000	——	2.590	25.000	271.000	14.000	——
7.300	——	——	6.000	99.000	0.210	11.000	288.000	0.000	0.120
69.700	——	0.468	52.000	59.000	0.130	13.000	237.000	0.000	0.090
96.900	——	0.149	22.000	110.000	0.240	24.000	474.000	2.000	0.130
124.000	——	0.148	27.000	109.000	0.500	27.000	496.000	2.000	0.130
7.500	——	——	24.000	33.000	0.860	8.000	78.000	14.000	0.380
86.500	——	——	33.000	22.000	0.140	14.000	359.000	4.000	0.100
45.000	——	——	9.000	——	0.890	41.000	687.000	15.000	——
21.600	——	——	8.000	——	1.160	20.000	252.000	20.000	——

(continued)

Food	Portion	Vitamin A (I.U.)*	Thiamine (mg.)	Riboflavin (mg.)	Niacin (mg.)	Vitamin B$_6$ (mg.)	Vitamin B$_{12}$ (mcg.)	Folate (mcg.)
Fruits and Fruit Juices—continued								
Peaches								
Canned/heavy syrup	1 cup	849.000	0.028	0.061	1.570	0.049	0.000	8.200
Canned/water	1 cup	1298.000	0.020	0.046	1.270	0.046	0.000	8.200
Raw, sliced	1 cup	910.000	0.029	0.070	1.680	0.031	0.000	5.800
Raw, unpeeled	1	465.000	0.015	0.036	0.861	0.016	0.000	3.000
Pears								
Bartlett, raw, unpeeled	1	33.000	0.033	0.066	0.166	0.030	0.000	12.100
Canned/heavy syrup	1 cup	0.000	0.026	0.056	0.617	0.036	0.000	3.000
Canned/juice	1 cup	14.000	0.027	0.027	0.496	——	0.000	0.000
Canned/water	1 cup	0.000	0.020	0.024	0.132	0.034	0.000	3.000
Persimmon, Japanese, raw	1	3640.000	0.050	0.034	0.168	——	0.000	12.600
Pineapple								
Bits, canned/juice	1 cup	95.000	0.238	0.048	0.710	——	0.000	0.000
Bits, canned/syrup	1 cup	37.00	0.229	0.063	0.736	0.189	0.000	11.900
Bits, canned/water	1 cup	37.000	0.229	0.064	0.733	0.182	0.000	11.900
Juice, canned	1 cup	12.000	0.138	0.055	0.643	0.240	0.000	57.800
Raw, diced	1 cup	35.000	0.143	0.056	0.651	0.135	0.000	16.400
Plantains, cooked	1 cup	1400.000	0.071	0.080	1.160	0.370	0.000	40.000
Plums								
Japanese hybrid, raw	1	213.000	0.028	0.063	0.330	0.053	0.000	1.450
Purple, canned/juice	1 cup	2542.000	0.058	0.149	1.190	——	0.000	——
Purple, canned/syrup	1 cup	668.000	0.041	0.098	0.751	0.70	0.000	6.500
Purple, canned/water	1 cup	2276.000	0.052	0.102	0.921	0.067	——	6.600
Pomegranate, raw	1	——	0.046	0.046	0.462	0.162	0.000	——
Prunes								
Dried, cooked	½ cup	324.500	0.026	0.106	0.765	0.231	0.000	0.050
Dried, uncooked	¼ cup	799.800	0.033	0.065	0.790	0.106	0.000	1.475
Quince, raw	1	37.000	0.018	0.028	0.184	0.037	0.000	——
Raisins, seedless	¼ cup	2.750	0.057	0.032	0.297	0.090	0.000	1.200
Raspberries, raw	1 cup	16.000	0.037	0.111	1.110	0.070	0.000	6.000
Rhubarb, cooked, w/sugar	½ cup	110.000	0.025	0.070	0.400	0.027	0.000	7.150
Strawberries, whole, raw	1 cup	41.000	0.030	0.098	0.343	0.088	0.000	26.400
Tangerine, raw, peeled	1	773.000	0.088	0.018	0.134	0.056	0.000	17.100

Vitamin C (mg.)	Vitamin D (I.U.)	Vitamin E (I.U.)	Calcium (mg.)	Copper (mcg.)	Iron (mg.)	Magnesium (mg.)	Potassium (mg.)	Sodium (mg.)	Zinc (mg.)
7.100	—	—	8.000	131.000	0.690	13.000	235.000	16.000	0.220
7.000	—	—	6.000	132.000	0.770	12.000	241.000	8.000	0.220
11.200	—	0.253	9.000	116.000	0.190	11.000	334.000	1.000	0.230
5.700	—	0.130	5.000	59.000	0.100	6.000	171.000	0.000	0.120
6.600	—	1.222	19.000	188.000	0.410	9.000	208.000	1.000	0.200
2.900	—	0.380	12.000	125.000	0.560	11.000	165.000	13.000	0.210
4.000	—	—	21.000	131.000	0.710	17.000	238.000	10.000	0.220
2.500	—	—	9.000	124.000	0.520	9.000	130.000	5.000	0.210
12.600	—	—	13.000	190.00	0.260	15.000	270.000	3.000	0.180
23.800	—	0.373	34.000	215.000	0.700	35.000	304.000	4.000	0.240
19.000	—	0.380	36.000	260.000	0.980	40.000	266.000	3.000	0.290
18.900	—	0.367	37.000	258.000	0.980	44.000	313.000	3.000	0.290
26.700	—	—	42.000	225.000	0.650	34.000	334.000	2.000	0.290
23.900	—	0.231	11.000	171.000	0.570	21.000	175.000	1.000	0.120
16.800	—	—	3.000	102.000	0.890	49.000	716.000	8.000	0.200
6.300	—	0.688	2.000	28.000	0.070	4.000	113.000	0.000	0.060
7.000	—	—	25.000	136.000	0.840	20.000	389.000	3.000	0.270
1.100	—	—	24.000	95.000	2.170	13.000	234.000	50.000	0.190
6.700	—	—	17.000	97.000	0.400	13.000	314.000	2.000	0.190
9.400	—	—	5.000	—	0.460	0.000	399.000	5.000	—
3.100	—	—	24.000	205.000	1.175	21.500	354.000	2.000	2.250
1.350	—	—	20.500	173.000	0.998	18.250	300.000	1.500	0.213
13.800	—	—	10.000	120.000	0.640	7.000	181.000	4.000	—
1.200	—	0.380	17.750	112.000	0.755	12.000	272.300	4.250	0.095
30.800	—	0.550	27.000	91.000	0.700	22.000	187.000	0.000	0.570
8.000	—	0.402	105.500	26.000	0.800	16.200	274.000	2.500	0.108
84.500	—	0.267	21.000	73.000	0.570	16.000	247.000	2.000	0.190
25.900	—	—	12.000	24.000	0.090	10.000	132.000	1.000	—

(continued)

Food	Portion	Vitamin A (I.U.)*	Thiamine (mg.)	Riboflavin (mg.)	Niacin (mg.)	Vitamin B_6 (mg.)	Vitamin B_{12} (mcg.)	Folate (mcg.)
■ **Grains and Grain Products** (*See also* Breads; Cereals)								
Barley								
Cooked	1 cup	——	0.108	0.080	2.790	0.160	——	1.780
Pearl, light, uncooked	1 cup	0.000	0.240	0.100	6.200	0.448	0.000	40.000
Bulgur, dry, commercial	1 cup	0.000	0.530	0.180	7.400	——	——	——
Corn fritters	3	420.000	0.180	0.210	1.800	——	——	——
Cornmeal, unbolted, dry	1 cup	620.000	0.460	0.130	2.400	0.305	0.000	29.300
Flour								
Buckwheat, light, sifted	1 cup	0.000	0.080	0.040	0.400	0.566	0.000	43.100
Soybean, low-fat	1 cup	70.000	0.730	0.320	2.300	——	——	——
Wheat, enriched,								
unsifted	1 cup	0.000	0.800	0.500	6.600	0.075	0.000	26.300
Whole wheat, stirred	1 cup	0.000	0.230	0.130	1.800	0.083	0.000	15.600
Macaroni, cooked, firm	1 cup	0.000	0.230	0.130	1.800	0.083	0.000	15.600
Noodles, egg, enriched,								
cooked	1 cup	110.000	0.220	0.130	1.900	0.141	0.000	19.200
Pancakes								
Buckwheat, mix	3	180.000	0.120	0.150	0.600	0.171	1.065	8.910
Plain, home recipe	3	90.000	0.180	0.210	1.500	0.171	1.065	8.910
Rice								
Brown, long-grain,								
cooked	1 cup	0.000	0.180	0.040	2.700	——	——	——
White, instant	1 cup	0.000	0.210	0.000	1.700	0.056	0.000	16.500
White, long grain,								
cooked	1 cup	0.000	0.230	0.020	2.100	0.871	0.000	22.600
Wild, cooked	1 cup	——	0.066	0.110	1.600	0.170	——	25.400
Spaghetti, cooked, firm	1 cup	0.000	0.230	0.130	1.800	0.083	0.000	15.600
Taco shell	1	——	0.032	0.017	0.189	——	0.000	——
Tortilla, corn	1	——	0.048	0.030	0.384	0.091	0.000	5.700
■ **Meats**								
Bacon								
Canadian, pork, grilled	1 slice	0.000	0.192	0.046	1.610	0.105	0.180	1.000
Pork, broiled or fried	3 slices	0.000	0.132	0.054	1.392	0.051	0.330	0.999
Beef								
Arm roast, cooked	3 oz.	——	0.058	0.201	2.672	0.240	2.490	8.000
Brisket, lean, braised	3 oz.	——	0.006	0.185	3.189	0.260	2.170	7.000
Hamburger, patty,								
extra-lean, broiled	3 oz.	——	0.051	0.230	4.216	0.230	1.840	8.000

Vitamin C (mg.)	Vitamin D (I.U.)	Vitamin E (I.U.)	Calcium (mg.)	Copper (mcg.)	Iron (mg.)	Magnesium (mg.)	Potassium (mg.)	Sodium (mg.)	Zinc (mg.)
0.000	—	—	14.900	137.000	1.760	29.800	126.000	12.200	1.080
0.000	—	0.060	32.000	—	4.200	74.000	320.000	6.000	—
0.000	—	0.156	53.000	—	8.200	—	459.000	—	—
3.000	—	—	66.000	—					
0.000	—	0.273	24.000	156.000	2.200	—	346.000	1.000	—
0.000	—	0.468	11.000	700.000	1.000	47.000	314.000	0.000	—
0.000	—	—	231.000	—	8.000	—	1636.000	1.000	—
0.000	—	0.075	20.000	239.000	3.600	31.300	119.000	2.000	0.800
0.000	—	0.039	14.000	26.000	1.400	26.000	103.000	1.000	0.700
0.000	—	0.039	14.000	26.000	1.400	26.000	103.000	1.000	0.700
0.000	—	—	16.000	270.000	1.400	43.200	70.000	3.000	—
0.000	0.000	—	177.000	—	1.200	15.390	198.000	480.000	0.576
0.000	0.000	—	81.000	60.000	1.200	15.390	99.000	480.000	0.576
0.000	—	1.982	23.000	—	1.000	—	137.000	0.000	—
0.000	—	0.271	5.000	169.000	1.300	13.200	—	13.000	0.700
0.000	—	0.337	21.000	210.000	1.800	16.400	57.000	6.000	0.700
—	—	—	22.900	147.000	0.800	40.600	128.000	29.200	1.270
0.000	—	0.116	14.000	—	1.400	24.700	103.000	1.000	0.700
—	—	—	15.600	35.000	0.286	11.400	—	—	0.142
0.000	—	—	42.000	90.000	0.570	19.500	52.200	53.400	0.426
5.000	8.320	—	2.500	13.000	0.190	5.000	90.500	360.000	0.395
6.390	9.000	0.148	2.001	33.000	0.309	5.010	92.100	303.000	0.618
0.000	—	—	9.000	112.000	2.610	17.000	207.000	51.000	5.730
0.000	—	—	5.000	102.000	2.360	20.000	244.000	61.000	5.850
0.000	—	—	6.000	60.000	2.000	18.010	266.000	59.000	4.630

(continued)

Meats—continued

Food	Portion	Vitamin A (I.U.)*	Thiamine (mg.)	Riboflavin (mg.)	Niacin (mg.)	Vitamin B$_6$ (mg.)	Vitamin B$_{12}$ (mcg.)	Folate (mcg.)
Beef—continued								
Hamburger, patty, lean, broiled	3 oz.	——	0.043	0.179	4.386	0.220	2.000	8.00
Hamburger, w/bacon and cheese	1	368.000	0.150	0.270	4.890	0.240	1.800	25.500
Heart, simmered	3 oz.	0.000	0.119	1.309	3.462	0.180	12.160	2.001
Liver, pan-fried	3 oz.	30689.000	0.179	3.519	12.274	1.221	95.030	187.100
Rib Roast, lean, roasted	3 oz.	——	0.070	0.179	3.497	0.260	2.480	7.000
Round steak, lean and fat, broiled	3 oz.	——	0.077	0.175	3.181	0.380	2.340	8.000
Sirloin steak, lean and fat, broiled	3 oz.	——	0.095	0.224	3.289	0.330	2.260	8.000
Tenderloin, lean and fat, cooked	3 oz.	——	0.099	0.230	3.072	0.340	2.080	6.000
Tip round, lean only, roasted	3 oz.	——	0.083	0.228	3.179	0.340	2.460	7.000
Bologna, pork	1 slice	——	0.120	0.036	0.897	0.060	0.210	1.000
Corned beef, canned	3 oz.	0.000	0.018	0.126	2.067	0.120	1.380	——
Corned beef hash, canned	1 cup	——	0.020	0.200	4.600	——	——	——
Deviled ham, canned	1 oz.	0.000	0.044	0.022	0.436	0.092	0.198	——
Frankfurters								
With bun	1	0.000	0.197	0.230	3.050	0.000	0.000	0.000
Without bun	1	——	0.113	0.068	1.500	0.080	0.740	2.000
Ham								
Canned, 13% fat, roasted	3 oz.	——	0.699	0.221	4.508	0.255	0.899	4.253
Extra-lean, 5% fat, roasted	3 oz.	0.000	0.644	0.172	3.420	0.340	0.553	3.038
Lean only, roasted	3 oz.	——	0.578	0.216	4.271	0.395	0.595	3.038
Lunch meat, regular, 11% fat	1 slice	0.000	0.244	0.071	1.490	0.100	0.240	1.000
Lamb								
Chop, lean and fat, broiled	3 oz.	——	0.105	0.182	3.918	0.234	1.720	2.552
Leg, lean and fat, roasted	3 oz.	——	0.130	0.230	4.703	0.234	1.831	2.552

Vitamin C (mg.)	Vitamin D (I.U.)	Vitamin E (I.U.)	Calcium (mg.)	Copper (mcg.)	Iron (mg.)	Magnesium (mg.)	Potassium (mg.)	Sodium (mg.)	Zinc (mg.)
0.000	—	—	9.000	56.000	1.790	18.000	256.000	65.000	4.560
1.500	—	0.119	116.000	120.000	2.740	34.500	339.000	660.000	5.250
1.201	—	—	5.003	629.000	6.380	22.000	198.100	54.000	2.660
19.410	—	—	9.000	2400.000	5.343	20.010	309.000	90.000	4.630
0.000	—	—	9.000	83.000	2.220	21.000	320.000	63.000	5.900
0.000	—	—	6.000	82.000	2.050	21.000	311.000	51.000	3.510
0.000	—	—	9.000	116.000	2.560	24.000	306.000	53.000	4.880
0.000	—	—	7.000	142.000	2.760	23.000	323.000	52.000	4.280
0.000	—	—	5.000	106.000	2.500	23.000	328.000	55.000	6.010
8.100	0.000	0.021	3.000	17.000	0.180	3.000	65.000	272.000	0.470
1.200	—	—	—	54,000	1.770	12.000	116.100	855.000	3.030
—	—	0.098	29.000	—	4.400	—	440.000	1188.000	—
—	13.520	0.000	2.181	—	0.654	3.685	—	348.900	0.519
0.000	19.100	0.171	27.100	107.000	1.530	13.100	140.000	636.000	2.050
15.000	20.300	0.119	6.000	50.000	0.660	6.000	95.000	639.000	1.050
11.910	22.110	0.355	7.290	111.000	1.166	14.580	303.800	800.100	2.126
17.860	22.110	0.355	6.683	67.000	1.258	12.150	244.200	1023.000	2.448
—	—	0.355	6.075	74.000	0.796	18.830	269.100	1129.000	2.187
8.000	0.000	—	2.000	30.000	0.280	5.000	94.000	373.000	0.610
—	0.000	0.203	7.645	137.000	0.956	14.430	191.100	59.250	3.345
—	0.000	0.064	9.005	50.000	1.401	17.010	241.000	59.030	3.502

(continued)

Food	Portion	Vitamin A (I.U.)*	Thiamine (mg.)	Riboflavin (mg.)	Niacin (mg.)	Vitamin B$_6$ (mg.)	Vitamin B$_{12}$ (mcg.)	Folate (mcg.)
Meats—continued								
Lamb—continued								
Shoulder, lean and fat, roasted	3 oz.	——	0.110	0.200	4.002	0.234	1.831	2.552
Liverwurst/liver sausage, pork	1 slice	——	0.049	0.185	——	0.030	2.420	5.000
Pepperoni, pork/beef	1 slice	——	0.018	0.014	0.273	0.010	0.140	——
Pork								
Chop, lean and fat, broiled	3 oz.	7.260	0.716	0.305	4.481	0.322	0.840	4.149
Loin, lean, roasted	3 oz.	5.989	0.770	0.222	4.642	0.380	0.509	0.997
Sausage, link, cooked	1	——	0.096	0.033	0.587	0.040	0.220	——
Sausage, link, Italian	1	——	0.417	0.156	2.790	0.220	0.870	——
Sausage, patty, cooked	1	——	0.200	0.069	1.220	0.090	0.470	——
Sausage, Polish, cooked	1 oz.	——	0.014	0.004	0.098	0.005	0.027	——
Spareribs, braised	3 oz.	8.984	0.347	0.323	4.642	0.299	0.919	3.983
Tenderloin, lean, roasted	3 oz.	5.989	0.797	0.332	3.983	0.359	0.470	5.001
Rabbit, stewed, no skin	3 oz.	——	0.043	0.061	9.599	——	——	——
Salami, dry or hard, pork	1 slice	——	0.093	0.033	0.560	0.060	0.280	——
Veal								
Cutlet, medium fat, broiled	3 oz.	——	0.060	0.210	4.603	——	1.361	——
Rib, no bone, roasted	3 oz.	——	0.110	0.260	6.604	——	1.401	——
Venison, roasted	3 oz.	0.000	0.315	0.238	6.294	——	——	——
■ Miscellaneous								
Gelatin, dry	1 envelope	——	0.000	0.000	0.000	0.000	——	——
Ketchup	1 tbsp.	210.000	0.010	0.010	0.200	0.016	0.000	0.750
Mustard, yellow, prepared	1 tbsp.	——	——	——	——	——	——	——
Olives, green, pickled, canned	2	20.000	——	——	——	——	0.000	0.080
Pickle relish, sweet	1 tbsp.	——	——	——	——	——	——	——
Pickles								
Cucumber, dill, medium	1	70.000	0.000	0.010	0.000	0.005	0.000	0.650

Vitamin C (mg.)	Vitamin D (I.U.)	Vitamin E (I.U.)	Calcium (mg.)	Copper (mcg.)	Iron (mg.)	Magnesium (mg.)	Potassium (mg.)	Sodium (mg.)	Zinc (mg.)
—	0.000	0.203	9.005	—	1.001	14.510	206.100	59.030	3.502
—	2.600	0.094	5.000	—	1.150	—	—	215.000	—
—	—	0.013	1.000	0.000	0.080	1.000	19.000	112.000	0.140
0.207	0.000	0.203	5.186	76.000	0.685	20.740	297.700	56.010	2.085
0.299	0.000	0.201	5.001	59.000	0.928	17.970	305.500	59.000	1.938
0.000	0.000	0.031	4.000	20.000	0.160	2.000	47.000	168.000	0.330
1.300	—	0.159	16.000	54.000	1.010	12.000	204.000	618.000	1.590
0.000	23.000	0.064	9.000	40.000	0.340	5.000	97.000	349.000	0.680
0.025	—	0.067	0.375	3.000	0.041	0.375	6.744	24.850	0.055
—	—	0.201	39.830	120.000	1.578	20.960	455.200	56.900	2.546
0.299	0.000	0.504	6.978	135.000	1.309	20.960	455.200	56.900	2.546
—	—	0.507	17.620	—	1.276	0.000	312.900	34.630	—
—	6.000	0.016	1.000	20.000	0.130	2.000	—	226.000	0.420
—	0.000	0.064	9.005	213.000	2.702	15.310	258.200	68.040	3.502
—	0.000	0.064	10.010	213.000	2.902	17.010	259.200	68.040	3.502
0.000	—	—	17.010	—	2.977	24.660	285.800	59.540	—
4.000	—	—	0.000	—	0.400	—	180.000	8.000	—
2.000	—	—	3.000	32.000	0.100	3.600	54.000	156.000	0.034
—	—	0.393	12.000	—	0.300	6.000	21.000	195.000	—
—	—	—	4.000	—	0.100	—	3.500	161.600	—
—	—	—	3.000	—	0.100	—	—	124.000	—
4.000	0.000	—	17.000	—	0.700	7.800	130.000	928.000	0.176

(continued)

Food	Portion	Vitamin A (I.U.)*	Thiamine (mg.)	Riboflavin (mg.)	Niacin (mg.)	Vitamin B$_6$ (mg.)	Vitamin B$_{12}$ (mcg.)	Folate (mcg.)
Miscellaneous—continued								
Pickles—continued								
Cucumber, fresh-pack	4	40.000	0.000	0.000	0.000	0.004	0.000	0.300
Sweet/gherkin, small	1	10.000	0.000	0.000	0.000	0.001	0.000	0.150
Vinegar, cider	1 tbsp.	——	——	——	——	0.000	——	——
Yeast, brewer's, dry	1 tbsp.	0.000	1.250	0.340	3.000	0.200	0.000	313.000
■ Nuts and Seeds								
Almond butter, plain	4 tbsp.	0.000	0.084	0.392	1.840	0.048	0.000	41.600
Coconut milk, raw	1 cup	0.000	0.062	0.000	1.820	——	0.000	——
Nuts								
Almonds, shelled, slivered	¼ cup	0.000	0.061	0.224	0.967	0.033	0.000	16.880
Brazil nuts, dried, shelled	¼ cup	——	0.350	0.043	0.568	0.088	0.000	1.400
Cashews, dry-roasted	¼ cup	0.000	0.069	0.069	0.480	0.088	0.000	23.700
Chestnuts, roasted	1 oz.	0.998	0.043	0.026	0.425	——	0.000	——
Coconut, raw, shredded	¼ cup	0.000	0.013	0.004	0.108	0.011	0.000	5.275
Filberts/hazelnuts, dried, chopped	½ cup	19.250	0.144	0.032	0.325	0.176	0.000	20.650
Macadamia nuts, dried	¼ cup	0.000	0.117	0.037	0.717	——	0.000	——
Mixed nuts, dry-roasted	¼ cup	5.250	0.069	0.069	1.610	0.102	0.000	17.250
Peanuts, Spanish, dried	¼ cup	0.000	0.242	0.048	5.175	0.108	0.000	36.750
Pecans, halves, dried	¼ cup	34.500	0.229	0.035	0.240	0.051	0.000	10.570
Pistachios, dry-roasted	¼ cup	——	0.135	0.079	0.450	——	0.000	——
Walnuts, black, dried, chopped	¼ cup	92.500	0.068	0.034	0.216	——	——	——
Peanut butter, smooth	4 tbsp.	——	0.096	0.068	8.600	0.248	0.000	52.400
Seeds								
Pumpkin or squash seeds, dried	¼ cup	131.300	0.073	0.111	0.602	0.031	0.000	——
Sesame seeds, dried, whole	¼ cup	3.250	0.285	0.089	1.625	0.285	0.000	34.750
Sunflower seeds, dried	¼ cup	18.000	0.822	0.090	1.620	0.452	0.000	85.000
Sesame butter (tahini)	4 tbsp.	——	0.732	0.284	3.272	——	0.000	——

Vitamin C (mg.)	Vitamin D (I.U.)	Vitamin E (I.U.)	Calcium (mg.)	Copper (mcg.)	Iron (mg.)	Magnesium (mg.)	Potassium (mg.)	Sodium (mg.)	Zinc (mg.)
2.000	0.000	——	10.000	——	0.600	——	——	200.000	0.080
1.000	0.000	——	2.000	——	0.200	0.150	——	128.000	0.020
——	0.000	——	1.000	——	0.100	——	15.000	0.125	0.020
0.000	——	——	17.000	——	1.400	18.400	152.000	9.000	——
0.400	——	8.702	172.000	576.000	2.360	192.000	484.000	8.000	1.960
6.700	——	——	39.000	638.000	3.940	89.000	630.000	37.000	1.610
0.173	0.000	10.281	76.500	270.000	1.053	85.000	210.500	3.175	0.840
0.250	0.000	3.342	61.500	6520.000	1.190	78.750	210.000	0.500	1.605
0.000	——	0.291	15.500	760.000	2.055	89.000	193.500	5.250	1.917
——	——	0.212	4.991	110.000	0.429	25.950	134.800	0.998	0.260
0.650	0.000	0.209	3.000	87.000	0.485	6.500	71.250	4.000	0.220
0.300	0.000	10.169	54.000	435.000	0.940	82.000	128.000	0.750	0.690
——	——	——	23.500	99.000	0.808	38.750	123.300	1.500	0.572
0.150	——	——	24.000	438.000	1.267	77.000	204.300	4.000	1.303
0.000	——	4.247	21.250	365.000	1.178	65.500	261.800	5.750	1.195
0.525	0.000	1.247	9.750	320.000	0.575	34.500	105.800	0.250	1.477
——	——	2.485	22.500	387.000	1.015	41.500	310.500	2.000	0.435
——	0.000	0.390	18.000	320.000	0.960	63.000	163.800	0.500	1.070
0.000	0.000	6.675	20.000	376.000	1.160	112.000	440.000	300.000	1.880
——	——	——	14.750	477.000	5.175	184.500	278.500	6.000	2.575
0.000	——	1.219	351.000	1470.000	5.250	126.300	168.500	4.000	2.800
——	——	26.716	42.000	630.000	2.438	127.300	248.000	1.000	1.822
0.000	——	——	256.000	968.000	5.360	56.000	248.000	68.000	2.760

(continued)

Food	Portion	Vitamin A (I.U.)*	Thiamine (mg.)	Riboflavin (mg.)	Niacin (mg.)	Vitamin B$_6$ (mg.)	Vitamin B$_{12}$ (mcg.)	Folate (mcg.)
■ Peas and Beans (Legumes)								
Beans								
Great Northern, dry, cooked	1 cup	2.000	0.280	0.104	1.205	0.207	0.000	180.900
Kidney, red, canned	1 cup	0.000	0.269	0.225	1.167	0.056	0.000	129.400
Lima, boiled, drained	½ cup	315.000	0.119	0.082	0.885	0.164	0.000	——
Navy pea, dry, cooked	1 cup	3.000	0.368	0.111	0.966	0.298	0.000	254.600
Cowpeas, black-eyed, boiled	1 cup	26.000	0.345	0.094	0.846	0.171	0.000	355.500
Lentils, whole, cooked	1 cup	15.000	0.335	0.145	2.099	0.352	0.000	357.900
Peas								
Green, frozen, boiled, drained	½ cup	534.000	0.226	0.080	1.185	0.090	0.000	46.900
Green, raw	1 cup	998.000	0.414	0.206	3.260	0.264	0.000	102.000
In pods, raw	1 cup	211.000	0.218	0.116	0.870	0.232	0.000	——
Split, dry, cooked	1 cup	14.000	0.372	0.110	1.744	0.094	0.000	127.300
Soybean(s)								
Curd (tofu)	4 oz.	95.200	0.091	0.058	0.21	0.053	0.000	16.800
Dry, cooked	1 cup	50.000	0.380	0.160	1.100	——	——	——
Green, boiled, drained	1 cup	281.000	0.468	0.279	2.250	——	0.000	——
Kernels, roasted	¼ cup	54.000	0.027	0.039	0.475	0.081	0.000	61.000
■ Poultry								
Chicken								
Breast, no skin, roasted	3 oz.	17.800	0.059	0.097	11.670	0.504	0.287	2.967
Breast, w/skin, roasted	3 oz.	78.970	0.056	0.102	10.800	0.469	0.278	2.604
Liver pâté, canned	2 tbsp.	188.000	0.014	0.364	1.954	——	——	——
Liver, simmered	3 oz.	13930.000	0.130	1.488	3.785	0.498	16.460	654.300
Leg, no skin, roasted	3 oz.	53.720	0.064	0.197	5.372	0.313	0.278	7.162
Leg, w/skin, roasted	3 oz.	114.900	0.058	0.181	5.267	0.276	0.261	5.968
Thigh, no skin, roasted	3 oz.	55.610	0.062	0.196	5.545	0.294	0.262	6.542
Wing, roasted	3 oz.	135.100	0.035	0.110	5.653	0.350	0.250	2.501
Wing, steamed	3 oz.	112.700	0.034	0.087	3.934	0.191	0.149	2.126
Duck								
No skin, roasted	3 oz.	65.810	0.221	0.400	4.329	0.212	0.339	8.467
With skin, roasted	3 oz.	179.000	0.148	0.229	4.108	0.156	0.252	5.566
Goose								
No skin, roasted	3 oz.	——	0.078	0.332	3.468	0.396	——	——
With skin, roasted	3 oz.	59.450	0.065	0.275	3.544	0.318	——	1.868

Vitamin C (mg.)	Vitamin D (I.U.)	Vitamin E (I.U.)	Calcium (mg.)	Copper (mcg.)	Iron (mg.)	Magnesium (mg.)	Potassium (mg.)	Sodium (mg.)	Zinc (mg.)
2.300	—	—	121.000	437.000	3.770	88.000	692.000	4.000	1.550
2.900	—	—	62.000	384.000	3.220	73.000	658.000	873.000	1.410
8.600	—	0.000	27.000	260.000	2.085	63.000	484.500	14.500	0.670
1.600	—	—	128.000	537.000	4.510	107.000	669.000	2.000	1.930
0.600	—	—	42.000	458.000	4.290	96.000	476.000	6.000	2.200
2.900	0.000	0.000	37.000	497.000	6.590	71.000	731.000	4.000	2.500
7.900	—	0.143	19.000	111.000	1.260	23.000	134.000	70.000	0.750
62.400	—	—	38.000	274.000	2.300	52.000	380.000	8.000	1.940
87.000	—	0.282	62.000	330.000	3.010	35.000	290.000	6.000	—
0.800	—	—	22.000	355.000	2.520	71.000	710.000	4.000	1.960
0.100	—	—	392.000	216.000	6.003	33.600	135.520	7.840	0.896
0.000	—	—	131.000	—	4.900	—	972.000	4.000	—
30.600	—	—	261.000	—	4.500	—	—	—	—
0.600	—	—	37.250	287.000	1.202	46.500	397.000	1.000	0.977
0.000	—	0.444	12.860	42.000	0.880	24.720	217.600	62.300	0.850
0.000	—	0.444	12.150	43.000	0.903	23.430	208.300	59.880	0.868
2.600	—	0.107	2.000	—	2.380	—	—	—	—
13.490	56.980	—	12.150	315.000	7.229	17.620	119.100	43.130	3.688
0.000	—	0.444	10.740	68.000	1.110	20.590	205.900	77.890	2.426
0.000	—	0.444	10.440	66.000	1.134	19.400	191.000	73.860	2.208
0.000	—	0.444	9.813	69.000	1.112	19.630	202.800	75.240	2.192
0.000	—	0.444	12.510	48.000	1.076	17.510	155.100	70.040	1.551
0.000	—	0.444	10.630	38.000	0.957	12.760	119.100	57.410	1.382
0.000	—	0.444	10.010	196.000	2.290	16.930	214.400	55.030	2.213
0.000	—	0.444	9.574	193.000	2.293	13.800	173.700	50.540	1.581
0.000	—	—	12.090	235.000	2.439	21.300	329.700	64.330	—
0.000	—	—	11.430	225.000	2.406	18.570	279.800	59.670	—

(continued)

Food	Portion	Vitamin A (I.U.)*	Thiamine (mg.)	Riboflavin (mg.)	Niacin (mg.)	Vitamin B$_6$ (mg.)	Vitamin B$_{12}$ (mcg.)	Folate (mcg.)
Poultry—continued								
Turkey								
Breast, no skin, roasted	3 oz.	0.000	0.037	0.111	6.379	0.475	0.328	5.281
Dark meat, no skin,								
roasted	3 oz.	0.000	0.053	0.211	3.104	0.304	0.316	7.898
Light meat, no skin,								
roasted	3 oz.	0.000	0.052	0.110	5.814	0.456	0.316	4.860
Turkey roll, light and dark	1 slice	——	0.026	0.081	1.360	——	——	——
■ Sauces and Gravies								
Sauces								
Barbecue	1 tbsp.	135.600	0.005	0.003	0.141	0.012	0.000	——
Chili, bottled	1 tbsp.	210.000	0.010	0.010	0.200	——	——	——
Marinara, canned	½ cup	1202.000	0.057	0.074	1.990	——	0.000	——
Soy	1 tbsp.	0.000	0.009	0.023	0.605	0.031	0.000	1.900
Spaghetti, canned	½ cup	1528.000	0.069	0.074	1.875	——	0.000	——
Tabasco	1 tsp.	——	0.000	0.010	0.000	——	——	——
Tartar, regular	1 tbsp.	30.000	0.000	0.000	0.000	——	——	——
Teriyaki, bottled	1 tbsp.	0.000	0.005	0.013	0.229	0.018	0.000	3.600
Tomato, canned, salt								
added	½ cup	1200.000	0.081	0.071	1.410	——	0.000	——
White, medium,								
enriched	2 tbsp.	143.800	0.015	0.054	0.088	0.008	——	——
Gravies								
Beef, canned	2 tbsp.	0.000	0.009	0.011	0.192	0.003	0.029	0.000
Chicken, canned	2 tbsp.	110.000	0.005	0.013	0.132	0.003	——	——
Mushroom, canned	2 tbsp.	0.000	0.010	0.019	0.200	0.006	0.000	——
■ Snacks								
Corn chips	1 oz.	——	0.048	0.026	0.553	——	0.000	——
Popcorn, popped, plain	1 cup	——	——	0.010	0.100	0.012	0.000	——
Potato chips, salt added	1 oz.	0.000	0.043	0.000	1.191	0.142	0.000	12.760
Pretzels, Dutch, twisted	1 oz.	0.000	0.089	0.071	1.240	0.005	0.000	4.536
■ Soups								
Beef								
Broth, canned,								
w/water	1 cup	0.000	0.005	0.050	1.870	——	——	——

Vitamin C (mg.)	Vitamin D (I.U.)	Vitamin E (I.U.)	Calcium (mg.)	Copper (mcg.)	Iron (mg.)	Magnesium (mg.)	Potassium (mg.)	Sodium (mg.)	Zinc (mg.)
0.000	—	0.115	10.560	59.000	1.301	24.740	247.900	44.190	1.473
0.000	—	0.811	27.340	136.000	1.987	20.660	246.600	66.830	3.797
0.000	—	0.115	16.400	36.000	1.142	23.690	258.800	54.070	1.731
—	—	—	9.000	21.000	0.380	5.000	77.000	166.000	0.570
∙1.094	—	—	3.000	—	0.141	0.000	27.190	127.000	—
2.000	—	—	3.000	—	0.100	—	56.000	201.000	—
15.950	—	—	22.000	177.000	1.000	29.500	530.500	786.000	0.335
0.000	—	—	3.000	18.000	0.490	8.000	64.000	1029.000	0.036
13.950	—	—	35.000	142.000	0.810	30.000	478.500	618.000	0.265
—	0.000	—	—	—	—	—	3.000	22.000	—
0.000	—	—	3.000	—	0.100	—	11.000	98.000	—
0.000	—	—	4.000	18.000	0.310	11.000	41.000	690.000	0.018
15.050	—	—	17.000	240.000	0.940	23.000	454.000	740.500	0.300
0.250	—	—	36.000	—	0.063	4.688	43.500	99.500	0.065
0.000	0.000	0.000	1.750	29.000	0.204	0.000	23.630	14.630	0.291
0.000	—	—	6.000	30.000	0.140	—	32.500	171.900	0.239
0.000	—	—	2.125	30.000	0.196	—	31.630	169.900	0.209
—	—	—	—	40.000	—	21.860	—	—	0.434
0.000	—	—	1.000	20.000	0.200	—	—	0.000	0.500
11.770	—	1.795	7.088	57.000	0.340	17.010	368.600	133.200	0.298
0.000	—	0.064	7.088	43.000	0.354	6.804	37.210	457.100	0.307
0.000	—	—	15.000	—	0.410	—	130.000	782.000	—

(continued)

Food	Portion	Vitamin A (I.U.)*	Thiamine (mg.)	Riboflavin (mg.)	Niacin (mg.)	Vitamin B$_6$ (mg.)	Vitamin B$_{12}$ (mcg.)	Folate (mcg.)
Soups—continued								
Beef—continued								
Broth, dehydrated	1 cube	——	0.007	0.009	0.119	——	——	——
Chunky, canned	1 cup	2611.000	0.058	0.151	2.710	0.132	0.610	13.400
With noodles, canned, w/water	1 cup	629.000	0.068	0.059	1.070	0.037	0.200	4.400
Chicken								
Broth, canned	1 cup	0.000	0.010	0.071	3.350	0.024	0.240	——
With dumplings, canned	1 cup	518.000	0.017	0.072	1.750	0.036	0.160	——
With noodles, canned, w/water	1 cup	711.000	0.053	0.060	1.390	0.027	——	2.200
Clam chowder								
Manhattan, canned, w/water	1 cup	920.000	0.063	0.049	1.340	0.083	2.190	9.500
New England, canned, w/milk	1 cup	164.000	0.067	0.236	1.030	0.126	10.300	9.700
Cream of asparagus, canned, w/milk	1 cup	599.000	0.102	0.275	0.880	0.064	——	——
Cream of chicken, canned, w/milk	1 cup	715.000	0.074	0.258	0.923	0.067	——	7.700
Cream of mushroom, canned, w/milk	1 cup	154.000	0.077	0.280	0.913	0.064	——	——
Cream of potato, canned, w/milk	1 cup	443.000	0.082	0.236	0.642	0.089	——	9.200
Split pea, canned, w/water	1 cup	444.000	0.147	0.076	1.480	0.068	0.000	2.500
Tomato, canned/ w/milk	1 cup	849.000	0.134	0.248	1.520	0.164	0.440	20.900
Vegetable beef, canned, w/water	1 cup	1891.000	0.037	0.049	1.030	0.076	0.310	10.600
Vegetarian, canned, w/water	1 cup	3005.000	0.053	0.046	0.916	0.055	0.000	10.600
■ Sugars and Sweets								
Candy								
Caramel, plain, chocolate	1 oz.	0.000	0.010	0.051	0.101	——	——	——
Fudge, chocolate, plain	1 oz.	0.000	0.010	0.030	0.101	——	——	——

Vitamin C (mg.)	Vitamin D (I.U.)	Vitamin E (I.U.)	Calcium (mg.)	Copper (mcg.)	Iron (mg.)	Magnesium (mg.)	Potassium (mg.)	Sodium (mg.)	Zinc (mg.)
—	—	—	—	—	0.080	2.000	15.000	864.000	0.008
7.000	—	—	31.000	240.000	2.320	—	336.000	867.000	2.640
0.300	—	—	15.000	139.000	1.100	6.000	99.000	952.000	1.540
0.000	—	—	9.000	124.000	0.510	2.000	210.000	776.000	0.249
0.000	—	0.000	15.000	123.000	0.620	4.000	116.000	861.000	0.366
0.200	—	—	17.000	195.000	0.780	5.000	55.000	1107.000	0.395
3.200	—	—	34.000	148.000	1.890	10.000	262.000	1808.000	0.927
3.500	—	—	187.000	139.000	1.480	23.000	300.000	992.000	0.799
3.900	—	—	175.000	139.000	0.870	20.000	359.000	1041.000	0.925
1.300	—	—	180.000	139.000	0.670	18.000	273.000	1046.000	0.675
2.300	—	—	178.000	139.000	0.590	20.000	270.000	1076.000	0.640
1.100	—	—	166.000	263.000	0.540	17.000	323.000	1060.000	0.675
1.400	—	—	22.000	369.000	2.280	48.000	399.000	1008.000	1.320
67.700	0.000	—	159.000	263.000	1.820	23.000	450.000	932.000	0.290
2.400	—	—	17.000	183.000	1.110	6.000	173.000	957.000	1.550
1.400	—	—	21.000	123.000	1.080	7.000	209.000	823.000	0.460
0.000	—	0.073	42.530	—	0.405	1.013	54.680	74.930	—
0.000	—	0.295	22.280	—	0.304	12.760	42.530	54.680	—

(continued)

Food	Portion	Vitamin A (I.U.)*	Thiamine (mg.)	Riboflavin (mg.)	Niacin (mg.)	Vitamin B₆ (mg.)	Vitamin B₁₂ (mcg.)	Folate (mcg.)
Sugars and Sweets—continued								
Candy—continued								
Milk chocolate								
w/almonds	1 oz.	70.880	0.020	0.122	0.203	—	—	—
Milk chocolate								
w/peanuts	1 oz.	50.630	0.071	0.071	1.418	—	—	—
Honey, strained/								
extracted	1 tbsp.	0.000	0.000	0.010	0.100	0.004	0.000	—
Jam/preserves, regular	1 tbsp.	0.000	0.000	0.010	0.000	0.004	0.000	1.600
Jelly, regular	1 tbsp.	0.000	0.000	0.010	0.000	—	—	—
Marshmallows	1 oz.	0.000	0.000	0.000	0.000	—	—	—
Molasses, cane,								
blackstrap	1 tbsp.	—	0.020	0.040	0.400	0.040	0.000	—
Sugar								
Brown, pressed down	1 tbsp.	0.000	0.001	0.004	0.025	—	—	—
White, granulated	1 tbsp.	0.000	0.000	0.000	0.000	—	—	—
White, powdered,								
sifted	1 tbsp.	0.000	0.000	0.000	0.000	—	—	—
Syrup, maple	1 tbsp.	0.000	—	—	—	—	—	—
■ Vegetables								
Alfalfa sprouts, raw	1 cup	51.000	0.025	0.042	0.159	0.011	0.000	12.200
Amaranth, boiled,								
drained	½ cup	1828.000	0.013	0.089	0.369	—	0.000	—
Artichoke, boiled,								
drained	1	172.000	0.068	0.059	0.709	0.104	0.000	53.400
Asparagus, spears, boiled	½ cup	746.000	0.089	0.109	0.945	0.127	0.000	88.000
Beet greens								
Boiled, drained	½ cup	3672.000	0.084	0.208	0.360	0.095	0.000	—
Raw	1 cup	2318.000	0.038	0.084	0.152	0.040	0.000	—
Beets, sliced, boiled,								
drained	½ cup	11.000	0.025	0.012	0.232	0.027	0.000	45.200
Broccoli								
Boiled, drained	½ cup	1099.000	0.064	0.161	0.590	0.154	0.000	53.500
Raw	½ cup	1356.000	0.058	0.104	0.562	0.140	0.000	62.400
Brussels sprouts, boiled	½ cup	561.000	0.083	0.062	0.473	0.139	0.000	46.800
Cabbage								
Bok choy, raw,								
shredded	1 cup	2100.000	0.028	0.049	0.350	—	0.000	—

Vitamin C (mg.)	Vitamin D (I.U.)	Vitamin E (I.U.)	Calcium (mg.)	Copper (mcg.)	Iron (mg.)	Magnesium (mg.)	Potassium (mg.)	Sodium (mg.)	Zinc (mg.)
0.000	10.130	0.465	65.810	——	0.506	0.000	126.600	23.290	——
0.000	10.130	0.465	49.610	——	0.405	0.000	139.700	19.240	——
0.000	0.000	——	1.000	8.000	0.100	0.630	11.000	1.000	0.020
0.000	0.000	0.027	4.000	62.000	0.200	——	18.000	2.000	——
1.000	0.000	0.024	4.000	16.000	0.300	0.900	14.000	3.000	——
0.000	——	——	5.063	——	0.506	——	2.025	11.140	0.010
——	0.000	0.122	137.000	284.000	3.200	52.000	585.000	18.000	——
0.000	0.000	——	11.690	48.000	0.469	——	47.310	4.125	——
0.000	0.000	——	0.000	2.000	0.000	——	0.000	0.120	0.006
0.000	0.000	——	0.000	1.000	0.006	——	0.188	0.052	——
0.000	——	——	33.000	——	0.200	2.000	26.000	3.000	——
2.700	——	——	10.000	52.000	0.320	9.000	26.000	2.000	0.300
27.150	——	——	138.000	——	1.490	36.500	423.000	14.000	——
8.900	——	0.340	47.000	73.000	1.620	47.000	316.000	79.000	0.430
18.200	——	2.652	22.000	90.000	0.590	17.000	279.000	4.000	0.430
17.950	——	1.624	82.500	181.000	1.370	48.500	654.000	173.000	0.360
11.400	——	——	46.000	72.000	1.260	28.000	208.000	76.000	0.140
4.675	——	0.039	9.000	48.000	0.525	31.000	266.000	42.000	0.215
49.000	——	0.532	89.000	54.000	0.890	47.000	127.000	8.000	0.120
82.000	——	0.603	42.000	40.000	0.780	22.000	286.000	24.000	0.360
48.400	——	0.983	28.000	65.000	0.940	16.000	247.000	17.000	0.250
31.500	——	——	74.000	——	0.560	13.000	176.000	45.000	——

(continued)

Food	Portion	Vitamin A (I.U.)*	Thiamine (mg.)	Riboflavin (mg.)	Niacin (mg.)	Vitamin B₆ (mg.)	Vitamin B₁₂ (mcg.)	Folate (mcg.)
Vegetables—continued								
Cabbage—continued								
Common, boiled,								
drained	½ cup	62.500	0.042	0.040	0.165	0.047	0.000	14.700
Common, raw,								
shredded	1 cup	113.000	0.045	0.027	0.270	0.086	0.000	51.000
Red, raw, shredded	1 cup	28.000	0.035	0.021	0.210	0.147	0.000	14.500
Sauerkraut, canned	½ cup	21.000	0.025	0.026	0.169	0.154	0.000	3.525
Carrots								
Juice, canned	1 cup	63350.000	0.226	0.136	0.950	0.534	0.000	9.400
Sliced, boiled, drained	½ cup	19150.000	0.027	0.044	0.395	0.192	0.000	10.800
Whole, raw, scraped	1	20250.000	0.070	0.042	0.668	0.106	0.000	10.100
Cauliflower								
Boiled, drained	½ cup	9.000	0.039	0.032	0.342	0.125	0.000	31.700
Raw, chopped	1 cup	16.000	0.076	0.057	0.633	0.231	0.000	66.100
Celery								
Pascal, raw, diced	1 cup	152.000	0.036	0.036	0.360	0.036	0.000	10.600
Pascal, raw, stalk	1	51.000	0.012	0.012	0.120	0.012	0.000	3.600
Celery cabbage, raw	1 cup	912.000	0.030	0.038	0.304	0.176	0.000	59.800
Chives, raw, chopped	1 tbsp.	192.000	0.003	0.005	0.021	0.005	0.000	——
Coleslaw	½ cup	408.000	0.040	0.040	0.176	0.080	0.016	16.800
Collards, boiled, drained	½ cup	2109.000	0.016	0.041	0.224	0.040	0.000	6.200
Corn								
Cream style, sweet,								
canned	½ cup	124.000	0.032	.068	1.230	0.081	0.000	57.500
Kernels, frozen, boiled	½ cup	204.000	0.057	0.060	1.050	0.082	0.000	16.700
Sweet, on cob, boiled	1 ear	167.000	0.166	0.055	1.240	0.046	0.000	35.700
Cress, garden, raw	1 cup	4650.000	0.040	0.130	0.500	0.124	0.000	——
Cucumber, raw, sliced	1 cup	46.000	0.032	0.020	0.312	0.054	0.000	14.400
Dandelion greens, boiled	½ cup	6145.000	0.069	0.092	——	——	0.000	——
Eggplant, boiled, drained	½ cup	30.500	0.037	0.010	0.288	0.042	0.000	6.900
Endive, raw, chopped	1 cup	1026.000	0.040	0.038	0.200	0.010	0.000	71.000
Garlic, clove, raw	1	0.000	0.006	0.003	0.021	——	0.000	0.100
Gingerroot, raw, sliced	1 tbsp.	0.000	0.002	0.002	0.042	0.010	0.000	——
Jerusalem artichokes, raw	1 cup	30.000	0.300	0.090	1.950	——	0.000	——
Kale								
Chopped, boiled	½ cup	4810.000	0.035	0.046	0.325	0.090	0.000	8.650
Raw, chopped	1 cup	5963.000	0.074	0.087	0.670	0.182	0.000	19.600

Vitamin C (mg.)	Vitamin D (I.U.)	Vitamin E (I.U.)	Calcium (mg.)	Copper (mcg.)	Iron (mg.)	Magnesium (mg.)	Potassium (mg.)	Sodium (mg.)	Zinc (mg.)
17.600	—	1.803	23.950	21.000	0.283	10.900	148.500	13.800	0.116
42.600	—	2.235	42.300	21.000	0.504	13.500	221.000	16.200	0.162
39.900	—	0.209	36.000	68.000	0.350	11.000	144.000	7.000	0.150
17.400	—	—	36.000	114.000	1.735	15.500	200.500	780.500	0.220
21.000	—	—	58.000	114.000	1.140	34.000	720.000	72.000	0.440
1.800	—	0.486	24.000	105.000	0.480	10.000	177.000	52.000	0.230
6.700	—	0.472	19.000	34.000	0.360	11.000	233.000	25.000	0.140
34.300	—	0.028	17.000	56.000	0.260	7.000	200.000	4.000	0.150
71.500	—	0.045	29.000	32.000	0.580	14.000	355.000	15.000	0.180
7.600	—	0.644	44.000	42.000	0.580	14.000	340.000	106.000	0.200
2.500	—	0.215	14.000	14.000	0.190	5.000	114.000	35.000	0.070
20.500	—	0.134	58.000	27.000	0.230	10.000	181.000	7.000	0.170
2.400	—	—	2.000	3.000	0.050	2.000	8.000	0.000	—
20.800	1.560	—	32.000	16.000	0.400	8.000	112.000	16.000	0.160
9.300	—	—	74.000	143.000	0.390	10.500	88.500	18.000	0.610
5.900	—	0.076	4.000	67.000	0.490	22.000	172.000	365.000	0.680
2.100	—	0.037	2.000	27.000	0.250	15.000	114.000	4.000	0.280
4.800	—	0.083	2.000	41.000	0.470	24.000	192.000	13.000	0.370
34.600	—	0.522	40.000	—	0.660	0.000	304.000	8.000	—
4.800	—	0.232	14.000	42.000	0.280	12.000	156.000	2.000	0.240
9.450	—	1.959	73.500	—	0.945	0.000	122.000	23.000	—
0.650	—	0.022	2.500	52.000	0.170	6.500	119.000	1.500	0.070
3.200	—	—	26.000	50.000	0.420	8.000	158.000	12.000	0.400
0.900	—	0.000	5.000	8.000	0.050	1.000	12.000	1.000	—
0.300	—	—	1.000	0.000	0.030	2.500	25.000	0.750	—
6.000	—	0.425	21.000	—	5.100	26.000	—	—	—
26.650	—	7.748	47.000	102.000	0.585	11.500	148.000	15.000	0.155
80.400	—	—	90.000	194.000	1.140	23.000	299.000	29.000	0.290

(continued)

Food	Portion	Vitamin A (I.U.)*	Thiamine (mg.)	Riboflavin (mg.)	Niacin (mg.)	Vitamin B_6 (mg.)	Vitamin B_{12} (mcg.)	Folate (mcg.)
Vegetables—continued								
Kohlrabi								
Boiled, drained	½ cup	29.000	0.033	0.016	0.322	——	——	——
Raw	1 cup	50.000	0.070	0.028	0.560	0.210	0.000	——
Leeks								
Boiled, drained	1	57.000	0.032	0.025	0.248	——	0.000	30.100
Raw	1	118.000	0.074	0.037	0.496	——	0.000	79.500
Lettuce								
Iceberg, raw, chopped	1 cup	182.000	0.025	0.017	0.103	0.022	0.000	30.800
Loose-leaf, raw	1 cup	1045.000	0.028	0.044	0.220	0.030	0.000	76.000
Romaine, raw, shredded	1 cup	1456.000	0.056	0.056	0.280	——	0.000	76.000
Mushrooms								
Boiled, drained	½ cup	0.000	0.059	0.234	3.478	0.072	0.000	14.300
Raw, chopped	1 cup	0.000	0.072	0.314	2.880	0.068	0.000	14.800
Mustard greens, boiled, drained	½ cup	2122.000	0.029	0.044	0.303	0.000	0.000	——
Okra, boiled, drained	½ cup	460.000	0.106	0.044	0.695	0.150	0.000	36.500
Onions								
Mature, boiled, drained	½ cup	0.000	0.044	0.008	0.084	0.189	0.000	13.300
Mature, raw, chopped	1 cup	0.000	0.102	0.017	0.170	0.267	0.000	33.800
Young, green	1	250.000	0.004	0.007	0.001	——	0.000	0.685
Parsley, raw, chopped	1 cup	3328.000	0.048	0.064	0.448	0.096	0.000	117.100
Parsnips, sliced, boiled, drained	½ cup	0.000	0.065	0.040	0.565	0.073	0.000	45.400
Peppers								
Hot, chili, raw	1 tbsp.	72.250	0.009	0.000	0.089	0.026	0.000	2.188
Hot, red, dried	1 tsp.	1300.000	0.000	0.020	0.200	——	0.000	——
Sweet, green, boiled, drained	1	283.000	0.039	0.026	0.265	0.079	0.000	7.200
Sweet, green, raw	1	392.000	0.063	0.037	0.407	0.121	0.000	12.500
Sweet, red, raw	1	4218.000	0.063	0.037	0.407	0.121	0.000	12.500
Potato(es)								
Mashed, w/milk and butter	½ cup	177.500	0.088	0.042	1.135	0.235	0.000	8.350
Skin, baked	1 oz.	——	0.035	0.030	0.870	0.174	0.000	6.110
Strips, frozen, french-fried	10	0.000	0.060	0.020	1.150	0.120	0.000	8.300
Whole, w/skin, baked	1	——	0.216	0.067	3.320	0.701	0.000	22.200

Vitamin C (mg.)	Vitamin D (I.U.)	Vitamin E (I.U.)	Calcium (mg.)	Copper (mcg.)	Iron (mg.)	Magnesium (mg.)	Potassium (mg.)	Sodium (mg.)	Zinc (mg.)
44.550	—	—	20.500	116.000	0.330	15.500	280.500	17.000	—
86.800	—	—	34.000	196.000	0.560	27.000	490.000	28.000	—
5.200	—	1.699	37.000	—	1.360	18.000	108.000	13.000	—
14.900	—	1.699	73.000	—	2.600	35.000	223.000	25.000	—
2.150	—	0.328	10.500	17.000	0.275	4.950	86.900	4.950	0.121
9.900	—	0.328	37.400	—	0.770	6.050	145.000	4.950	0.121
13.400	—	0.334	20.000	—	0.620	4.000	162.000	4.000	—
3.250	—	0.097	6.500	390.000	1.365	6.500	279.500	0.000	0.650
2.400	—	0.083	4.000	78.000	0.860	8.000	260.000	2.000	0.344
17.700	—	2.093	51.500	—	0.490	10.500	141.500	11.000	—
13.100	—	—	50.000	69.000	0.360	46.000	257.000	4.000	0.440
6.000	—	0.188	29.000	42.000	0.210	11.000	159.000	8.000	0.190
14.300	—	0.785	42.500	68.000	0.629	17.000	264.000	3.400	0.306
2.250	—	0.009	3.000	—	0.095	1.000	12.800	0.200	0.022
57.600	—	1.669	83.200	32.000	3.968	25.600	345.600	25.600	0.448
10.100	—	1.155	29.000	108.000	0.450	23.000	287.000	8.000	—
22.750	—	—	1.625	16.000	0.112	2.375	31.880	0.625	0.029
0.000	—	—	5.000	—	0.300	3.400	20.000	20.000	0.054
81.300	—	0.739	3.000	52.000	0.640	7.000	94.000	2.000	0.090
94.700	—	0.749	4.000	76.000	0.940	10.000	144.000	2.000	0.130
141.000	—	—	—	—	0.940	10.000	144.000	2.000	0.130
6.450	—	0.063	27.000	144.000	0.275	18.500	303.500	309.500	0.290
3.813	—	—	9.776	232.000	1.994	12.220	162.300	5.866	0.137
5.500	—	0.149	4.000	80.000	0.670	11.000	229.000	15.000	0.210
26.100	—	0.091	20.000	616.000	2.750	55.000	844.000	16.000	0.650

(continued)

Food	Portion	Vitamin A (I.U.)*	Thiamine (mg.)	Riboflavin (mg.)	Niacin (mg.)	Vitamin B$_6$ (mg.)	Vitamin B$_{12}$ (mcg.)	Folate (mcg.)
Vegetables—continued								
Potato salad	½ cup	261.500	0.097	0.075	1.115	0.177	0.193	8.400
Pumpkin, boiled, drained,								
mashed	½ cup	1326.000	0.038	0.096	0.505	——	0.000	——
Pumpkin pie mix, canned	½ cup	11205.000	0.022	0.160	0.505	——	0.000	——
Radishes								
Daikon, sliced, boiled	½ cup	0.000	0.000	0.017	0.111	——	0.000	——
Raw	4	1.200	0.000	0.008	0.056	0.012	0.000	4.880
Rutabagas, boiled,								
drained	½ cup	0.000	0.061	0.031	0.535	0.077	0.000	13.200
Shallots, raw	1 tbsp.	——	0.006	0.002	0.020	——	0.000	——
Snap beans								
Green, boiled	½ cup	416.500	0.047	0.061	0.384	0.035	0.000	20.800
Wax, boiled	½ cup	416.500	0.047	0.061	0.384	0.035	0.000	20.800
Spinach								
Boiled, drained	½ cup	7370.000	0.086	0.213	0.441	0.218	0.000	131.000
Raw, chopped	1 cup	3760.000	0.044	0.106	0.406	0.110	0.000	108.000
Squash								
Acorn, baked	½ cup	439.000	0.171	0.014	0.905	0.199	0.000	19.200
Butternut, baked	½ cup	7175.000	0.074	0.018	0.995	0.127	0.000	19.650
Hubbard, boiled,								
mashed	½ cup	4726.000	0.050	0.033	0.394	0.122	0.000	11.500
Summer, boiled, sliced	½ cup	258.500	0.040	0.037	0.462	0.059	0.000	18.100
Zucchini, raw, sliced	1 cup	442.000	0.091	0.039	0.520	0.116	0.000	28.800
Sweet potatoes								
Baked, peeled	1	24880.000	0.083	0.145	0.689	0.275	0.000	25.700
Boiled, mashed	½ cup	27970.000	0.087	0.230	1.050	0.400	0.000	18.150
Swiss chard								
Boiled, drained	½ cup	2747.000	0.030	0.075	0.315	0.000	0.000	——
Raw	1 cup	1188.000	0.014	0.032	0.144	0.000	0.000	——
Tomato(es)								
Juice, canned	1 cup	1351.000	0.114	0.075	1.640	0.270	0.000	48.400
Juice, canned, low-								
sodium	1 cup	1356.000	0.114	0.076	1.640	0.270	0.000	48.400
Paste, canned, salt								
added	1 tbsp.	404.100	0.025	0.031	0.527	0.062	0.000	——
Red, canned, stewed	½ cup	707.500	0.059	0.045	0.910	——	0.000	3.700
Red, raw	1	1530.000	0.081	0.068	0.810	0.065	0.000	12.700

Vitamin C (mg.)	Vitamin D (I.U.)	Vitamin E (I.U.)	Calcium (mg.)	Copper (mcg.)	Iron (mg.)	Magnesium (mg.)	Potassium (mg.)	Sodium (mg.)	Zinc (mg.)
12.450	——	——	24.000	148.000	0.815	19.500	317.500	661.500	0.390
5.750	——	1.863	18.500	——	0.700	11.000	282.000	1.500	——
4.750	——	——	49.500	92.000	1.435	21.500	186.000	280.500	0.360
11.100	——	——	12.500	——	0.110	6.500	209.500	9.500	——
4.120	——	——	3.600	8.000	0.052	1.600	41.600	4.400	0.052
18.600	——	0.191	36.000	31.000	0.400	18.000	244.000	15.000	0.260
0.800	0.000	0.031	4.000	——	0.120	——	33.000	1.000	——
6.050	——	0.019	29.000	65.000	0.800	16.000	186.500	2.000	0.225
6.050	——	0.271	29.000	65.000	0.800	16.000	186.500	2.000	0.225
8.850	——	2.518	122.000	157.000	3.210	78.500	419.000	63.000	0.685
15.800	——	1.535	56.000	72.000	1.520	44.000	312.000	44.000	0.300
11.050	——	0.183	45.000	88.000	0.955	43.500	448.000	4.500	0.175
15.450	——	0.183	42.000	67.000	0.610	29.500	291.500	3.500	0.135
7.700	——	0.212	11.500	56.000	0.335	16.000	252.000	6.000	0.110
5.000	——	0.262	24.000	93.000	0.320	22.000	173.000	1.000	0.355
11.500	——	0.232	20.000	74.000	0.550	28.000	322.000	3.000	0.260
28.000	——	7.748	32.000	237.000	0.520	23.000	397.000	12.000	0.330
27.950	——	11.175	35.000	264.000	0.915	16.000	301.000	21.000	0.435
15.750	——	1.959	51.000	97.000	1.980	75.000	480.500	156.500	——
10.800	——	0.805	18.000	40.000	0.640	30.000	136.000	76.000	——
44.500	——	0.797	21.900	245.000	1.410	26.700	535.000	877.000	0.340
44.600	——	0.800	20.000	246.000	1.420	28.000	536.000	24.400	0.360
6.938	——	——	5.731	97.000	0.489	8.375	152.600	129.400	0.131
16.900	——	0.419	42.000	143.000	0.930	14.500	305.500	323.500	0.210
23.800	——	0.684	9.450	104.000	0.648	14.900	279.000	10.800	0.149

(continued)

Food	Portion	Vitamin A (I.U.)*	Thiamine (mg.)	Riboflavin (mg.)	Niacin (mg.)	Vitamin B₆ (mg.)	Vitamin B₁₂ (mcg.)	Folate (mcg.)
Vegetables—continued								
Turnip greens, boiled	½ cup	3959.000	0.033	0.052	0.296	0.130	0.000	85.500
Turnips, boiled, drained, diced	½ cup	0.000	0.021	0.018	0.233	0.053	0.000	7.200
Vegetable juice, canned	1 cup	2831.000	0.104	0.068	1.760	0.339	——	0.000
Water chestnuts, Chinese, canned	½ cup	2.800	0.008	0.017	0.252	——	0.000	——
Watercress, raw	1 cup	1598.000	0.031	0.041	0.068	0.044	0.000	——

SOURCE: Table prepared by Diane L. Drabinsky, Registered Dietitian, of the Rodale Food Center.

NOTES:

Values for chromium, iodine and selenium have been omitted. Present technology cannot yet distinguish between biologically available factors and inorganic forms of chromium. The iodine and selenium content of food varies considerably, depending on soil content or animal diets, so only limited data are available for those nutrients.

Where a dash appears, no data are available; food may or may not contain this nutrient.

*For fruits and vegetables, vitamin A value reflects the amount of vitamin A derived from the yellow, orange and green pigments in these foods.

Vitamin C (mg.)	Vitamin D (I.U.)	Vitamin E (I.U.)	Calcium (mg.)	Copper (mcg.)	Iron (mg.)	Magnesium (mg.)	Potassium (mg.)	Sodium (mg.)	Zinc (mg.)
19.750	——	2.421	99.000	182.000	0.575	16.000	146.500	20.500	0.100
9.050	——	0.36	17.150	54.000	0.172	6.250	105.500	39.000	——
67.000	——	——	26.600	486.000	1.020	26.600	467.000	883.000	0.484
0.910	——	——	2.800	70.000	0.610	3.500	82.500	5.600	0.266
14.600	——	0.507	40.800	32.000	0.068	7.140	112.000	13.900	——

Index

Note: Page numbers in **boldface** type refer to entire chapters; page numbers in *italics* refer to tables.

Rodale Press, Inc., publishes PREVENTION®, the better health magazine.
For information on how to order your subscription,
write to PREVENTION®, Emmaus, PA 18098.